Holism in Ancient Medicine and Its Reception

Studies in Ancient Medicine

VOLUME 53

The titles published in this series are listed at *brill.com/sam*

Holism in Ancient Medicine and Its Reception

Edited by

Chiara Thumiger

TUTA SUB AEGIDE PALLAS · 1683 ·

BRILL

LEIDEN | BOSTON

Cover illustration: Image by Christoph Geiger.

Library of Congress Cataloging-in-Publication Data

Names: Thumiger, Chiara, editor.
Title: Holism in ancient medicine and its reception / edited by Chiara Thumiger.
Description: Leiden ; Boston : Brill, [2021] | Series: Studies in ancient medicine, 09251421 ; 53 | Includes bibliographical references and index.
Identifiers: LCCN 2020040624 (print) | LCCN 2020040625 (ebook) | ISBN 9789004443082 (hardback) | ISBN 9789004443143 (ebook)
Subjects: LCSH: Holistic medicine. | Medicine—History.
Classification: LCC R733 .H64 2021 (print) | LCC R733 (ebook) | DDC 610—dc23
LC record available at https://lccn.loc.gov/2020040624
LC ebook record available at https://lccn.loc.gov/2020040625

Typeface for the Latin, Greek, and Cyrillic scripts: "Brill". See and download: brill.com/brill-typeface.

ISSN 0925-1421
ISBN 978-90-04-44308-2 (hardback)
ISBN 978-90-04-44314-3 (e-book)

This book is printed on acid-free paper and produced in a sustainable manner.

Contents

Acknowledgments

I would like to thank the Wellcome Trust for sponsoring the conference where this volume originated, along with the Institute of Classical Studies in London, which hosted the event in September 2017, and Greg Woolf for his support as Director. Above all else, I am grateful once again to the Wellcome Trust for generously funding my fellowships in the Department of Classics and Ancient History at the University of Warwick at the time when this project began, as well as during the preparation of this volume. I would also like to thank the Excellence Cluster ROOTS at Kiel University, with which I have been affiliated during the final phases of preparation of the manuscript, for its generous help and backing. I am grateful to all the participants in the original conference for both their written contributions and their constructive discussion there. Simon Swain was very helpful and positive about this project from the start, and offered precious advice before and during the preparation of the volume. The authors and I also benefitted immensely from the comments and constructive criticism offered by numerous readers and peer-reviewers, which have made a great difference in matters large and small. Among them, it is a particular pleasure to mention the anonymous reader at Brill who offered insightful advice, and Philip van der Eijk for his constant interest in the project and support. S. Douglas Olson's editorial expertise was vital in converting the various individual manuscripts into their final published form. Finally, Giulia Moriconi, Dinah Rapliza and the rest of the team at the press deserve warm thanks for their assistance throughout.

Chiara Thumiger

Abbreviations

CMG *Corpus Medicorum Graecorum*

CML *Corpus Medicorum Latinorum*
Leipzig and Berlin, Teubner, Akademie-Verlag and de Gruyter; texts available online at: http://cmg.bbaw.de/epubl/online/editionen.html

AHw W. von Soden (ed.). *Akkadisches Handwörterbuch*. Wiesbaden: Otto Harrassowitz (1965, 1972, and 1974)

AMT R. Campbell Thompson (ed.) *Assyrian Medical Texts from the Originals in the British Museum*. London: Milford (1923).

BAM Prefix to cuneiform hand copies numbered consecutively across vols. 1–6 of F. Köcher, *Die babylonisch-assyrische Medizin in Texten und Untersuchungen.* Berlin: De Gruyter (1963–1980)

CAD *The Assyrian Dictionary of the Oriental Institute of the University of Chicago*. Chicago: The Oriental Institute of the University of Chicago (1956–2011)

CT *Cuneiform Texts from Babylonian Tablets, &c. in the British Museum*. London: British Museum (1896–)

IG I^3 *Inscriptiones Graecae I: Inscriptiones Atticae Euclidis anno anteriores*. Ed. D. Lewis and J. Jeffery. 3rd edn. Berlin. De Gruyter (1981, 1994)

I.Métr. *Metrical Inscriptions of Graeco-Roman Egypt*. Ed. E. Bernand, *Inscriptions métriques de l'Egypte gréco-romaine*. Paris (1969).

K. K. G. Kühn (ed.) *Claudii Galeni Opera Omnia*, 22 vols., Leipzig (1821–33)

L. É. Littré (ed.) *Oeuvres complètes d'Hippocrate*. Paris: J. B. Baillière (1839–61)

LBAT T. G. Pinches and J. N. Strassmaier, *Late Babylonian Astronomical and Related Texts*. Providence: Brown University Press (1955)

STT Prefix to cuneiform hand copies numbered consecutively across O. R. Gurney and J. J. Finkelstein, *The Sultantepe Tablets*, vol. 1. London: Percy Lund, Humphries and Co. Ltd. (1957) and O. R. Gurney and P. Hulin, *The Sultantepe Tablets*, vol. 2. London: Percy Lund, Humphries and Co. Ltd. (1964)

Notes on Contributors

Hynek Bartoš
is an Associate Professor in the Faculty of Humanities at the Charles University in Prague. He is the author of *Philosophy and Dietetics in the Hippocratic On Regimen* (Brill 2015) and a range of essays on the history of ancient Greek philosophy and medicine. Most recently, he co-edited (with C. G. King) the volume *Heat, Pneuma, and Soul in Ancient Philosophy and Science* (CUP 2020).

Sean Coughlin
is Research Fellow at the Collaborative Research Centre SFB 980 Episteme in Bewegung funded by the German Research Foundation (DFG) at the Institute for Classical Philology, Humboldt-Universität zu Berlin. He was previously a Research Fellow at Excellence Cluster Topoi and a Visiting Research Fellow at Einstein Centre Chronoi (Berlin), the Research Training Group "Philosophy, Science and the Sciences" (Berlin), and the Martin Buber Society of Fellows (Jerusalem). He is co-editor with David Leith and Orly Lewis of *The Concept of Pneuma after Aristotle* (Berlin: Edition Topoi, 2020) and he publishes on topics in Ancient Greek philosophy, science, and medicine.

Elizabeth Craik
formerly professor at Kyoto University, is now honorary professor in the School of Classics, University of St Andrews. She has in recent years published editions, with commentaries, of several Hippocratic texts (*Places in Man, On Sight, On Anatomy, On Glands*) and a complete scholarly guide to the Hippocratic Corpus (*The Hippocratic Corpus: Content and Context*), as well a range of articles.

Brooke Holmes
is Robert F. Goheen Professor in the Humanities at Princeton University. She is the author of *The Symptom and the Subject: The Emergence of the Physical Body in Ancient Greece* (2010) and *Gender: Antiquity and its Legacy* (2012), in addition to being the co-editor of five volumes, most recently *Antiquities beyond Humanism* (2019) and the exhibition project *Liquid Antiquity* (2017). From 2012 to 2020 she directed the programme Postclassicisms and co-authored *Postclassicisms* (2020). She is finishing a book entitled *The Tissue of the World: Life, Nature, and Sympathy*.

Helen King
is a historian of medicine and the body. She retired from The Open University in 2017. Since then she has held a one-year post at Gustavus Adolphus College, MN, to promote interdisciplinary approaches to history. Her earlier career included visiting roles at the Peninsula Medical School and the universities of Vienna, Texas, Notre Dame and British Columbia. She has published on aspects of medicine from classical Greece to the nineteenth century and her most recent book, *Hippocrates Now*, was published in 2019. She is currently working on a history of the female body for Profile Books.

Giouli Korobili
is a Marie Skłodowska-Curie Post-doctoral Fellow at the University of Utrecht. She studied Classical Philology and Philosophy at the National and Kapodistrian University of Athens (BA), at the University of Ioannina (MA) and at Humboldt University of Berlin (Ph.D.). She has contributed to a number of collective volumes on Aristotle, ancient medicine and Byzantine Aristotelian commentators. She is currently revising her Ph.D. thesis on Aristotle's *On Youth and Old Age, on Life and Death, on Respiration* for publication.

David Leith
is Senior Lecturer in Classics at the University of Exeter. His research focuses on Graeco-Roman medicine, and especially its interactions with philosophy. He has published on the Hellenistic and Roman medical sects and their theories, especially Herophilus, Erasistratus, Asclepiades and the Methodists, and has edited fragments of medical papyri for *The Oxyrhynchus Papyri* series. He is currently preparing an edition, with essays and commentary, of the *testimonia* on Asclepiades of Bithynia.

Vivian Nutton
is emeritus professor of the history of medicine at UCL. He has written extensively on many aspects of the history of medicine from the Ancient Greeks to the seventeenth century. His recent books include *Ancient Medicine*, 2nd edition, 2013; *Johann Guinther and Andreas Vesalius, Principles of Anatomy according to Galen*, 2017; *An Autobibliography by John Caius*, 2018; and *Galen, a thinking Doctor in Imperial Rome*, 2020. His current project is a history of medicine in the sixteenth century. He is a Fellow of the British Academy, and a member of the Ancient Society of College Youths.

Julius Rocca
is a Research Fellow at the Institute for Classical Philology, Humboldt University, Berlin, holding an award from the Deutsche Forschungsgemeinschaft (DFG). He graduated in medicine and philosophy, and was awarded his Ph.D. at the University of Sydney. He has published in ancient medicine and philosophy and has held Wellcome Trust Awards in the UK and a Fellowship at the Center for Hellenic Studies, Washington, DC. Works include *Galen on the Brain* (Brill's Studies in Ancient Medicine Series: 2003), the edited volume *Teleology in the Ancient World* (Cambridge: 2017), and the chapter 'Galen and Middle Platonism: The Case of the Demiurge', in *Brill's Companion to the Reception of Plato in Antiquity* (2018).

William Michael Short
is Lecturer in Classics at the University of Exeter. His research interests rest at the intersection of language, culture, and cognition, and in this area he has pioneered an approach to ancient Roman culture inspired by Lakovian conceptual metaphor theory. Besides being author of numerous studies of individual metaphors in Latin and Greek, he is editor of *Embodiment in Latin Semantics*, which introduced cognitive semantics into Latin linguistics, and of *The World through Roman Eyes* (with M. Bettini), which showcases anthropological approaches to the ancient world, as well as of several other collective volumes in the field of 'cognitive' classics.

P. N. Singer
is a Research Fellow at Birkbeck, University of London. He took his Ph.D. at Cambridge University and has held research posts at Newcastle University and at the Humboldt Universität and Einstein Center Chronoi, Berlin. His research centres on ancient views of psychology and the mind, in both medical and philosophical writing, with a particular focus on Galen. He published the first major collection of texts by Galen in English translation (*Galen: Selected Works*, OUP, 1997) and co-edited and translated the first two volumes of the Cambridge Galen Translations (*Galen: Psychological Writings*, CUP, 2013; *Galen: Works on Human Nature, vol. I*, CUP, 2018). He is co-editor, with Chiara Thumiger, of *Mental Illness in Ancient Medicine: From Celsus to Paul of Aegina* (Brill, 2018), and author of a range of articles on psychology, the emotions, health, disease classification, pharmacology and physiology, as well as on Graeco-Roman commentary and editorial practices, and aspects of ancient Greek drama.

Konstantinos Stefou
studied Classics and Ancient Philosophy at the University of Ioannina. In April 2014 he completed his Ph.D. entitled *Early Greek Moral Values and Political Behaviour in Plato's Works*. He is currently a Post-doctoral Fellow at the Ionian University, Corfu, and an Adjunct Lecturer at the Democritus University of Thrace. He has authored a monograph and a number of papers on the Platonic Socrates and the so-called 'Socratic' dialogues. His research interests include ancient Greek and Roman literature, philosophy, historiography, oratory and rhetoric, and medicine.

Chiara Thumiger
Ph.D. (2004), Habil. (2017) is a Research Fellow at the Cluster of Excellence Roots, Kiel University. She is a classicist and historian of science. She has worked on a variety of medical themes and authors from the Hippocratic Corpus (her monograph *A History of the Mind and Mental Health in Classical Greek Medical Thought* was published in 2017) to the late-antique world and beyond (*Mental Illness in Ancient Medicine. From Celsus to Paul of Aegina*, 2018, co-edited with P. N. Singer). Most recently she has researched the history of the ancient disease *phrenitis*; the results of this work are now under submission in monographic form. She has also published on tragedy, ancient animals and the history of emotions.

Laurence Totelin
is Reader in Ancient History at Cardiff University. Her research focuses on the history of Greek and Roman botany, pharmacology, and gynaecology. Her publications include *Hippocratic Recipes: Oral and Written Transmission of Pharmacological Knowledge in Fifth- and Fourth-Century Greece* (Brill, 2009); with Gavin Hardy, *Ancient Botany* (Routledge, 2016); and edited with Rebecca Flemming, *Medicine and Markets in the Graeco-Roman World and Beyond: Essays in Honour of Vivian Nutton* (Classical Press of Wales, 2020).

Claire Trenery
is a Medieval historian based at Queen Mary University of London. She completed her Ph.D. at Royal Holloway in 2016 on the subject of madness in Medieval English miracle collections and published her first monograph, *Madness, Medicine and Miracle in Twelfth-Century England*, with Routledge in 2019. Her research explores how madness was distinguished and diagnosed as a condition of the mind and what effects it was thought to have on the bodies, minds and souls of sufferers whose miraculous encounters with madness were recorded by monks in large collections of miracles attributed to the saints.

John Z. Wee
read Assyriology and Classical History at Yale University (Ph.D., 2012), and is Assistant Professor at the University of Chicago (2015–). He is a historian of science, medicine, and mathematics in Mesopotamian and Graeco-Roman antiquity, and writes on the cultural histories of astronomical and medical ideas, scientific and mathematical language, and scholastic hermeneutics. Also from Brill are his monograph on *Knowledge and Rhetoric in Medical Commentary* (2019), a critical edition of *Mesopotamian Commentaries on the Diagnostic Handbook Sa-gig* (2019), and an edited volume of essays on *The Comparable Body* (2017).

Francis Zimmermann
teaches South Asian anthropology and history of science at the École des Hautes Études en Sciences Sociales, Paris. He has been combining the study of Sanskrit medical texts with ethnographic fieldwork in Kerala (South India) among learned practitioners of the local tradition of classical Ayurveda.

Introduction

Chiara Thumiger

As a term, 'holism' is a fairly recent arrival in the English language and in other modern languages that have taken over various forms of it from the English.[1] The contemporary use of the label began with the South African statesman and thinker Jan Christian Smuts, who adopted it in his wide-ranging 1926 *Holism and Evolution*, an exposition of what he saw as the 'synthetic tendency in the universe … the principle for the origin and progress of wholes in the universe', bringing together fields of inquiry as disparate as biology, politics, evolution and psychology.[2]

The book was perhaps not very influential in itself, but 'holism' became widely used in a variety of contexts and senses.[3] What the new term served to indicate, an approach to natural and human phenomena directed at the understanding and valorization of whole systems rather than particulars, was not in itself obviously novel at all. The new label became embedded within a longer history, whose modern intellectual phases are notably associated with Enlightenment vitalism.[4] The wider dialogue or opposition between a focus on the part(ial) or part(icular) and a notion of the whole or general, however, is a constant presence at various stages and levels in the history of Western thought, perhaps more than in other traditions. This broad opposition is widely disseminated in ancient science and philosophy (which reflected in various ways on cosmology, anthropology, psychology and metaphysics[5]), in

---

1 A glance at the classical languages already makes a semantic disjuncture evident, since the Greek for 'whole', ὅλος, can be only partially superimposed on Latin *universum* or *totus*. *Universum* conveys extension and replicability more than completeness, compactness and internal coherence, while *totus* suggests entirety as a merely quantitative and relative datum.

2 This work, with its environmental, psychological and biological scope, can be understood as background for Smuts' own political activity as a defender of human rights and ecological activist, based on a belief in natural law as the basis of civil law: see Anker (2001) 41–75 on the politics of Smuts' environmentalism in the context of 'paternalist ecology' (238–44).

3 Two years later the term was inserted into the *Encyclopedia Britannica*, described as 'a viewpoint additional and complementary to that of science.'

4 Harrington (1999) well describes the discontent with mechanicism and the demand for a 'reenchanted science' in German culture at the end of the nineteenth century.

5 See the treatment of the topic in Chiaradonna and Galluzzo (2013); the overview in D'Anna et al. (2019a); and the individual studies in D'Anna et al. (2019) on the topic of 'parts' and 'wholes' in modern thought after Montaigne.

DOI:10.1163/9789004443143_002

political theory from the Renaissance onwards,[6] and in the more recent history of the social sciences,[7] in which the term 'holism' finally established itself and its own brand of discussion of particulars and universals.

Today the terms 'holism' and 'holistic' evoke many varied associations. Some are technical: professional medical ideals,[8] lamenting disregard for the ill individual as 'whole' being and the interruption of the dialogue of information and negotiation between scientist-doctor and patient in modern medical practice (the 'disappearance of the sick man', in Jewson's formula[9]); biological theories; psychological and social doctrines.[10] Others involve 'complementary' (or 'alternative' or 'integrated') medicine, for which 'holism' implies a critique of mainstream bio-medicine as reductionist through reliance on an alternative system. There are also aspects of popular culture inspired by medical trends (anti-establishment postures, forms of anti-Western cultural critique, environmental and ecological concerns, popular trends).[11] Alongside these are negative paradigms of favoring the general at the expense of the individual: totalitarian conformity, the denial of idiosyncratic ambitions and individual rights, and a romantic reverence for an awe-inspiring, annihilating superior order with touches of the irrational, which in the early decades of the twentieth century found elements of complicity with Nazi ideology.[12] Academically, methodological forms of holism have been advocated mostly in social-historical or anthropological quarters, but there are important applications to aspects of the life sciences, as Sober makes clear by comparing methodological holism in sociology and in the discussion of group vs. individual selection in evolutionary biology.[13] How can such a multifarious category assist rigorous reflection on

6 In Guicciardini's famous formula, the contrast between *universale* and *particulare*, immutable nature vs. the uniqueness of the individual case; see Ginzburg (2018) 29–30 for an assessment of the tension between universal and individual in Machiavelli (and throughout the history of political theory), and the tradition of its 'contextualist' and 'universalist' interpretations.

7 See Gellner (1968) for an illustrative discussion, and 267–68 for reasonable assessment of methodological individualism vs. methodological holism in sociology and (social) history; the chapters in Brodbeck (1968) 239–336.

8 For surveys of these, see Rosenberg (1998); Laurence and Weisz (1998) 2–18; Poynton (1989).

9 Jewson (1976).

10 See Sober (1980); Weir (1985); Tennant (1986).

11 Various sub-cultural worlds, New Age and others, come into play here; see also Laurence and Weisz (1998) 6–8, 18.

12 See Laurence and Weisz (1998) 8–9; Harrington (1999), esp. 34–71, although with a balanced reevaluation of the traditional co-implications of vitalistic-holistic ideas and totalitarianism.

13 Sober (1980); Laurence and Weisz (1998) 5–6; Rosenberg (1985) 338–39.

the heritage of ancient thought and culture, and especially scientific thought and culture, or historical inquiry more widely?

Ancient medicine and philosophy, along with culture more generally, visibly thematized the concepts of 'part' and 'whole' in their theoretical reflections about nature, whether cosmologically or biologically. A famous Greek narrative about the origin of the world opens as follows: 'First of all, Chaos came into being.' Thus the beginning of the genealogy in Hesiod's *Theogony*[14] on the antecedent of all differentiations and plurality in the world: in the beginning was an opening, a *chaos*, a gaping ensemble of undistinguished being. Further down the genealogical line, the progressive division and individuation (between sexes, among classes of human beings, separating mortals and immortals) that are preconditions to the existence of the world we know are always brought about by conflict, a process of unavoidable deterioration and toil that culminates in the separation of the human race from the community of the gods. This story describes the fracturing of an original unity in both a cosmological and a cultural sense, a process we can locate within a Greek mythical pre-historic era, but which also works as archetypal 'pre-history' in an ideal sense. The marker of the premodern, for the anthropologist, is its inescapable 'monism': 'the native is a logical hoarder ... he is forever tying the threads, unceasingly turning over all the aspects of reality, whether physical, social or mental.'[15]

We easily recognize here the weight of wholeness (whether material, *chaos*; socio-historical, the community of human and divine; or biological, the original lack of sexual differentiation) as the perfect primeval state that characterizes most Western philosophical and metaphysical traditions. In ancient philosophy, this fundamental anteriority/superiority of the 'whole' assumes the shape of a competition between a monistic view of the *arche* (the fundamental substance/origin) of reality, which will ultimately prevail, and its pluralistic, and especially dualistic alternatives.[16] The contrasting pluralist

14 Hesiod, *Theogony* 116 ἤτοι μὲν πρώτιστα Χάος γένετ'.

15 Lévi-Strauss (1962/1966, 267), quoted by Latour (1993) 42. According to Latour in this work qualified actions of 'translation' (by which he meant the blending of concepts and cultural activities, creating forms of hybridism) are seminally opposed to those of 'purification' (by which he meant separation, distinction, specialisation) in defining premodernity and modernity, respectively. The psychological correlative to a 'native' (or premodern) exigency to reconstitute a unity, cosmological or ontological, is De Martino's concept of a 'crisis of presence' in ethnographic accounts, the 'risk of disintegration of the person's unitary being' (De Martino 1948/2007, 158–59, discussed by Chiaradonna and Marraffa 2018, 49–51).

16 The term 'monism' (like all such -isms of philosophical historiography) is also modern – allegedly first used by the eighteenth-century German philosopher Christian von Wolff in

view considers experienced reality fundamentally divided, whether through an opposition between mind and matter, body and soul, or mundane and divine (*dualism*), or as composed of a plurality of things of equal ontological weight (*pluralism*). The influence exerted by such oppositional 'one' vs. 'many' schemes – the problem of explaining plurality in the world and identifying mortality, materiality, imperfection and derivativeness with the ontological category of the plural – runs through many cosmological, biological, ethical and religious themes that require no more than a mention here: the various *archai* identified by pre-Socratic naturalist philosophy; Heraclitus' reference to a 'common account' of reality opposed to the 'own thinking' that people erroneously think they possess (D2); Eleatic monism and Parmenides' philosophy of the 'one';[17] the Pythagoreans' numerical representation of the world; Plato's identification of a sole source of Good and Being, to which the Ideas and everything that exists must refer (most evident in the *Republic*);[18] Aristotle's mission to accommodate the irreducible variety of the natural world; and the complexities of subsequent cosmologies in their attempts to account for the nature of the world on a materialistic basis, most influentially those of the Epicureans and Stoics.[19] The philosophical concept of the cosmos (κόσμος) as positive, as an expression (with various differences) of order, structure and design also belongs to this discussion.[20] Moreover, the idea of the universe as a purposeful whole obeying a comprehensive plan is fundamental in another influential ancient concept in the history of philosophy, that of a 'soul of the world' or *anima mundi*, originating in Plato's cosmology in the *Timaeus*. The *anima mundi* will be elaborated in important ways by Neoplatonic interpreters and beyond.[21] All these can be read on the premises of the seminal opposition between singularity and plurality, 'parts' and 'wholes',[22] with consequences

his *Logic* (1728). On the philosophical history, see Schaffer (2007/2018); Weir (2012a); and the entire volume (Weir 2012) for a cultural history of modern monism.

17 See Harriman (2019) 13–16 on Eleatic monism.

18 See Harte (2002) on the discussions about the relationship between parts and wholes in Plato's *oeuvre*.

19 See Gill (2006a) 209–22 for a discussion of these two systems; Holmes (2019) for the contacts between cosmology and biology in the Stoic notion of *sympathy*; Holmes and Coughlin in this volume.

20 See chapters in Hornky (2019), with Hornky (2019a), (2019b).

21 See Helmig (2020), (2020a); Miklós (2010) 1–8, and throughout for the legacy in German philosophy; Zachhuber (2020) for the possible combination with Aristotelian elements in the subsequent history of philosophy up to the eighteenth century.

22 The fundamental overview of mereology in ancient philosophy is offered by Barnes (1988/2011).

beyond cosmology.[23] Ancient religious traditions embodied the same tensions and existential uncertainties by depicting a polytheistic world of multiple divine entities overarched by a sovereign autocratic force, be it fate, eros or Zeus in abstract form.

Ancient ways of conceiving the human body and soul are model and matrix to these larger cosmological and ontological ideologies, as reflected by the core medical alternative between understanding the body as an ensemble of (co-working) parts to be independently analysed, or as a whole to be deciphered only as such.[24] Likewise, non-centripetal models of self can be reconstructed from ancient literature and philosophy, most evidently in archaic and tragic psychology.[25] Most notably, the question of the relationship between body and soul, psyche and matter, and their relations as parts of an assumed whole is variously approached by philosophers and doctors: the Platonic representation of the soul and its long heritage;[26] Aristotle's hylomorphic account of the soul;[27] the Stoic and Epicurean views of man as versions of psychosomatic unity;[28] the Galenic elaboration of the tripartite Platonic soul in its relationship with the body, especially in *De Placitis Hippocratis et Platonis*; even the various discussions in Christian theology about the nature of the divine trinity as unity or composition, as merely arithmetic plurality or as multiple

---

23 See Polito (2006) 286–90, nailing down through Galen's words (*De Nat.Fac.* 2.27–29) the fundamental schism in ancient philosophical history between 'those who posit that matter is a *continuum* and a *unity*' and 'advocate *intentionality* and *rationality* both at the level of nature and as a standard of human *knowledge* and *conduct*', and 'those who posit void and *particles*, and who explain life and *intelligence* in terms of the mechanical processes that inert matter undergoes, thus, in Galen's view, *abolishing human responsibility*' (my italics). This passage locates the opposition between unity and plurality at the core of ancient philosophy, and explicitly formulates the epistemological and ethical implications of the cosmological claim; on these, with a perspective on their heritage, see also Barnes (1988/2011a) 431–32.

24 See Gundert (1992) on the Hippocratics, and Lonie (1984) 137–40 on holistic images of the body in some Hippocratic texts; Von Staden on Celsus (2010) for discussion of what he sees as different 'stages' of medical thinking in this respect; Frey (2006) on the debate on the Aristotelian conception of the human living body vis-à-vis its matter and components; Gill (2006) on forms of 'mind-body holism' in Epicurean and Stoic thought.

25 See notably (if only representatively) the discussion of ancient 'selfhood' and modern individualism by Gill (1996); Remes and Sihvola (2008) and Chiaradonna and Maraffa (2018) 33–35 for the *status quaestionis*; n. 39 above.

26 On these, see Chiaradonna and Maraffa (2018), reading ancient and modern philosophical contributions vis-à-vis a 'unitary' self (or soul), especially 33–34; 36–41 on Plato; 45–46 on Plotinus.

27 See Frey (2006).

28 See Barnes (1990/2011b) 490–509; Gill (2006) 3–26 on Hellenistic and Roman philosophy, and Gill (2006a); (2010) 85–167 on psychology, and 229–43 on 'psychic parts and wholes.'

essence, and so on, is to an important extent articulated in the terms set by mereology in antecedent philosophy.[29]

The contact between natural philosophies and the reflections of medicine remains tangential, since the two domains of ancient science were always fundamentally distinct in purpose and practice, despite points of dialogue between them, and despite Galen famously boasting that 'the best doctor' – like himself – 'is also a philosopher.'[30] The history of monism in ancient cosmology as briefly sketched out above, and versions of 'holism' as a concept of medical interest, are thus comparable only in part, although the rich history of 'part' and 'whole' as metaphors outside medical discussions bears testimony to a common territory.[31] The authors of the *Corpus Hippocraticum* put forth a set of primarily non-anatomical, non-taxonomic models of health and pathology (often in competition with one another), holistic as such although not necessarily alternative to or competitive with any existing localized model. The therapeutic approaches in these classical sources, their etiological accounts and their reflections on patient cases follow similarly pragmatic lines, which holistic representations of the body in its active life serve better than theoretical abstractions do.[32] Examples of such delocalized, holistic themes are

29 Cf. Ramelli (2012) on this topic, with a focus on the concept of *hyposthasis*; Perilli (forthcoming) on *synarithmesis* in Galen and its echoes in the debate concerning the Trinity in early Christianity. It is also noteworthy that Galen's most explicit praise of nature and its 'demiurge' (*UP* 17.1, 446 3.7 Helmreich = IV.358 K.), evident in the teleological order shaping, for him, the animal bodies is offered at the end of his *De Usu Partium* (*On the Usefulness of Parts*). In this work the perfect adaptation of body parts to function and purpose, and to the qualities of the animal possessing them is expressed in terms of their being instrumental to the 'whole': 'the usefulness of them all (*scil.* the parts) is in relation to the soul' (χρεία δ' αὐτῶν ἁπάντων ἐστὶ τῇ ψυχῇ, *UP* 1.1, 1.13 Helmreich = III.1 K.).

30 On the territorial claims of philosophy and medicine in antiquity, see Levin (2014) on Plato; Polito (2016); Gill (2010).

31 For a confirmation of the antiquity and pervasiveness of this net of imagery, simply consider the principle of balance between elements and correct interaction between parts attested as early as Alcmaeon's doctrine on *isonomia tōn dunameōn*, 'balance of forces' (on which see Kouloumentas 2014). This image becomes highly influential as a bodily-medical metaphor in Graeco-Roman political theory – the 'whole' as ideal balance between parts in the correct state vs. the pathological predominance of one part or element, on which Coughlin (239–43) and Korobili and Stefou (201–3) in this volume have additional comments (see Brock 2000, 2006, and especially 2013, 69–70 on anatomical parts and wholes in Greek political imagery). Needless to say, balance as an ideal of well-being is widespread in medical systems, most often in association with humoural theories or fluid concepts of physiology; see the comparative discussion by Horden (2013) 3–7, as well as the individual chapters in that collection (Horden and Hsu 2013).

32 Gundert (1992); Pitman (2006); see Nutton (2013) 130–39 on the relatively late – Hellenistic – rise of anatomy.

the humours and their flux and balance, and the different individual 'constitutions' they determine in human beings, as Galen asserts in his *On Mixtures*; and the importance of respiration[33] or of the processes of air circulation and suffocation, especially (but not exclusively) in gynecological contexts,[34] as evident in the Hippocratic *On Breaths*. In addition, there is the devising of diffuse bodily features and physiological processes to account for vital functions, such as the elusive *poroi*, 'channels', mentioned in the Hippocratic *De Victu*, through which sensation is said to occur, or the *pēgai*, 'sources'; both reflect a 'composite' and delocalized, pluralistic conception of mental life comparable to the one most conspicuous in poetic accounts. Finally, one might mention the attention to non-localised indicators of well-being such as posture, movement and 'felt sense' of self, and the almost complete lack of literature on *loci* in this earlier phase of medicine.[35] All these features point towards a representation of the human body in which processes and fluid forces are at work, and holistic, non-localised explanatory models are resorted to, most famously represented by the image of the circle found at the beginning of *Places in Man*: 'there is no beginning in the body; but everything is alike beginning and end. For when a circle has been drawn, its beginning is not to be found.'[36] The so-called 'environmentalism' of classical medicine (perhaps less of a thematized doctrine than it is sometimes thought to be) echoes a similarly holistic representation of the refractions and influences between individual human beings and *milieu*. The complex theories of the effect of one's surroundings on bodily health (*Airs, Waters, Places* is the telling title of the main early source in this regard) extend to geographic settings, as well as to elements of weather and seasonal variation that permeate a number of clinical accounts. The so called 'constitutions' (*katastaseis*) described in Books 1 and 3 of the *Epidemics* are medical profiles, or accounts of predispositions to health-states directly

33 See Debru (1996) on respiration in Galen; Horden and Hsu (2013), with Horden's introduction on holistic paradigms; Horstmanshoff, King and Zittel (2012); Totelin (2016) on milk and flux in gynecology.

34 See King (1998) 80–84; Thumiger (2017) 103–8.

35 The principle is made eloquently explicit at *Places in Man* 1.1–4 (36 Craik = VI.276 L.): 'the beginning of ailments comes from the entire body alike … each part of the body at once transmits illness one to the other, whenever it arises in one place or another … The body is homogeneous (αὐτὸ ἑωυτῷ τωὐτόν ἐστι) and is composed of the same things, though not in uniform disposition, in its small parts and in its large; in parts above and parts below' (trans. Craik).

36 *Places in Man* 1 (36 Craik = VI.276 L.); see also *Regimen* 1.19 (138.27–9 Joly-Byl = VI.492–94 L.); *Nutr.* 23 (IX.106 L.). Lonie (1984) 139–40 analyses these and their philosophical parallels as examples of a combination of mechanicism and vitalism in Hippocratic medicine.

influenced by context.[37] The strongest expressions of environmental principles are found in the Hippocratics. But if we extend – as we should – the concept of environment to the chronological dimension and to seasonality (also important in classical medicine), other senses of a holistic sensibility emerge. As Coughlin shows,[38] the Pneumatists in particular elaborated the topic of the influence of seasons and weather on human health, and Galen as well, in his commentary on the Hippocratic *Airs, Waters, Places*, suggestively described the effect of the stability of seasons or lack thereof on human health as that between the correct tuning of the strings of an instrument and the harmony they can produce:

> When the mixture merges seasons with one another and the winter becomes warm and the summer cold, the effect of this goes counter to our nature; and because of these alterations, our nature is damaged and becomes weak. The strings [of a musical instrument] are an example of this: for when they are fitted as their working order requires, they produce a sound the listener enjoys. If one of the strings, the one called *hypatē* (the string touched by the index finger) is in the place of the string called *neatē* (that is, the string touched by the little finger), its tone has no harmony or sweetness. This is an example that explains the seasons and the health of our bodies in them.[39]

Holistic strategies, and above all else holistic questions, clearly continued to flourish in ancient medicine after the time of Hippocrates, due in part to the inspiration of natural philosophy, of biology and ethics. This happened in

37 See Nutton (2013) 75–86 on this aspect; but note already Vegetti (1965) 44 for accurate criticism of an ideal of Hippocratic doctrine as 'cosmically holistic', with an Eastern influence.

38 Coughlin (in preparation).

39 Commentary on 10,5, p. 48, 13–18 Diller, translated by G. Strohmaier, whom I thank for letting me use his forthcoming edition and translation into German (*Galeni in Hippocratis De Aere Aquis Locis Commentariorum Versionem Arabicam Primum Edidit, In Linguam Germanicam Vertit, Commentatus Est Gotthard Strohmaier*, CMG Suppl. Orientale V): 'Wenn die Mischung der Jahreszeiten gegeneinander versetzt und der Winter warm und der Sommer kalt wird, widerstreiten sie damit unseren Naturen, und diese nehmen durch diese Vorgänge Schaden und werden dabei geschwächt. Ein Beispiel dafür sind die Saiten. Denn wenn sie aufgezogen sind, wie es ihre Ordnung erfordert, kommt von ihnen ein Ton, an dem sich der Zuhörer erfreut. Wenn eine der Saiten an dem Platz einer anderen ist, also die Saite, die *hypatē* heißt – das ist die des Zeigefingers – an der Stelle der Saite, die *neatē* heißt – das ist die des kleinen Fingers – hat ihr Ton keinen Wohlklang und keine Süße. Das ist ein Beispiel, das die Jahreszeiten und die Gesundheit unserer Körper in ihnen veranschaulicht'.

concomitance with the development of the two most powerful tools of organization of knowledge in the Western medical tradition: anatomical studies, from the Alexandrian era onwards, and the rise of the great nosological categories, in the Imperial era.[40] Semi-metaphysical entities such as *pneuma*, a concept of Aristotelian origin with important medical currency;[41] the study of bodily connectives such as the nerves, the great development of the (post)-Hellenistic era;[42] theories regarding blood;[43] the reframing of humoural theories to account for states of disease in new, more articulated ways (Galen's theory of temperaments, *krasis*; the complexity of his physiology of respiration, treated by Debru[44]); a new holistic understanding of human mental health, combining the traditional materialism of Hippocratic medicine with the 'softer' psychological approach inspired by Hellenistic philosophies of the self, with the devising of a philosophical psycho-therapeutic medicine;[45] the principle of *sympatheia*[46] – all these complicate and strengthen the holistic element in the medicine of the Imperial age, posing questions and problems, and proposing solutions that return again and again in modern medical cultures. It is within this frame, for instance, that we can understand Soranus' discussion of pathology subdividing the kinds of affection (πάθος) which are against nature (like fever) into 'general and innate' (τὸ μὲν ὡς καθόλου καὶ γενικόν) and 'partial and secondary/acquired' (τὸ δὲ μερικὸν καὶ ὑποβεβηκός) – like what he treats as constriction and the disease *phrenitis* (or *lethargy*), respectively.[47] This clear distinction, absent from classical medicine, presupposes a notion of holism that is both organic (a *pathos* involving the whole body, not only a part) and transcends the individual case (a *pathos* innate to a category of human beings, as opposed to a state acquired by the living being).

---

40 Von Staden speaks of his passage as one from a 'Greek body' to a 'Roman body' (Von Staden 2010); see Roselli (2018) on nosology in ancient medicine.

41 See Lewis (2016) 215–310, and now the studies in Coughlin, Leith and Lewis (2020), 7–16 for the introduction; the classic study by Verbecke (1945).

42 See Rocca (2003) on Galen; Von Staden (2004) 155–61 on Herophilus.

43 See Lewis (2016) 215–310 on Praxagoras of Cos and the development of theories regarding blood vessels in Greek medicine; Boylan (2015) on the history of blood and blood circulation in ancient science.

44 Debru (1996).

45 For a survey, see Thumiger (2018); Gill (2018).

46 On which, see Holmes (2013), (2014), (2019).

47 Sor. *Gyn.* 3.1.2 (94,10–15 Ilberg), 'πάθος' δὲ λέγεται τὸ μὲν κατὰ φύσιν (οἷον τὸ συλλαμβάνειν καὶ ἀποτίκτειν καὶ γάλα ποιεῖν), τὸ δὲ παρὰ φύσιν (οἷον πυρέττειν) καὶ τοῦ παρὰ φύσιν τὸ μὲν ὡς καθόλου καὶ γενικόν (οἷον τὸ στεγνόν), τὸ δὲ μερικὸν καὶ ὑποβεβηκός (οἷον τὸ φρενιτικὸν ἢ ληθαργικόν).

Despite its evident importance, the weight and influence of 'holistic' engagement in the ancient beginnings of the history of science and its reception[48] have not been thematised in modern scholarship on ancient medicine, despite being common topics for historians of science generally.[49] Even when not declaring this openly, and while practicing historical and anthropological caution otherwise, the history of ancient science has most often focused on the developments and discoveries of the Graeco-Roman physicians through the demands and expectations of contemporary bio-medicine, i.e. of nosological taxonomy (the study of important 'diseases')[50] and of anatomical inquiry (the understanding of the ancient body with its parts, structures and functional 'seats' of this or that faculty). As a consequence, nosological entities, *loci affecti* and individual pathological data have tended to be isolated, if not in the ancient reality under reconstruction, then at least in the gaze and language of the historian working on ancient doctrines. The key tension between *localization* and *connectivity*, a fundamental one in the history of health, as neurology eloquently shows,[51] has seen localization prevail as the privileged frame of interpretation.[52] We should not ignore individual studies that examine non-localised features such as fluids and notably the humours[53] and interrogate ancient medical ideas from a variety of cultural-historical perspectives, posing larger philosophical questions that reestablish the deep intellectual affinities between modern and ancient science. But most scholarship on ancient medical doctrines has looked at parts, organs and diseases, or at authors, texts and medical schools. Ancient views about the overarching forces that superintend life and the systemic structures that shape the living body have been touched on only episodically.

48 Exceptions in a comparative spirit to this trend are Pitman (2006); Horstmanshoff, King and Zittel (2012); Horden and Hsu (2013).

49 But see now Holmes (forthcoming) on the Greek foundations in the discussions of vitalism in the history of biology, focusing on Canguilhelm. See also Lawrence and Weisz (1998) for an introduction to holism in interwar medicine, 6–9 on its affiliations to vitalism; Harrington (1999) 1–30 on vitalism and holism in German culture.

50 Such as gynecological diseases, malaria, melancholy and mania; see the discussion of (ancient) nosology in Thumiger/Singer (2018) 2–15, with a focus on the psychiatric sphere.

51 See Günther (2017) on the 'break with the localization project' at the roots of both modern neurology and psychoanalysis (7); Harrington (1999) 72–102; Huneman (2008a).

52 Salmón (2017) aims to redress a similar unbalance with reference to Medieval medicine in his exploration of the brain as actor within a 'holistic system' in Medieval medicine.

53 See again Horden and Hsu (2013), with the introduction; Horstmanshoff, King and Zittel (2012), with the discussion of the history of physiology by King (1–12); Debru (1996) on physiology.

On a parallel path, strands of the so-called 'alternative medicines' have chosen to reconnect their practices to (their version of)[54] the medical principles and practices of ancient Greece through reliance on a continuity within traditional Western medical systems seen as running alongside official and institutional medicine. Such readers have often established connections with non-Western traditions, as Pitman does in her analysis of Hippocratic medicine as 'holistic.'[55] This is not only a narrative of enrichment. Alongside the perceived debts of a more natural, 'human' approach to ancient approaches to health, an historian can only note the ancient roots of our own constraints and limitations: the normativity and politics of certain holisms also have ancient champions.[56] The holistic ideal of the healthy, handsome (young, male) body that is so significant in our tradition as to have become inconspicuous is also rooted in ancient aesthetic and medical understandings of the human. Only in recent years have disability studies and feminist scholarship begun to invent means to correct this hegemonic outlook and to explore alternative paths.[57]

Finally, there is a methodological holism that has long given form to the tradition of personalized forms of authority – a catalogue of influential figures, whose *corpora* of works are fetishized at the expense of more fluid epistemological histories. This tradition becomes coterminous with the published and transmitted doctrines of elite cultures, at the expense of popular bodies of knowledge that intersected with them and gave them flesh and blood, even if they were officially relegated to their margins or openly opposed.[58] The culmination of this tradition is its current, unchallenged status as ultimate 'scientific truth', which invests Western biomedicine with the merit and responsibility of deciphering and rescuing the 'health of the world' as a whole, inevitably

---

54 See King in this volume for a critical assessment of this attitude in contemporary popular culture; in an anthropological frame of discussion, see the critique by Zimmermann (1995), e.g. 145, of the 'artificial universalism' of the supporters of 'alternative medicines' (my translation).

55 Pitman (2006), with a detailed parallel to Āyurvedic medicine; Di Stefano (2006) for an example of discussion of 'complementary medicine' and the holistic ideal; Pitman (2014) 36–37 on holism and herbal medicine, 29–32 on holism traced back to ancient Greek medicine via complementary medicines; Griggs (1997), e.g. 14, for Hippocrates' 'emphasis on a balanced, wholistic approach to doctoring'; see also Lopez (2004) for reflection on philosophical aspects of Hippocratic doctrines in terms of 'pensiero olistico.'

56 See again Wohl (2019).

57 See Adams (2017) for a theoretically minded discussion; the explorations in Laes (2017), with (2017a); (2018) 1–22.

58 For recent discussion of the stratified nature of 'medical cultures' vis-a-vis the ancient world, see Oberhelman (2013); Harris (2016a).

surpassing any alternative tradition. This exclusivism is also a part, not always desirable, of the legacy of ancient medicine and its reception.

This volume cannot entirely escape the modes of scholarly discussion that characterise our field, and must accordingly focus on one particular set of ancient sources and themes within the ancient life sciences and their cultural parallels. The realms of politics, economy, sociology and social history, and linguistic and literary studies, all potentially relevant, are mostly ignored. The contributors tackle the topic of 'parts', 'wholes' and 'holism' as concept and topic from a variety of perspectives. They all concentrate on central questions in the history of science, in some cases choosing key authors or medical schools, in others a theme or element of debate. In a few cases, they explore the parallels and itineraries of reception beyond ancient Graeco-Roman cultures.

The chapters are accordingly organised in three sections: the first more theoretical and methodological; the second focusing on Graeco-Roman medicine and culture; and the third broadening the field to reception and cross-cultural considerations.

The first section, 'Holism: Methodological and Theoretical Perspectives', opens with a general study of 'Holism, parts, wholes', in which I attempt to trace the different senses in which holism, although an irreducibly elusive concept, has been central in a variety of fields of knowledge in European intellectual history, including medicine, science, philosophy and politics, but also in pillars of modernity such as psychology and psychoanalysis, reflections about gender, and ecology. Academically, it poses central questions about our own way of relating to the 'classical' past. The topic of our volume is of course much more narrowly defined. But it is fundamentally important to bear in mind the suggestive and complex histories of this term and theoretical instrument as we look for instances of it in the past from a modern standpoint. I distinguish here between a methodological holism (a holistic approach to the study of history and culture, in the first instance) and an ontological one (the active belief in the holistic nature of things), while highlighting the point of contact between the two. Most of the chapters will in fact adopt a composite attitude by probing the holistic features of aspects of ancient scientific thought, while at the same time engaging with it as project and value.

The other two chapters in this more theoretical section are examples of these two typologies. In 'Holism, Sympathy, and the Living Being in Ancient Greek Medicine and Philosophy', Brooke Holmes focuses on the concept and philosophical standing of 'sympathy' in human nature in a variety of elaborations from Plato to Galen, and along two different typologies or 'axes'. At the same time, she takes the opportunity to interrogate 'ancient holism' as an instance of modern reception of ancient Greek medicine and science, as well as of Greece as 'pure, unified form of life'. William Short, on the other hand, considers the emotions as a historical object of inquiry in a methodologically holistic perspective informed by embodied cognitivism. Short offers an instructive survey of recent historical approaches to this fundamental aspect of human psychology, currently a rich field of study in the broader field of classics ('"Holism" in Cognitive Approaches to the Ancient Emotions'), while showing the sense in which the claim of a fundamental mind-body holism holds as central to an understanding of human emotions as embodied and closely dependent on our interactions with the environment.

The second section poses more concretely and textually the question that informs the volume in a historical sense: 'Is Graeco-Roman Medicine Holistic?' These chapters, organised in part chronologically and in part thematically, share a focus on key figures, schools or intellectual approaches in ancient medical-biological thought. They discuss ancient responses to the question of wholes and parts in the nature of things and the human way of approaching them, beginning with the Hippocratic texts and proceeding to their philosophical contemporaries and heirs. Chapters 4 to 6 explore the history of ancient medicine from the Hippocratics to Galen in the broadest perspective. Hynek Bartoš delves into the fundamental example of the Hippocratic *De Victu*, a fascinating work that contains holistic views of the human body and its health in relation to a cosmic context ('Hippocratic Holisms'). This text, whose at times obscure and hermetic style has made access difficult for non-specialists, deserves to be better known and studied outside the restricted circles of ancient medical historians as a central contribution to ancient philosophy. David Leith offers a thorough discussion of the ancient school most readily associated with a holistic approach, the Methodists ('Holism and the Methodists'), a group of medical thinkers whose works survive to a large extent indirectly. Leith offers a rich selection of passages and comments on them vis-a-vis holism. On the one hand, he clarifies and nuances received narratives about Methodist approaches to localisation and therapy in medical practice, while on the other he places these thinkers in dialogue with other figures in the Greek medical tradition. P. N. Singer concentrates on Galen ('Is Graeco-Roman Medicine Holistic? Galen and Ancient Medical-Philosophical Debates'), reflecting on the meaning of the concept holism in the context of Imperial-age medicine and placing holistic themes and concerns in Galen in dialogue with other, less studied authors, both medical and philosophical, while framing it within Greek intellectual history from as early as Plato. The next two chapters are located earlier chronologically, considering sources outside medicine in the classical era – tragedy and

Plato, respectively. Elizabeth Craik's 'Holism of Body and Mind in Hippocratic Medicine and Greek Tragedy' brings to light the deep holistic interconnections between medical and poetic representations in Greek tragedy, while 'Plato's *Charmides* on Philosophy as Holistic Medical Practice' by Giouli Korobili and Konstantinos Stefou turns to a major philosophical source, Plato, and explores his reflections on medicine in a famous and intriguing passage in the *Charmides* where attention to 'parts' and 'wholes' serves as the kernel of a debate between different medical approaches.

Chapters 9–11, again primarily medical, share a concern for the materiality of human physiology in ancient thought. In this sense, physiological fluids occupy a central position in Hippocratic gynecology, as is shown by Laurence Totelin in her study of 'liquid' expressions of life in gynecological ideas (medical and non-medical), 'A Woman in Flux: Fluidity in Hippocratic Gynaecology.' Sean Coughlin takes the discussion to philosophical authors who had an important influence on the ancient medical debate, and sets out to reconstruct a key 'holistic' principle found in Greek thought from early natural philosophy to Aristotle and the Stoics: that of the 'cohesive cause' that holds a body's parts together, providing the condition for their forming a 'whole.' This chapter offers a careful survey of a set of underexplored sources in this respect (Empedocles, Anaximenes, Diogenes of Apollonia and others) and then assesses the Aristotelian position in dialogue with them and with Plato ('Cohesive Causes in Ancient Greek Philosophy and Medicine'). Julius Rocca, finally, offers a rich discussion of *pneuma*, a fundamental concept and physiological substance in Galen's thought (as well as earlier traditions). Rocca focusses on Galen's view of *pneuma* as a holistic concept and broadens his scope to explore the afterlife of the concept ('Pneuma as a Holistic Concept in Galen').

As I argue in more detail in Chapter 1, this project not only concedes the deep co-implications of modern and ancient, Western and non-Western approaches to holism, but also argues positively for the enduring relevance of such discussions to modern debates, while exposing the flaws of simplistic images of affiliation. In this spirit, the final section (Chapters 12–17), 'Medical Holism beyond the Graeco-Roman World', opens the floor to the heritage and reception of ancient discussions in later science and medicine, and to comparative material and non-Western perspectives. In 'Humoralism in Āyurvedic Medicine', Francis Zimmermann probes the commonalities between Indian and Greek medical systems in terms of doctrinal principles, representations of the functioning of the human body and even intellectual strategies, uncovering parallels between Hippocratic and Galenic positions (for example vis-a-vis humouralism and dietetics) and Sanskrit medical writings. John Z.

Wee explores in great detail evidence from the ancient Near East ('A Systemic Etiology of Sicknesses from Ancient Iraq: Organ Systems and the Functional Holism of the Babylonian Body') and the different kinds of 'holism' (bodily, environmental, cosmological) they embed in their medical systems, mindful of the role played by the modern scholarly gaze in interpreting the ancient data as homogenous antecedents to medical principles familiar to us. Vivian Nutton undertakes the interpretation of a fundamental feature of Greek medicine, and a delocalised one, the humours, as an expression of a specific disposition to health (a person's individual *krasis*) in opposition to environmental and thus collective patterns of epidemiology. Within this framework, Nutton addresses the conundrum of the ancients' lack of a thematised interest in the concept of infection, on the one hand, and of 'disease of specific groups' of the kind found in early modern medicine, on the other, placing the evidence in a historical perspective that takes us from the Hippocratics to the Renaissance ('Epidemic disease in a Humoral Environment; from *Airs, Waters and Places* to the Renaissance'). The compartmentalization we wished to avoid in this collection counts not only non-Western productions among its victims, but also expressions of human culture less shaped by narratives of scientific progress. Counterbalancing such tendency, Claire Trenery's study explores the legacy of ancient holism and Graeco-Roman medical doctrines more generally in Medieval spiritual approaches to human health. Through a variety of fascinating examples from English miracle texts, she illustrates how the 'materialistic', holistic basis of Hippocratic and Galenic medicine, inherited by Medieval intellectuals through Syriac, Arabic and Latin translations, was combined with religious ideas of insanity in the actions of celebrated saints and healers in western Christendom ('Mind-Body Interaction: The Influence of Ancient Ideas in Twelfth-Century England'). This section, along with the volume as a whole, concludes with a unique study that questions more radically the scope and legitimacy of a project such as ours: Helen King opens the door to a world rarely touched by scholarly attention, that of popular and lay reception of ancient medicine, especially in on-line communities ('"Treating the Patient, not just the Disease": Reading Ancient Medicine in Modern Holistic Medicine').

Holism emerges from this discussion not only as a project, a methodology and an interpretation of reality, but as a complex set of questions and strategies deeply imbedded in embodied human life and as a consequence in human culture and epistemology generally. These questions may change shape, take contradictory forms, reject ancient solutions or suggest new ones, while never permanently solving them. They may engender very different, even opposed intellectual and scholarly strategies for approaching other cultural traditions, whether ancient or modern. But the problem of embodied human existence, balanced between individuality and generality, animal and environment, 'parts' and 'wholes', is set to remain at the centre of medical, biological and philosophical reflection – indeed, of our entire experience as living beings.[59]

Acknowledgments

I am grateful to several readers who commented on this text. In particular, Simon Swain, Brooke Holmes, Helen King, and Sean Coughlin offered precious insights and suggested improvements on individual points. I would also like to thank S. Douglas Olson for his many comments and corrections to the draft at various stages. I owe gratitude as well to the Wellcome Trust, which funded me for the research project within which the present paper took shape.

Bibliography

Adams, E. 'Fragmentation and the Body's Boundaries: Reassessing the Body in Parts.' In *Ancient Anatomical Votives Past, Present and Future*, ed. J. Draycott and E.-J. Graham. London and New York: Routledge (2017) 193–213.

Anker, P. *Imperial Ecology: Environmental Order in the British Empire, 1895–1945*. Cambridge MA: Harvard University Press (2001).

Barnes, J. 'Bits and Pieces.' In *Method and Metaphysics: Essays in Ancient Philosophy I*. Oxford: Oxford University Press (1988/2011a) 429–83 (originally published in *Matter and Metaphysics*, ed. J. Barnes and M. Mignucci. Naples 1988, 224–94).

Barnes, J. 'Partial wholes.' In *Method and Metaphysics: Essays in Ancient Philosophy I*. Oxford: Oxford University Press (1990/2011b) 484–509 (originally published in *Social Philosophy and Policy*, 8 (1990) 1–23).

Boylan, M. *The Origins of Ancient Greek Science: Blood – A Philosophical Study*. London and New York: Routledge (2015).

Brock, R. 'Sickness in the Body Politic: Medical Imagery in the Greek Polis.' In *Death and Disease in the Ancient City*, ed. V. Hope and M. and E. Marshall. London & New York: Routledge (2000) 24–34.

Brock, R. 'The Body as Political Organism in Greek Thought.' In *Penser et représenter le corps dans l'antiquité*, ed. F. Prost and J. Wilgaux. Rennes: Presses Universitaires (2006) 351–59.

59 See Laurence and Weisz (1998) 16 on holism as an enduring 'barometer' in the history of the life sciences.

Brock, R. *Greek Political Imagery from Homer to Aristotle*. London: Bloomsbury (2013).
Brodbeck, M. *Readings in the Philosophy of the Social Sciences*. Cambridge MA: MIT Press (1968).
Chiaradonna, R. and G. Galluzzo (eds.) *Universals in Ancient Philosophy*. Pisa: Edizioni della Normale (2013).
Chiaradonna, R. and G. Galluzzo. 'Introduction.' In *Universals in Ancient Philosophy*, ed. R. Chiaradonna and G. Galluzzo. Pisa: Edizioni della Normale (2013a) 1–22.
Chiaradonna, R. 'Universals in Ancient Medicine.' In *Universals in Ancient Philosophy*, ed. R. Chiaradonna and G. Galluzzo. Pisa: Edizioni della Normale (2013b) 381–424.
Chiaradonna, R., and M. Maraffa. 'Ontology and the Self: Ancient and Contemporary Perspectives.' In *Ancient Ontologies: Contemporary Debates*. Discipline Filosofiche XXVIII I, ed. R. Chiaradonna, F. Forcignanò and F. Trabattoni. Macerata: Quidlibet (2018) 33–64.
Coughlin, S. *Athenaeus of Attalia: The Complete Fragments*. In preparation.
Coughlin, S., D. Leith, and O. Lewis (eds.) *The Concept of Pneuma after Aristotle*. Berlin Studies of the Ancient World 61. Berlin: Edition Topoi (2020).
D'Anna, G., E. Massimilla, F. Piro, M. Sanna and F. Toto (eds.) *Morfologie del Rapporto Parti-Tutto. Totalità e complessità nelle filosofie dell'età moderna*. Milan: Mimesis (2019).
D'Anna, G., E. Massimilla, F. Piro, M. Sanna and F. Toto. 'Prefazione.' In *Morfologie del Rapporto Parti-Tutto. Totalità e complessità nelle filosofie dell'età moderna*. Milan: Mimesis (2019a) 9–24.
De Martino, E. *Il Mondo Magico*. Torino: Bollati Boringhieri (1948/2007).
Debru, A. *Le corps respirant – La pensée physiologique chez Galien*. Leiden: Brill (2018).
Di Stefano, V. *Holism and Complementary Medicine. Origins and Principles*. Allen and Unwin: Crows Nest (2006).
Francia, S., and A. Stobart (eds.) *Critical Approaches to the History of Western Herbal Medicine from Classical Antiquity to the Early Modern Period*. London: Bloomsbury (2014).
Frey, C. 'Organic Unity and the Matter of Man.' *Oxford Studies in Ancient Philosophy*, 32 (2007) 167–204.
Gellner, E. 'Holism Versus Individualism.' In *Readings in the Philosophy of the Social Sciences*, ed. M. Brodbeck. Cambridge MA: MIT Press (1968) 254–68.
Gill, C. *Personality in Greek Epic, Tragedy and Philosophy*. Oxford: Clarendon Press (1996).
Gill, C. *The Structured Self in Hellenistic and Roman Thought*. Oxford: Oxford University Press (2006).
Gill, C. 'Psychophysical Holism in Epicureanism and Stoicism.' In *Common to Body and Soul: Philosophical Approaches to Explaining Living Behaviour in Graeco-Roman Antiquity*, ed. R. A. H. King. Berlin: De Gruyter (2006a) 209–31.

Gill, C. *Naturalistic Psychology in Galen and Stoicism*. Oxford: Oxford University Press (2010).

Gill, C. 'Philosophical Psychological Therapy – Did It Have Any Impact on Medical Practice?' In *Mental Illness in Ancient Medicine from Celsus to Paul of Aegina*, ed. C. Thumiger and P. N. Singer. Leiden: Brill (2018) 365–80.

Ginzburg, C. *Nondimanco. Machiavelli, Pascal*. Milan: Adelphi (2018).

Griggs, B. *Green Pharmacy: The History and Evolution of Western Herbal Medicine*. Rochester VT: Healing Arts Press (1997).

Gundert, B. 'Parts and Their Roles in Hippocratic Medicine.' *Isis*, 83.3 (1992) 453–65.

Günther, K. *Localization and Its Discontents. A Genealogy of Psychoanalysis and the Neuro Disciplines*. Chicago: University of Chicago Press (2015).

Harriman, B. *Melissus and Eleatic Monism*. Cambridge: Cambridge University Press (2018).

Harrington, A. *Reenchanted Science: Holism in German Culture from Wilhelm II to Hitler*. Princeton: Princeton University Press (1999).

Harris, W. V. (ed.) *Popular Medicine in Graeco-Roman Antiquity: Explorations. Columbia studies in the classical tradition*, 42. Leiden and Boston: Brill (2016).

Harris, W. V. 'Popular Medicine in the Classical World.' In *Popular Medicine in Graeco-Roman Antiquity: Explorations. Columbia Studies in the Classical Tradition*, 42, ed. W. V. Harris. Leiden and Boston: Brill (2016a) 1–64.

Harte, V. *Plato on Parts and Wholes: The Metaphysics of Structure*. Oxford: Clarendon Press (2002).

Helmig, C. (ed.) *World Soul – Anima Mundi. On the Origins and Fortunes of a Fundamental Idea*. Berlin: De Gruyter (2020).

Helmig, C. 'The World Soul in Antiquity and Beyond.' In *World Soul – Anima Mundi. On the Origins and Fortunes of a Fundamental Idea*, ed. C. Helmig. Berlin: De Gruyter (2020a) 1–26.

Holmes, B. 'Disturbing Connections: Sympathetic Affections, Mental Disorder, and Galen's Elusive Soul.' In *Mental Disorders in Classical Antiquity*, ed. W. V. Harris. Leiden: Brill (2013) 147–76.

Holmes, B. 'Proto-Sympathy in the Hippocratic Corpus.' In *Hippocrate et les hippocratismes: médecine, religion, société: Actes du XIVe Colloque International Hippocratique*, ed. J. Jouanna and M. Zink. Paris: Académie des Inscriptions et Belles Lettres (2014) 123–38.

Holmes, B. 'On Stoic Sympathy: Cosmobiology and the Life of Nature.' In *Antiquity beyond Humanism*, ed. E. Bianchi, S. Brill and B. Holmes. Oxford: Oxford University Press (2019) 239–70.

Holmes, B. 'Canguilhem and the Greeks: Vitalism between History and Philosophy.' In *Vitalism and the Contemporary Life Sciences*, ed. C. Donohue and C. Wolfe. New York: Springer (forthcoming).

Holmes, B., and C. Güthenke. 'Hyperinclusivity, Hypercanonicity, and the Future of the Field.' In *Marginality, Canonicity, Passion*, ed. M. Formisano and C. Kraus. Oxford: Oxford University Press (2018) 57–73.

Horden, P. 'Introduction.' In *The Body in Balance. Humoral Medicines in Practice*, ed. P. Horden and E. Hsu. Oxford: Berghahn (2013) 1–21.

Horden, P., and E. Hsu (eds.) *The Body in Balance. Humoral Medicines in Practice.* Oxford: Berghahn (2013).

Hornky, S. P. (ed.) *Cosmos in the Ancient World.* Cambridge: Cambridge University Press (2019).

Hornky, S. P. 'Introduction.' In *Cosmos in the Ancient World*, ed. S. P. Hornky. Cambridge: Cambridge University Press (2019a) 1–21.

Hornky, S. P. 'When Did kosmos Become the Kosmos.' In *Cosmos in the Ancient World*, ed. S. P. Hornky. Cambridge: Cambridge University Press (2019b) 22–41.

Horstmanshoff, M., H. King and C. Zittel (eds.) *Blood, Sweat, and Tears: The Changing Concepts of Physiology from Antiquity into Early Modern Europe. Intersections*, 25. Leiden and Boston: Brill (2012).

Hsu, E. 'What next?' In *The Body in Balance. Humoral Medicines in Practice*, ed. P. Horden and E. Hsu. Oxford: Berghahn (2013) 259–80.

Huneman, P. '"Animal Economy" – Anthropology and the Rise of Psychiatry from the 'Encyclopédie' to the Alienists.' In *Anthropology of the Enlightenment*, ed. L. Wolff and M. Cipolloni. Stanford: Stanford University Press (2008) 262–76.

Jewson, J. D. 'The Disappearance of the Sick-Man from Medical Cosmology, 1770–1870.' *Sociology*, 10.2 (1976) 225–44.

King, H. *Hippocrates' Woman*. London: Routledge (1998).

King, H. *The One-Sex Body on Trial: The Ancient and Early Modern Evidence*. London: Routledge (2012).

Kouloumentas, S. 'The body and the polis: Alcmaeon on Health and Disease.' *British Journal for the History of Philosophy*, 22.2 (2014) 867–87.

Laes, C. (ed.) *Disability in Antiquity*. London: Routledge (2017).

Laes, C. 'Introduction.' In *Disability in Antiquity*. London: Routledge (2017a) 1–21.

Laes, C. *Disabilities and the Disabled in the Roman World: a Social and Cultural History*. Cambridge: Cambridge University Press (2018).

Latour, B. *We Have Never Been Modern*. Trans. C. Porter. Cambridge MA: Harvard University Press (*Nous n'avons jamais été modernes: Essai d'anthropologie symmetrique*, 1991).

Lawrence, C., and G. Weisz. 'Medical Holism: the Context.' In *Greater than the Parts: Holism in Biomedicine 1920–50*, ed. C. Lawrence and G. Weisz. Oxford: Oxford University Press (1998) 1–22.

Lévi-Strauss, C. *The Savage Mind*. Chicago: University of Chicago Press (1962/1966).

Levin, S. B. *Plato's Rivalry with Medicine: A Struggle and Its Dissolution*. Oxford: Oxford University Press (2014).

Lewis, O. *Praxagoras of Cos on Arteries, Pulse and Pneuma: Fragments and Interpretation*. Leiden: Brill (2017).

Lonie, I. M. 'Hippocrates the Iatromechanist.' *Medical History*, 25 (1981) 113–50.

Miklós, V. *Anima Mundi: The Rise of the World Soul Theory in Modern German Philosophy*. Dordrecht: Springer (2010).

Nutton, V. *Ancient Medicine*. London: Routledge (2013).

Oberhelman, S. M. *Dreams, Healing, and Medicine in Greece: From Antiquity to the Present*. Farnham and Burlington VT: Ashgate (2013).

Perilli, L. 'Synarithmesis. Trinitarian Arithmetics, Early Christianity and Medicine in the Second Century CE.' Forthcoming.

Pitman, V. *The Nature of the Whole. Holism in Ancient Greek and Indian Medicine*. Delhi: Motilal Banarsidass Publishers (2006).

Pitman, V. 'Early Greek Medicine: Evidence of Models, Methods and Materia Medica.' In *Critical Approaches to the History of Western Herbal Medicine from Classical Antiquity to the Early Modern Period*. London: Bloomsbury (2014) 27–46.

Polito, R. 'Matter, Medicine, and the Mind: Asclepiades vs. Epicurus.' *Oxford Studies in Ancient Philosophy* 30 (2006) 285–335.

Polito, R. 'Competence Conflicts Between Philosophy and Medicine: Caelius Aurelianus and the Stoics on Mental Diseases.' *Classical Quarterly*, NS 66 (2016) 358–69.

Poynton, J. C. 'Holistic Thinking in Medicine: Pitfalls and Possibilities.' *Holistic Medicine*, 4.3 (1989) 137–44.

Ramelli, I. L. E. 'Origen, Greek Philosophy, and the Birth of the Trinitarian Meaning of "Hypostasis".' *Harvard Theological Review*, 105.3 (2012) 302–50.

Remes, P. and J. Sihvola (eds.) 'Introduction.' *Ancient Philosophies of the Self*. Dordrecht: Springer (1998) 1–10.

Rocca, J. *Galen on the Brain: Anatomical Knowledge and Physiological Speculation in the Second Century AD*. Leiden: Brill (2003).

Roselli, A. 'Nosology.' In *The Cambridge Companion to Hippocrates*, ed. P. E. Pormann. Cambridge: Cambridge University Press (2018) 80–199.

Rosenberg, C. E. 'Holism in Twentieth-Century Medicine.' In *Greater than the Parts: Holism in Biomedicine 1920–50*, ed. C. Lawrence and G. Weisz. Oxford: Oxford University Press (1998) 335–55.

Salmón, Fernando. 'Explorando el cerebro: La transmisión y desarrollo de un sistema médico holístico en los siglos XIII y XIV.' *Romance Philology*, 71 (2017) 623–42.

Schaffer, J. 'Monism'. *The Stanford Encyclopedia of Philosophy* (Winter 2018 Edition). Ed. Edward N. Zalta (2007/2018). Available at https://plato.stanford.edu/archives/win2018/entries/monism/, retrieved May 2020).

Smuts, J. C. *Holism and Evolution*. New York: The MacMillan Company (1926).

Sober, E. 'Holism, Individualism, and the Units of Selection.' *Proceedings of the Biennial Meeting of the Philosophy of Science Association,* (1980) 93–121.

Tennant, N. W. 'Reductionism and Holism in biology.' In *A History of Embryology*, ed. T. J. Horder, J. A. Witkowski and C. C. Wylie. Cambridge: Cambridge University Press (1986) 407–33.

Thumiger, C. 'Therapy of the Word and other Psychotherapeutic Approaches in Ancient Greek Medicine.' In *Other Psychotherapies*. Special issue of *Transcultural Psychiatry*, ed. R. G. White, C. McGeachan, G. Miller and S. Xenophontos (2018).

Thumiger, C., and G. Petridou. 'Introduction.' In *Homo Patiens. Approaches to the Patient in the Ancient World*, ed. G. Petridou and C. Thumiger. Leiden: Brill (2015) 1–22.

Totelin, L. M. V. 'Motherhood in Flux: Greek Nymphs, Breastfeeding, and Ancient Gynaecology.' In *Maternità e Politeismi. Motherhood(s) and Polytheisms*, ed. F. P. Guignard, G. Pedrucci and M. Scapini. Bologna: Patron Editore (2017) 359–70.

Vegetti, M. 'Il pensiero di Ippocrate.' Introduzione alle *Opere di Ippocrate*. Torino: UTET (1965) 9–63.

Verbecke, G. *L'évolution de la Doctrine du pneuma: du Stoicisme a S. Augustin*. Paris: Desclée de Brouwer (1945).

Von Staden, H. *Herophilus: The Art of Medicine in Early Alexandria*. Cambridge: Cambridge University Press (2004).

Von Staden, H. 'How Greek was the Latin body? The Parts and the Whole in Celsus' *Medicina*.' In *Body, Disease and Treatment in a Changing World: Latin Texts and Contexts in Ancient and Medieval Medicine: Proceedings of the Ninth International Conference*, ed. D. R. Langslow and B. Maire. Lausanne: Éditions BHMS (2010) 3–23.

Weir, A. 'Against Holism.' *The Philosophical Quarterly*, 35 (1985) 225–44.

Weir, T. H. (ed.) *Monism: Science, Philosophy, Religion, and the History of a Worldview.* London: Palgrave (2012).

Weir, T. H. 'The Riddles of Monism: an Introductory Essay.' In *Monism: Science, Philosophy, Religion, and the History of a Worldview*, ed. T. H. Weir. London: Palgrave (2012a) 1–44.

Wohl, V. 'Afterword.' In *Cosmos in the Ancient World*, ed. S. P. Hornky. Cambridge: Cambridge University Press (2019) 295–303.

Zachhuber, J. 'World Soul and Celestial Heat. Platonic and Aristotelian Ideas in the History of Natural Philosophy.' In *World Soul – Anima Mundi. On the Origins and Fortunes of a Fundamental Idea*, ed. C. Helmig. Berlin: De Gruyter (2020) 335–53.

Primary Texts: Editions and Translations Used

De Aere Aquis Locis. Hippokrates über die Umwelt (= CMG 1,1,2). Ed. and trans. by H. Diller. Berlin (1970).

Galeni in Hippocratis De Aere Aquis Locis Commentariorum Versionem Arabicam Primum Edidit, In Linguam Germanicam Vertit, Commentatus Est Gotthard Strohmaier (= CMG Suppl. Orientale V). Ed. and trans. by G. Strohmaier. Berlin (forthcoming).

PART 1

Holism: Methodological and Theoretical Perspectives

CHAPTER 1

Holism, Parts, Wholes

Chiara Thumiger

Abstract

'Holism', strangely enough, given the absolute quality it indicates, is a concept that can only be grasped through negative examples: what it is contrary to, the paradigms to which it constitutes an alternative. Definitions of 'holism' thus usually involve the interdependence among the parts composing an individual object; their relationship with that object as their container and sum; its insertion within a context, environmental or cosmic; and crucially, the existence of an additional *quid* which defines that object as a totality independent of its components – the idea that 'the whole is greater than the sum of its parts.'

In all these senses, the significance of the relationship between 'parts' and 'whole' can be much broader than the medical and anatomical discussions with which we would most immediately associate it, and which are under the spotlight in this volume. The breadth and malleability of the concept are key to a cultural history which is extremely long, despite the fact that 'holism' itself, like many such labels, can easily be seen as anachronistic if applied to the pre-modern world. This chapter aims to offer a glimpse of this long history and to illustrate the relevance of the Graeco-Roman past to our understanding of the idea of holism, and to its various manifestations throughout the centuries which separate us from the ancients.

1 The Challenges of Holism

The fact that 'holism' still lacks the status of a univocal, free-standing item in cultural history or philosophy is due to more essential reasons than those implied by its recent history and current popularity, with their sometimes imprecise and amateurish usages. A double challenge to defining the concept is posed by it being inherently relative and by its involvement in the idea of value.

First of all, 'holism' has a situated quality that resists any attempt at precision, a circumstance that far exceeds the contingent datum of the recent coinage of the name itself. The impossibility of a univocal 'holism' is due to the truism that 'whole' and 'parts' are relative, non-neutral entities. What we consider a whole, which 'parts' we choose to highlight, and 'what we let into

© CHIARA THUMIGER, 2021 | DOI:10.1163/9789004443143_003

the whole',[1] are key, ideologically loaded variables, the product of arbitrary choices. What a holistic view should entail is thus bound to remain a matter of perspective.

This takes us to the second point: the concept is marred by a component of evaluation, be it ethical or epistemological, which compromises a neutral discussion of holism. 'Whole' enjoys an inherent superiority to 'parts', so that the negotiation of the second with the first has the connotation of a transaction in value. There thus appears to be a philosophical, ethical and aesthetic anteriority of wholeness so implicit in our mentality that we feel no need even to argue for it. In part, as cognitivists would frame the issue, the human preference for wholeness must be grounded in self-evident considerations of biological survival: integrity and fulfillment versus mutilation and loss are obvious embodied experiences of advantage, seen in everyday events such as eating and growth, or in familiar contrasting forms of deterioration such as wounds and decline through age.[2] It is suggestive in this regard to recall that the English term 'health' is connected to the Germanic-Old English *hael*,[3] 'whole' (cf. the English cognate 'hale' in 'hale and hearty'), as the use of 'wholesomeness' (in German *heil*) for 'health' indicates; already in Latin, the direct cognation between *saluus* ('safe', 'saved', 'healthy') and Greek *holos* ('whole') is telling. This immediate positivity of 'whole' applies to cosmological conceptions and sociological and political models, as much as to intuitions about the wellbeing of individual bodies. Ancient studies offer a good example of how the aspiration to entirety is so ingrained in our view of goodness that we can fail to notice how it shapes and biases the history of ideas about the human body as well as many other domains as a consequence.[4] When Bruno Snell famously focused part of his historical anthropology on the Homeric inability (on his reading of the evidence) to perceive the body 'as a whole' rather than as the sum of its components ('nicht *als Einheit*, sondern *als Vielheit*'[5]) as a symptom of a historically located mindset and a defective view of personal identity, he was anachronistically projecting on the ancient material his own expectations of wholeness and integrity – most of all, of a *certain kind* of wholeness and integrity.[6]

1 Thus Holzhey and Gragnolati (2017a) 7–8.

2 These are 'basic dimensions of our experience' for Lakoff and Johnston (1980) 82: as human beings, we 'experience ourselves as having parts (arms, legs, etc.) that we can control independently' and 'impose a part-whole structure on events and activities. And, in the case of participants, we distinguish *kinds* of parts.'

3 As noted by Pitman (2006) xi.

4 Disability studies (on theoretical ground opened up by feminist scholarship) has been challenging these assumptions and thematising alternative angles; see Adams (2017).

5 Snell (1946) 17.

6 Cf. also Adkins (1970). For a critique, see Renehan (1981), and most extensively Gill (1996) 29–41.

Notwithstanding its relativity as a concept, holism maintains its efficacy and perspicuity. Consider the following passage:

> But of course it is reason, that the whole is bigger than its parts! Otherwise, how is it that when the heart is heated or made cold, *melancholia* or *phrenitis* are caused and the reasoning of the soul is destroyed, but if the hand or foot is inflamed, nothing of the kind happens?
>
> κοινὴ γάρ ἐστιν ἔννοια, τὸ ὅλον μεῖζον εἶναι τοῦ μέρους. ἔπειτα πῶς τῆς μὲν καρδίας μᾶλλον ἐκθερμαινομένης ἢ ψυχομένης μελαγχολίαι γίνονται καὶ φρενίτιδες καὶ τῆς ψυχῆς ἀπόλλυται τὸ φρονεῖν, τῆς δὲ χειρὸς ἢ τοῦ ποδὸς φλεγμαίνοντος οὐδὲν τοιοῦτον πάσχει;

Thus wrote the fourteenth-century orthodox theologian Johannes VI Cantacuzenus, summing up an entire system of thought inherited from antiquity and using it for the purpose of theological argument.[7] What is worth noting are the implications of the medical imagery used by a high-Medieval author: the writer's point – that it is obviously the case that 'the whole is bigger, and better, than its parts' – is illustrated via a corporal allegory. The whole (the ensouled human individual) is greater than the sum of its more trivial parts (feet, hands, limbs, etc.). Damage to one of the latter does not affect the overarching 'reasoning of the soul', which resides on a superior, 'holistic' level; damage to the heart (here 'holistically' conceived of as the governing seat of the soul), on the other hand, causes diseases of greater import (*melancholy* or *phrenitis*) that affect the reasoning faculties.

Modern readers immediately understand this schematic image and the message that lies behind it. The intelligibility of the passage rests on a number of less-than-straightforward assumptions rooted in ancient medical and philosophical ideas about human beings, and on a specific conviction about the *whole* and the *parts* of things: first, the well-known vitalistic point that the living whole is larger than and superior to its parts[8] to the extent that it includes an animate force of some kind, just as the governing soul is superior to the inert matter of the body's limbs. Second, that certain elements in an individual qualify as 'parts' (hands, feet), whereas others, although at first glance equally parts of it, are its culmination and in a more abstract sense its holistic container or ruler (the soul), i.e. that there is a hierarchy among parts. Finally, and self-evidently, that the whole is superior to its parts. These ideas are easily understood by a modern reader. But they are understood precisely

7 *Disputatio cum Paulo Patriarcha Latino epistulis septem tradita*, *Ep.* 3.4.34–38.
8 Itself not a straightforward notion: see Coughlin in this volume, 239–42.

because this presentation is in line with a long tradition of medical ideas that goes back to ancient science and philosophy, combined with a highly influential concept of the living body as hierarchically organized that was ratified by the early encounter between philosophy (Platonic, Aristotelian and then Stoic) and medicine.

This Medieval example exposes a relevant fact: all reflections on holism have in one way or another the (human, animated) body at their centre, whether as concrete object of knowledge and intervention or as key figural referent. Holism, one might argue, is inherently body-centred, and as such literally or metaphorically medical. It is really only conceivable as a product of thinking by human beings in terms of the human body and the connections around, within and through it.[9] This embodied analogy sustains holism as a productive scientific and cultural tool: it comes as no surprise that holistic models and images are to be seen everywhere in the life sciences, from the study of mimicry as a network of communication events reverberating through the natural world,[10] to the notion of 'rhythms' as key to understanding the brain's internal structures and organized working,[11] to 'synchrony' as a biological force relevant to disparate fields such as technology, finance, molecular biology, physics, music, demographics, sociology and psychology.[12] Our understanding of universals and particulars is set out in terms of the human bodies we individually possess, through which we relate to a 'natural world' surrounding us.

2 A Case Study: Holism and the Sexed Body

An eloquent example of the centrality of the (human) body vis-à-vis holism as an equivocal notion *and* a naturalizing force with a long history behind it is the

9 Even when superseded by the artifices of a 'post-human' move of decentration within a holistic programme, the individual body remains in the middle – as in Coccia's ecological proposal in his recent *Life of Plants* (2018), where an account of the world as *mélange* dominated by non-animal forms of life is holistically construed, but the most animal (even mammal, lungs-possessing) experience of *breathing* remains at the centre.

10 Maran (2017) for a discussion of a semiotic interpretation of mimicry.

11 Buzsaki (2011).

12 For example, Jackson et al. (2018). On the origins of these models in Montpellier vitalism, see Wolfe (forthcoming) 156–57: he mentions (and interprets in the sense of an 'extended mechanicism') the images of the bee swarm or the flock of cranes to represent the coherent system of a living organism. On vibrational models for the nervous system as made of 'resonances' (my translations); see also Huneman (2008) on the eighteenth-century vitalistic label 'animal economy' for such connections. A varied exploration of the more general category of 'sympathy' is offered by Schliesser (2015).

imperative of a complementarity of sexes (and of the intrinsic goodness of this complementarity) incarnated by the Platonic *androgynos*. When Plato chose the two-sexed 'hermaphrodite'[13] (a four-legged, four-armed, two-faced creature with two sets of genitals) as the representation of a perfect primeval creature endowed with extraordinary strength,[14] he conjured up a representation of the two sexes as 'parts', and as exclusive parts composing a 'fitted'

13 In regard to sexed body(-ies) and their tradition, Laqueur (1990) proposed that until modern times a two-bodies sexual model was not recognised. According to him, the ancients conceived rather of a 'one-sex' body for both genders, with the female genitalia being an introverted or under-developed version of the male (in varying forms). See the definitive critique of this misrepresentation in King (2013).

14 'For 'man-woman' (ἀνδρόγυνον) was then a unity in form no less than name, composed of both sexes and sharing equally in male and female ... the form of each person was *round all over* (στρογγύλον), with back and sides encompassing it every way; each had four arms, and legs to match these, and two faces perfectly alike on a *cylindrical* neck (πρόσωπα δύ' ἐπ' αὐχένι κυκλοτερεῖ, ὅμοια πάντῃ). There was one head (κεφαλὴν ... μίαν) to the two faces, which looked opposite ways; there were four ears, two sets of genitals, and all the other parts, as may be imagined, in proportion ... They were *globular* in their shape (περιφερῆ) ... Now they were of surprising strength and vigour (τὴν ἰσχὺν δεινὰ καὶ τὴν ῥώμην), and so grand in their ambitions (τὰ φρονήματα μεγάλα) that they even conspired against the gods ... Then Zeus, putting all his wits together, spoke at length and said: 'I think I can contrive that men, without ceasing to exist, shall cease from their iniquity through a lessening of their strength. I propose now to slice every one of them in two (διατεμῶ δίχα), so that while making them weaker, we shall find them more useful by reason of their multiplication; and they shall walk erect upon two legs. If they continue turbulent and do not choose to keep quiet, I will do it again,' said he; 'I will slice every person in two, and then they must go their ways on one leg, hopping.' So saying, he sliced each human being in two ... Now when our first form had been cut in two, each half in longing for its fellow would come to it again (ποθοῦν ἕκαστον τὸ ἥμισυ τὸ αὑτοῦ συνῄει); and then would they fling their arms about each other and in mutual embraces yearn to be grafted together (ἐπιθυμοῦντες συμφῦναι), till they began to perish of hunger and general indolence, through refusing to do anything apart. And whenever on the death of one half the other was left alone, it went searching and embracing to see if it might happen on that half of the whole woman which now we call a woman, or perchance the half of the whole man. In this plight they were perishing away, when Zeus in his pity provided a fresh device. He moved their genitals to the front – for until then they had these, like all else, on the outside, and did their begetting and bringing forth not on each other but on the earth, like crickets. These parts he now shifted to the front, to be used for propagating on each other – in the female member by means of the male; so that if in their intercourses a man should happen on a woman, there might be conception and continuation of their kind; and also, if male met with male, they might have satisfaction of their union and relief, and so might turn their hands to their labors and their interest to ordinary life. Thus from ancient times is mutual love ingrained in mankind, recreating our original nature and endeavoring to combine two in one and heal human nature (ἔστι δὴ οὖν ἐκ τόσου ὁ ἔρως ἔμφυτος ἀλλήλων τοῖς ἀνθρώποις καὶ τῆς ἀρχαίας φύσεως συναγωγεὺς καὶ ἐπιχειρῶν ποιῆσαι ἓν ἐκ δυοῖν καὶ ἰάσασθαι τὴν φύσιν τὴν ἀνθρωπίνην)' (Pl. *Smp.* 189e–91d).

whole – even 'rounded', 'globular' – as if in perfect accomplishment of a lost nature, a representation that would be massively influential and eventually naturalized in our tradition:[15] eros in its highest form becomes the desire to 'return to one', to recompose the lost unity. To challenge and demystify this dominant holistic view, we do not need to reach for the champions of contemporary gender theory; only compare and contrast the *androgynos* with the famous prehistoric 'Venus of Lespugue' (fig. 1.1, 1.2) (whose age is established at 25,000 years), a formidable ivory figurine representing a fertility-like female figure with prominent breasts and buttocks, and/or, when one looks at it from a different perspective, a set of male genitals.[16] As in the case of the Platonic mythological figure, here too the two sexes are associated. But unlike there, the holistic image is created by aggregation rather than perfect fit: the male and the female merge into a blend in which only by the angle from which it is viewed could each component be distinguished, both separate and exposed, by means of an optical trick, as one and the same thing. This visual example effectively exposes our two challenges: holism is unstable – what 'parts'? and especially what kind of 'wholes'? This permanent instability of metaphorical 'holism' and 'whole' results in moral fuzziness and ambivalence: forms of oppressive normativity can lie both, as Queer critiques would posit, with the binary, cis-gendered, heterosexual myth of the aspiration to entirety, a sexed being's search for his or her complement in a lost 'whole';[17] and from a different angle, for some feminist critics, with the 'reduction to body parts' as dismissive of 'the whole of the person', one of the main figures of objectification to which the female is seen as subjected (e.g. in pornography).[18] In addition, we must

15 Lucretius vividly challenges this erotic ideal in his disenchanted description of the bodies of the lovers desperately struggling to melt into one another in search of an unattainable fusion (*De Rerum Natura* 4.1108–13): *adfigunt avide corpus iunguntque salivas / oris et inspirant pressantes dentibus ora, / ne quiquam, quoniam nihil inde abradere possunt / nec penetrare et abire in corpus corpore toto; nam facere inter dum velle et certare videntur*. Gender theory's unveiling of the constructedness of gender(s) and of sex(es) – impossible to survey even cursorily here – can be in this sense read as demystification of a kind of holistic ideal (see Butler (1990) 1.5, 'Identity, sex and the metaphysics of substance' for key points).

16 See Barrow (2018) 5, exposing how the phallic component in these European Paleolithic figurines subverts their traditional interpretation as 'emblems of female fertility representative of a single religion of the 'Mother Goddess' in a matriarchal society'; Joyce (2008) for the full argument in comparative anthropology (esp. chapters 1 and 2), 6–18 for the set of questions.

17 In this spirit, the category 'holism' as biologically associated with 'reproductive sex' is suspicious if not entirely negative in Haraway (2004), e.g. 38.

18 See Langton (2009) 228–29; McKinnon (1987) 76.

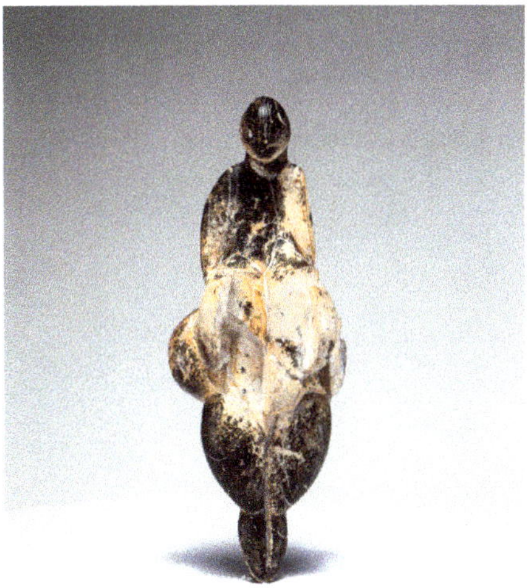

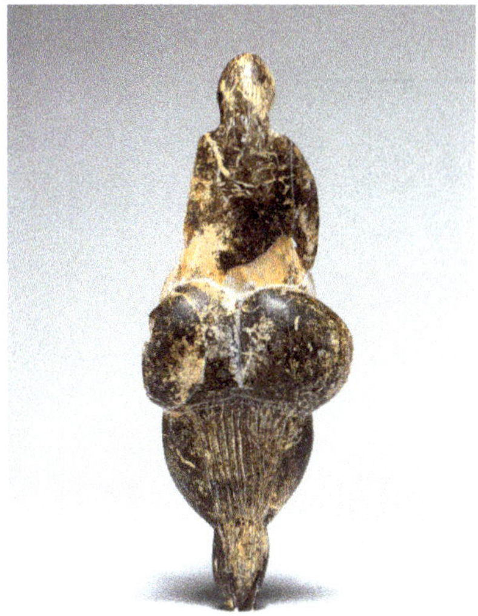

FIGURE 1.1 FIGURE 1.2
Vénus de Lespugue, paléolithique supérieur, ivoire de mammouth, France
MUSÉUM NATIONAL D'HISTOIRE NATURELLE, PARIS

confront the normative power imparted by the iconography of wholeness, of which the passage from the *Symposium*, with its immense cultural afterlife, is a trite but powerful example.[19]

These two points, relativity and involvement with value, so evident in the traditional image of the two sexes as coordinated parts yearning for erotic composition, make analysis of the heritage of holism rich and problematic in many ways. Our exploration must be of a meta-scholarly kind, in the sense that the object of scrutiny is simultaneously 'ontological' – the idea that something should be intrinsically holistic (e.g. health, as holistic by its nature) and methodological (e.g. believing in a holistic approach to ancient history and to holism

19 Irigaray's statement of the female as 'the sex which is not one' is all the more powerful against these classical intimations of holism (Irigaray 1985); see Gragnolati and Holzhey (2017a) 8; Braidotti (2011) 110–12 on the non-binary, composite sexuality in the insect world as exemplary model of 'nature's queerness' (with my paraphrase). Dworkin (1974) 162 criticizes the misinterpretations of androgynous myths as 'upholding patriarchal notions of sexual polarity, duality, male and female as opposite and antagonistic'; cf. Paglia (1990) 3–6, returning to the Platonic imagery of 'roundedness' – while undermining it – to celebrate the Venus of Willendorf (fig. 3) as 'solipsist, navel-gazing … Femaleness is self-referential and self-replicating … the egg-shaped Venus thinks in circles.'

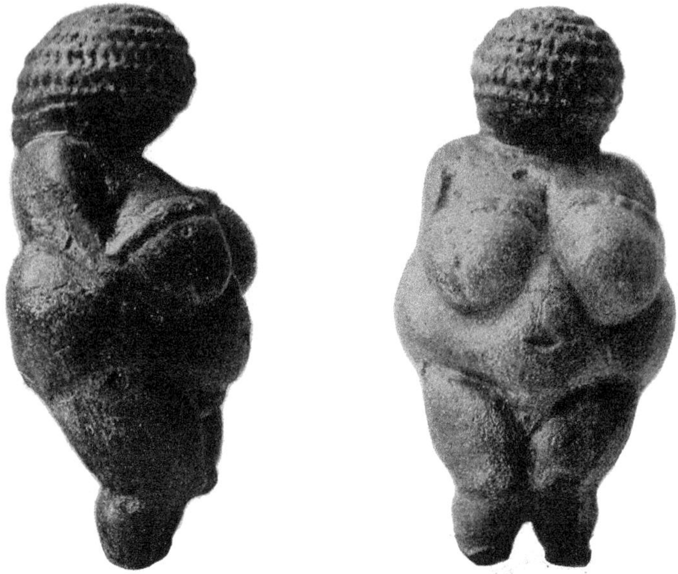

FIGURE 1.3 A female Paleolithic figurine, Venus of Willendorf

itself). This intertwinement between the ontological claim or faith and the methodology is fundamental in the case of holism.[20] The implications and the cultural and scholarly domains touched by the two are so numerous and varied that the risk is dispersion and dilution of the concept through its numerous reverberations.[21] I thus begin with a schematic sketch of the territory covered by 'holism' in Western culture as generally defined above – whether terminologically explicit or not – before moving on to individual questions.

3 Ontological Holism

The most direct instance of ontological holism is the biological notion according to which a defining quality of animate life, and especially of animal (and

---

20 This is Sober's distinction: (1980) 104–5.

21 Horden (2013) 18 faces a similar issue (and turns it into a positive occasion) vis-à-vis the many implications of a concept germane to our 'holism', 'balance', across different medical systems: 'balance must therefore be an abstraction, partially detectable only by its opposite.' Compare also Horky (2019a) 15–19, and especially 23–26 in his approach to the idea of 'cosmos' in ancient philosophy and in philosophical historiographies.

human) embodied life, is that it forms a whole that can only be properly understood as a living system, not as a mere conglomerate of parts that mechanically suffice to determine life. On a medical level, for ontological holism the body is an 'organism', interacting parts that form a complex system, establishing a continuum between the two opposites of mind and body, itself a concept with a complex history in our culture and philosophy, beginning with Aristotle and developing in modern biology.[22] To this quintessential pair, other homologous pairs are juxtaposed (reason and emotions, cognition and sensation, and so forth).[23]

In the Western biological and medical tradition, this strand of holism (which, in practical terms, addresses the body diagnostically and therapeutically as an organic whole) was at various times seen as deeply rooted in aspects of Graeco-Roman medicine, as different generations of biological and medical thinkers interpreted them. This is most evidently the case with the reception of ancient medicine, in particular Hippocratic,[24] by various generations of European vitalism and elaborations on animistic views of nature,[25] whose key phase is associated with the *École de médecine de Montpellier* in the eighteenth century,[26] and which experienced an important revival in the middle decades of the twentieth century with various forms of neo-vitalism.[27]

On a further and more comprehensive level, ontological holism identifies deeper (symbolic and analogical,[28] as well as substantial or mechanical) relationships that hold together not only beings within themselves, but also beings as 'microcosm' and as macrocosmic containers, or forming a *milieu*. The earliest theorised concept in this respect is that of the *anima mundi*, which

---

22 See Smith (2011) 97–234.

23 On pairing and the positing of extreme alternatives in Greek thought, see the classic Lloyd (1966).

24 Cf. Temkin (1991) 8–15 for an appraisal of this 'Hippocratic holism'; Williams (2009) 595, 609–10; Williams (2001).

25 See Lonie (1980) on the potential for both mechanicism and vitalism as appearing in Hoffman's reading of Hippocrates; Wolfe (forthcoming) 154.

26 Cf. Waisse (2011); Wolfe and Terada (2008) on the holistic concept of 'animal economy' in Montpellier vitalism; Wolfe (2008) 461; (2017).

27 See Lawrence and Weisz (1998), esp. 2–5; Rosenberg (1998) for an overview of medical holism; Harrington (1999); Poynton (1989) 141–42; Normandin and Wolfe (2013a) on contemporary vitalisms (and the collection in Normandin and Wolfe (2013)); Wolfe (2019) 307–41 on the twentieth century and returns to holism in biology.

28 For a discussion of the metaphorical connections between human micro- and macrocosm in ancient science, see Taub (2012), and the discussions in Wee (2017), especially Nyord (2017); comparatively Hsu (2013) 269–74 for 'microcosm-macrocosm homologies' in various medicines.

originates in Plato's *Timaeus*.[29] Here animal or ecological communities, the environment, the universe as a whole come into play.[30] In political or sociological contexts, on the other hand, holism puts forth a claim for interconnections among individuals and things and the society that derives from them as defining components of human reality.

In this way, the biological and medical are the most powerful archetypes of ontological holism, shaping other domains in turn. In modern Western intellectual life, the demands and failures of holistic ideals have exerted a powerful influence on the realm of psychology, and above all else on psychoanalysis from its origins to its French post-war developments.[31] The integrity of identity as ideal is overt in Freudian therapy, with its reconstitution of the legitimate, hegemonic, active 'I' in mediation between and supervision of the excesses of its components and bodily drives, which Freud names *superego* and *id*: 'wo es war, soll ich werden.' This fundamental role of integrity is difficult to overestimate, despite the continuous demystification and complications disrupting its itinerary towards attainment.[32] A holistic engagement also played a major role in the thought of the other founder of the psychoanalytic movement, Carl Gustav Jung. In contrast to Freud, Jung elaborated an extended theory of the human mind as participating in a collective unconscious (as well as possessing an individual one), in which an archetypical level of reality, a 'collective psyche', arises. This move strongly inserted man into a cosmic order and a metaphysical narrative, with points of contact with various spiritualist and vitalist environments ranging as wide as alchemy, Oriental religions and quantum physics.[33] Lacanian psychology best illustrates the heritage of these divergences in the history of psychoanalysis. Lacan emphasized the contradictions

29 See above (pp. 4–5); Helmig (2020a), Miklós (2010) 1–8 on the ancient idea and its legacy in the history of philosophy.

30 The two aspects are obviously interrelated in vitalistic accounts; cf. Canguilhelm (2008) 111 'from a biological point of view, one must understand that the relationship between the organism and the environment is the same as that between the parts and the whole of an organism'; also, Laurence and Weisz (1998) 16. Vegetation is mostly excluded from these accounts, as noted by Coccia (2018) in his suggestive exploration of the world of vegetation as one of fluidity, 'a metaphysics of mixture'.

31 The inclusion of psychological aspects into the sphere of action of medical care can also be seen as having its roots in vitalism: Huneman (2008, 2008a).

32 For an early critique of this 'fetishism of the individual', one might turn to avant-garde twentieth-century experiences and theatre, especially surrealism; see Thumiger (2009) for a discussion in dialogue with and in opposition to ancient concepts of the (theatrical) person.

33 See McMillan, Main and Henderson (2020); Main, Henderson and McMillan (2019) on Jung and 'holism.'

in the Freudian project and centered his analysis on subverting the individual subject and fragmentating its delusory mirage of 'completeness': the full image of oneself in the mirror is dreamt of in vain by the child and never fully attained by the adult.[34] Mental life as a consistent course of action is irreparably and *a-priori* compromised by the plural, fragmented nature of our relation to the objects in the world and of our bodily responses to them. Post-Freudian thinkers Deleuze and Guattari push the bodily metaphor of holism further, factoring in the concept of a multi-layered 'body without organs' (to borrow Artaud's words[35]) and rejecting a consistent 'one body image' as foundation of personal experience.[36]

In all the directions briefly surveyed above, human positioning vis-à-vis 'wholeness' and 'partiality' assumes fluctuating definitions, playing now the negative, now the positive role: the individual can be idealized as 'whole' to reconstruct, but can also be negatively opposed to a greater, cosmic 'whole', or demystified by the complex ensemble of ever-changing embodied human experiences.[37] It is thus appropriate that for our purposes 'holism' should serve as a level of discussion, aural and dialectical, rather than as positive doctrine.

Something closer to a positive doctrine of holism appears in a separate chapter in the history of psychology, which from its beginning was characterized by a much stronger scientific background: Gestalt psychology, whose founders, Max Wertheimer, Wolfgang Köhler and Kurt Koffka, claimed precisely that human mental life differs from the collection or sum of its sensations and cognitions. In a phenomenological spirit, *Gestalttheorie* also foregrounds human mental life as *experience*: perceiving and learning are based on 'common images' that are inherent in the objects we experience, and arise through the spontaneous organization of thought into structures as economical and simple as possible;[38]

34 See for example Lacan (1973/1978) 190 for discussion of Freudian love as 'sexual passion for the *gesamt ich*', 196–200; (1977). For an interdisciplinary take on this long line of thinking about the human self and personal identity, see Tallon Russell (2009), a critique of the Western tradition of 'oneness' regarding the self, especially in Christian theology.

35 From his last radio piece (Artaud 1947).

36 Deleuze (1997) 15–20; Deleuze and Guattari (1983) 20–27, also 34–39 and 56–66. Deleuze (2004) 101 dreams of a holistic new dimension of the schizophrenic body, an organism without parts which operates entirely by 'insufflation, respiration, evaporation and fluid transmission.'

37 See McMillan (2018) for a discussion of 'organicism and holistic relations' in Jung and Deleuze and their sources.

38 Laurence and Weisz (1998) 6–8. On the *Gestalt*, Ash (1998); Harrington (1999) 103–39; Canguilhelm (2008) 110, recognising the debts of his own reflections on the interaction between living being and environment 'as a whole to total objects' to *Gestalttheorie*; Poynton (1989) 139–41.

these can be deconstructed and studied. Thus Gestaltist thinkers too critique the idea of cognition as *a priori* and isolated within the individual, grounding their theory of perception and mental life in the 'experienced world.' When recent developments in embodied cognition and phenomenology refer to 'common structures' and 'cognitive models', basing their universalizing move on the study of human motor-sensory functions, the intellectual contributions of these earlier lines of research are easy to recognise, despite the radical differences in scientific or cultural premises and objectives – most of all in the pursuit of 'universally human' paradigms of embodied psychology.[39]

Non-Western cultures and their influence, finally, should not be omitted from this overview, although extraneous to the terms of the internal discussion and disagreement that characterize Western psychology. They are relevant, first of all, in a comparative spirit, by virtue of the richness of these traditions, as well in regard to the mind-body question and to relations between micro- and macrocosm. When it comes to views of personhood and psychology, comparative perspectives help us relativise our own psychological fundamentals, those we have seen at work within the history of psychoanalysis. As Dumont first showed, proposing a notion of human subjects as naturally composite 'dividuals', as he referred to them, indivisibility, impenetrability and unity seem to be specific modern Western requirements or expectations of personhood and views of self.[40]

There is another fundamental sense in which non-Western cultures are an inescapable part of the discussion when we consider 'holism': their perspective is also relevant as a point of reception by Western audiences, as recurring incarnations of an ideal of lost completeness, a desirable 'elsewhere' often colored by Orientalism.[41] Eastern religious and spiritual systems, with their medical and therapeutic practices (Buddhist, Āyurvedic, Chinese), conspicuously refer to a holistic understanding of the human body and its life cycles, as

39 Only an episodic selection of current directions in this sense, in which holism is positively applied to embodied cognition and phenomenology: Frisch (2014) n. 3 on the connections between holism, phenomenology, Gestalt and cognitive embodiment; Clark (2010) for the classic account of 'extended mind'; Cornejo (2008) for a reading of holism vis-à-vis intersubjectivity and phenomenology; see also Short in this volume.

40 Cf. Dumont (1965). This plural conception of personhood in Indian culture was then influentially applied by Strathern to Melanesian society: Strathern (1988) 13, 15 for the explanation; Smith (2012) for a survey of the influences of these discussions.

41 See Slingerland (2019) on China and the 'othering' potential of the unscrutinised attribution of the 'holistic' label to non-Western cultures (1–64, and 1–21 for the broader intellectual context); Zimmermann (1995), esp. 1–26 on 'les poisons de l'ethnicité' with reference to the construct of 'alternative', 'traditional' Eastern medicines in Western merchandise and medical cultures.

well as to a metaphysical belief in the universe as a system of interconnected strands, as illustrated by Zimmerman in his classic study of 'ecological' aspects of Hindu medicine.[42]

4 Methodological Holisms

'A fox knows many things, the hedgehog one important thing', as Berlin's use of the ancient animal fable has it: one can approach knowledge by tackling several partial, illuminating details, or by focusing on a single defining idea.[43] So too the ontological opposition between 'wholes' and 'parts' is reflected in a variety of scholarly and historiographical postures.[44] In studies of the ancient world (as in cultural studies generally), anti-canonical approaches (interdisciplinarity, reception and comparativism, for example) can be seen as holistic sets of demands in themselves that employ holistic tools (whether diachronically or synchronically) variously aimed at comprehensiveness, multiple perspectives, relativism or demystification of the particular situated datum as such. A holistic methodology *qua* holistic recognizes the need to place historical or anthropological evidence within its net of interconnections, whether bio-genetic, geographical, economic, social, cultural, traditional or even logical.

On the other hand, the canonical, Classicist[45] approach to antiquity (most visibly in its Romantic idealization) comes with a hegemonic mission which is also of a holistic kind: the reduction to meaning, the explanation, the categorization, the fitting within an order, historiographic or critical, that allows a tradition to be organized and controlled. The very concept of *tradition* – a package handed over, *traditum*, to us – is in this light a holistic profession of faith.[46] Many of our historiographic strategies are based on versions of holistic fantasies of exhaustiveness, where the wholes of philological *corpora*, of

42 Zimmermann (1988/1992). See e.g. Pitman (2006); Horden (2013); Hsu (2013); in this volume, Zimmermann on Āyurvedic, and Wee on ancient Near Eastern systems.

43 Isaiah Berlin's essay (1953), whose title quotes Archilochus fr. 201 West.

44 Rosenberg (1998) 338 distinguishes two categories of what we are calling 'methodological' holism: 'metahistorical', reading health and disease of humanity in terms of its distant past, in an evolutionary perspective; or historiographical – for example, reference to Hippocratism as an ideal of medical practice, on which see Sturdy (1998).

45 As implied by the evaluative and political implications of the term 'Classics' itself: see the reflections on the 'historic connection between socio-economic hierarchies ('class')' and also the differences between the cultural and imaginative lives of people in different 'classes' offered by Hall and Stead (2020).

46 The concept of 'tradition' as preservation of cultural material unchanged has longed been challenged; see the seminal discussion by Pouillon (1977).

opera omnia, of individual thinkers recomposed from *fragments*[47] to their *whole* are painstakingly pursued with an eye to the ultimate goal of complete reconstruction.[48]

The negative aspects of this attitude are more evident in some areas than others. Critics may denounce these historiographic attitudes as grounded in oppression and in a conservative safeguarding of a cultural *status quo* representing a tradition drawn 'from above' and run through by grand unifying narratives, held together by relations of power. The focus on the particular, the individual, the minority case, then, perhaps emerges as a more truthful form of inquiry, which finally rescues the subaltern and marginalized historical actors from death by statistical reduction, as in the micro-historical genre pioneered by Ginzburg and others in a Marxist spirit: the story of an otherwise unknown sixteenth-century Italian miller, in this way, can become a window open to the socio-cultural reality and religiosity of an entire era.[49] The difficulties for scholars of antiquity, as they face these two sets of alternative 'holisms', defy an easy choice and impose a composite strategy.[50]

The irreducible burden of truth carried by the particular is evident in medical literature in the highest degree. Indeed, medicine *is* the model environment from which casuistry originates and finds full legitimization. Medical and biological realities are of course expressed through statistical 'big data', but they also dwell in irreducible casuistic particulars, as Forrester argued in a seminal article.[51] In its own way, then, biomedicine with its reductionism is also holistic in its project – arguably impoverishing – of reducing human data to a homogeneity of average outcomes and statistics. This is very far from the 'positive' holistic connotations of complementary medicines, but it responds to the same exigency of exhaustiveness.[52] The methodological dialectic or tension between universalisation and particular is unresolved in the life sciences, as it is in Western thought generally.

---

47 On the cultural history of fragment collection, see the introduction to Most (1997); Most (2009) 18–19.

48 With reference to classics, see Holmes 48–55 in this volume, and Holmes (forthcoming); Holmes and Güthenke (2018).

49 Ginzburg (1976/1980). On microhistory as 'history from below', Port (2010); see for example Ginzburg (1976/1980) *preface*; Ginzburg, Tedeschi and Tedeschi (1993); Ginzburg (2018).

50 As proposed by Holmes and Güthenke (2018).

51 Forrester (1996); see also Asper (2019) 1–3; Langholf (1990) 194–208 on cases and types in the *Epidemics*, and Wee (2015) on 'minority reporting'; Chiaradonna (2013b) on universals in ancient medicine, especially 382–91 on Aristotle's views of generalisation in medicine; Thumiger and Petridou (2015) in general on patient-perspective as individualizing force in medical accounts.

52 On patient cases and big data, see Graumann and Thumiger (2019).

In all these methodological stances and scholarly strategies, *holism* has the potential to incarnate an ideal, an abstract target. The most famous and in-the-face examples of militant commitment to holism are found in forms of ecology, alternative medicine and totalitarian politics.[53] Ultimately, however, it is implicit in the ideological superiority of 'whole' that works as a fundamental premise in most levels of cultural and scientific discussion we have explored, and one cannot help but think that the longing for a lost wholeness (which is at least in part a universal human experience) is *also*, to an important extent, a specific Western malaise, which haunts the history of the 'classical tradition':[54] a kind of existential holism, of *Sehnsucht* for a primeval totality of which we contemporaries have only pieces at our disposal. This trope of classical antiquity as an inheritance of ruins and fragments is a recurring one (of Romantic origin) in the disillusion twentieth-century modernist poets express at our civilization, which for them '(unlike that '*organic world of antiquity*'?) ... is all *in bits, in fragments*.'[55] This loss, and the presence-through-absence that defines the aesthetics of ruins,[56] inspires both awe and despair, and moral engagement with the destiny of annihilated things. Again, the element of value is never absent from this particular discussion of parts and wholes.[57]

This long intellectual survey sheds some light on the value of reflection on holism as a medical-historical project: the uncovering of a permanent, if ever-changing dialectic in human science and culture by examining ancient examples and their legacy. The relationship between mind and body in ancient philosophy, biology and medicine; the reception and manipulation of ancient (medical) traditions; the discussion of the human place in the cosmic order; the pragmatics and ethics of human intervention of any kind (political, therapeutic, economic, ecological): all these are implicated in the histories surveyed above, and in turn inform the way we operate as historians of medicine and readers of the ancient world.

---

53 Relevant to our discussion, Wohl (2019) 232 has important remarks about the normativity of the ideal of *kosmos* proposed by Greek thought and its later tradition as sustaining 'a political ontology of the whole, an aesthetics of politics that privileges unity, coherence, stability, and centripedality', to which dissonant, pluralistic models are opposed – '*chaosmos*' (300); see p. 300 n. 5 on reactionary politics and holism.

54 That is, *one* Classical tradition – see Stead and Hall (2020), above n. 45; Stead and Hall (2020a).

55 Silk, Gildenhard et al. (2014) 50, my italics. On this chapter of the classical tradition, exemplified through the words of Ezra Pound and T. S. Eliot, see Silk, Gildenhard et al. (2014) 49–51; Kahane (2011a), (2011b) on ruins as a form of discourse in our relationship to the classical past; Settis (2011) on ruinism as 'peculiar to Western culture.'

56 Settis (2011).

57 Kahane (2011a) 635–36 on 'ruins and responsibility.'

Acknowledgments

I am again grateful to colleagues for the many suggestions and the constructive criticism on this text; to Simon Swain, Brooke Holmes, Helen King and Sean Coughlin in particular; and to S. Douglas Olson for his invaluable help with linguistic aspects of the presentation. I also express my gratitude to the Wellcome Trust, which funded this research.

Bibliography

Adams, E. 'Fragmentation and the Body's Boundaries: Reassessing the Body in Parts.' In *Ancient Anatomical Votives Past, Present and Future*, ed. J. Draycott and E.-J. Graham. London: Routledge (2017) 193–213.

Adkins, A. W. H. *From the Many to the One*. London: Constable (1970).

Artaud, A. 'To Have Done with the Judgment of God.' In *Selected Writings*, ed. S. Sontag. Berkeley: University of California Press (1976) (originally published as *Pour en finir avec le judgement de dieu*, 1947).

Asper, M. 'Introduction.' In *Cases and Anecdotes*, ed. M. Asper. Berlin: De Gruyter (2019) 1–7.

Asper, M. (ed.) *Cases and Anecdotes*. Berlin: De Gruyter (2019) 31–48.

Barrow, R. J. *Gender, Identity and the Body in Greek and Roman Sculpture*. Cambridge: Cambridge University Press (2018).

Berlin, I. *The Hedgehog and the Fox*. London: Weidenfeld & Nicolson (1953).

Braidotti, R. *Nomadic Theory: The Portable Rosi Braidotti*. New York: Columbia University Press (2011).

Butler, J. *Gender Trouble: Feminism and the Subversion of Identity*. London: Routledge (1990).

Buzsaki, G. *Rhythms of the Brain*. Oxford: Oxford University Press (2011).

Canguilhelm, G. *Knowledge of Life*. Trans. S. Geroulanos and D. Ginsburg. New York: Fordham University Press (2008) (originally published as *La connaissance de la vie*, 1952).

Cantor, D. (ed.) *Reinventing Hippocrates*. London: Ashgate (2001).

Clark, A. *Supersizing the Mind: Embodiment, Action, and Cognitive Extension*. Oxford: Oxford University Press (2010).

Coccia, E. *The Life of Plants: A Metaphysics of Mixture*. Cambridge: Polity Press (2019).

Cornejo C. 'Intersubjectivity as Co-Phenomenology: from the Holism of Meaning to the Being-In-The-World-With-Others.' *Integr. Psychol. Behav. Sci.*, 42.2 (2008) 171–78 doi: 10.1007/s12124-007-9043-6.

Deleuze, G. *Logic of Sense*. Trans. M. Lester and C. J. Stivale. London: Continuum (2004) (originally published as *Logique du sens*, 1969).

Deleuze, G. *Essays Critical and Clinical*. Trans. D. W. Smith and M. A. Greco. Minneapolis: University of Minnesota Press (1997) (originally published as *Critique et Clinique*, 1993).
Deleuze, G., and F. Guattari. *Anti-Oedipus. Capitalism and Schizophrenia*. Trans. R. Hurley, M. Seem and H. R. Lane. Minneapolis: University of Minnesota Press (1983) (originally published as *Capitalisme et schizophrénie. L'Anti-Oedipe*, 1972).
Dumont, L. 'The Modern Conception of the Individual: Notes on its Genesis and that of Concomitant Institutions.' *Contributions to Indian Sociology*, 8 (1965) 13–61.
Dworkin, A. *Woman Hating*. New York: E. P. Dutton (1974).
Forrester, J. 'If P, Then What? Thinking in Cases.' *History of the Human Sciences*, 9.3 (1996) 1–25.
Frisch, S. 'How Cognitive Neuroscience Could be More Biological – and What It Might Learn from Clinical Neuropsychology.' *Front. Hum. Neurosci.*, 21 July 2014 https://doi.org/10.3389/fnhum.2014.00541.
Gill, C. *Personality in Greek Epic, Tragedy and Philosophy*. Oxford: Clarendon Press (1996).
Ginzburg, C. *Nondimanco. Machiavelli, Pascal*. Milan: Adelphi (2018).
Ginzburg, C. *The Cheese and the Worms: The Cosmos of a Sixteenth-Century Miller*. Trans. J. Tedeschi and A. Tedeschi. Baltimore: The Johns Hopkins University Press (1980) (originally published as *Il Formaggio e i Vermi*, 1976).
Ginzburg, C., J. Tedeschi and A. C. Tedeschi. 'Microhistory: Two or Three Things That I Know about It.' *Critical Inquiry*, 20.1 (1993) 10–35.
Graumann, L. A., and C. Thumiger. 'Children and the Art of Medical Storytelling: Contemporary Practice and Hippocratic Case-Taking Compared.' In *Cases and Anecdotes*, ed. M. Asper. Berlin: De Gruyter (2019) 31–48.
Hall, E., and H. Stead. *A People's History of Classics. Class and Greco-Roman Antiquity in Britain and Ireland 1689 to 1939*. London: Routledge (2020).
Hall, E., and H. Stead. 'Approaching Classical Reception through the Frame of Social Class.' In *Framing Reception Studies*, ed. E. Hall and H. Stead. Leiden: Brill (2020a).
Haraway, D. 'A Manifesto for Cyborgs: Science, Technology and Socialist Feminism in the 1980s'. In *The Haraway Reader*. New York and London: Routledge (2004) 7–45.
Harrington, A. *Reenchanted Science: Holism in German Culture from Wilhelm II to Hitler*. Princeton: Princeton University Press (1999).
Helmig, C. (ed.) *World Soul – Anima Mundi. On the Origins and Fortunes of a Fundamental Idea*. Berlin: De Gruyter (2020).
Helmig, C. 'The World Soul in Antiquity and Beyond.' In *World Soul – Anima Mundi. On the Origins and Fortunes of a Fundamental Idea*, ed. C. Helmig. Berlin: De Gruyter (2020a) 1–26.
Holmes, B., and C. Güthenke. 'Hyperinclusivity, Hypercanonicity, and the Future of the Field.' In *Marginality, Canonicity, Passion*, ed. M. Formisano and C. Kraus. Oxford: Oxford University Press (2018) 57–73.

Holmes, B. 'Canguilhem and the Greeks: Vitalism between History and Philosophy.' In C. Donohue and C. Wolfe (eds.), *Vitalism and the Contemporary Life Sciences*. New York: Springer (forthcoming).

Holzhey, C. F. E., and M. Gragnolati (eds.) *De/Constituting Wholes. Towards Partiality Without Parts*. Vienna: Turia + Kant (2017).

Holzhey, C. F. E., and M. Gragnolati. 'Beginnings: Constituting Wholes, Haunting, Plasticity.' In *De/Constituting Wholes. Towards Partiality Without Parts*, ed. C. F. E. Holzhey and M. Gragnolati. Vienna: Turia + Kant (2017a) 7–30.

Horden, P. 'Introduction.' In *The Body in Balance. Humoral Medicines in Practice*, ed. P. Horden and E. Hsu. Oxford: Berghahn (2013a) 1–21.

Horden, P., and E. Hsu (eds.) *The Body in Balance. Humoral Medicines in Practice*. Oxford: Berghahn (2013).

Hornky, S. P. (ed.) *Cosmos in the Ancient World*. Cambridge: Cambridge University Press (2019).

Hornky, S. P. 'Introduction.' In *Cosmos in the Ancient World*, ed. S.P. Hornky. Cambridge: Cambridge University Press (2019a) 1–21.

Hornky, S. P. 'When did Kosmos Become the Kosmos.' In *Cosmos in the Ancient World*, ed. S. P. Hornky. Cambridge: Cambridge University Press (2019b) 22–41.

Horstmanshoff, M., H. King and C. Zittel (eds.) *Blood, Sweat, and Tears: The Changing Concepts of Physiology from Antiquity into Early Modern Europe. Intersections, 25*. Leiden and Boston: Brill (2012).

Hsu, E. 'What next?' In *The Body in Balance. Humoral Medicines in Practice*, ed. P. Horden and E. Hsu. Oxford: Berghahn (2013) 259–80.

Huneman, P. 'Montpellier Vitalism and the Emergence of Alienism in France: The Case of the Passions.' *Science in Context*, 21.4 (2008) 615–47.

Huneman, P. "Animal Economy' – Anthropology and the Rise of Psychiatry from the 'Encyclopédie' to the Alienists." In *Anthropology of the Enlightenment*, ed. L. Wolff and M. Cipolloni. Stanford: Stanford University Press (2008a) 262–76.

Irigaray, L. 'The Sex that is Not One.' In *The Sex that is not One*. Trans. C. Porter and C. Burke. New York: Cornell University Press (1977/1985) 23–34.

Jackson, J. C., J. Jong et al. 'Synchrony and Physiological Arousal Increase Cohesion and Cooperation in Large Naturalistic Groups.' *Scientific Reports*, 8,127 (2018) 127.

Joyce, R. A. *Ancient Bodies, Ancient Lives: Sex, Gender, and Archaeology*. New York: Thames & Hudson (2008).

Kahane, A. 'Antiquity and the Ruin: Introduction.' *European Review of History*, 18 (2011a) 631–44.

Kahane, A. 'Image, Word and the Antiquity of Ruins.' *European Review of History*, 18 (2011b) 829–50.

King, H. *The One-Sex Body on Trial: The Ancient and Early Modern Evidence*. London: Routledge (2013).

King, R. A. H. 'Introduction.' In *Common to Body and Soul. Philosophical Approaches to Explaining Living Behaviour in Greco-Roman Antiquity*, ed. R. A. King. Berlin: De Gruyter (2006) 1–12.
Lacan, J. *The Four Fundamentals of Psychoanalysis*. Trans. A. Sheridan. New York: W. W. Norton (1978) (originally published as *Le Seminaire de Jacques Lacan, Livre XI, 'Les quatre concepts fondamentaux de la psychanalyse*, 1973).
Lacan, J. 'The Subversion of the Subject and the Dialectic of Desire in the Freudian Unconscious.' Trans. A. Sheridan in *Écrits: A Selection*. New York: W. W. Norton and Co. (1977).
Lakoff, G., and M. Johnson. *Metaphors We Live By*. Chicago: University of Chicago Press (1980).
Langholf, V. *Medical Theories in Hippocrates. Early Texts and the 'Epidemics.'* Berlin: De Gruyter (1990).
Langton, R. *Sexual Solipsism: Philosophical Essays on Pornography and Objectification*. Oxford: Oxford University Press (2009).
Laqueur, Thomas. *Making Sex: Body and Gender from the Greeks to Freud*. Cambridge: Cambridge University Press (1990).
Lawrence, C., and G. Weisz. 'Medical Holism: the Context.' In *Greater than the Parts: Holism in Biomedicine 1920–50*, ed. C. Lawrence and G. Weisz. Oxford: Oxford University Press (1998) 1–22.
Lloyd, G. E. R. *Polarity and Analogy. Two Types of Argumentation in Early Greek Thought*. Cambridge: Cambridge University Press (1966).
Lonie, I. M. 'Hippocrates the Iatromechanist.' *Medical History*, 25 (1981) 113–50.
MacKinnon, C. *Feminism Unmodified*. Cambridge, MA and London: Harvard University Press (1987).
Main, R., D. Henderson and C. Mcmillan (eds.) *Jung, Deleuze, and the Problematic Whole*. London: Taylor & Francis (2020).
Maran, T. *Mimicry and Meaning: Structure and Semiotics of Biological Mimicry*. Berlin: Springer (2017).
McMillan, C., R. Main and D. Henderson (eds.) *Holism: Possibilities and Problems*. London: Routledge (2019).
McMillan, C. 'Jung and Deleuze: Enchanted Openings to the Other: a Philosophical Contribution.' *International Journal of Junghian Studies*, DOI: 10.1080/19409052.2018.1505236.
Most, G. W. (ed.) *Collecting Fragments-Fragmente Sammeln. Aporemata* 1. Göttingen: Vandenhoeck & Ruprecht (1997).
Most, G. W. 'On Fragments.' In *The Fragment: an Incomplete History*, ed. Willian Tronzo. Getty Research Institute (2009) 9–22.
Normandin, S., and C. T. Wolfe (eds.) *Vitalism and the Scientific Image in Post-Enlightenment Life Science, 1800–2010*. Berlin: Springer (2013).

Normandin, S., and C. T. Wolfe. 'Vitalism and the Scientific Image: an Introduction.' In *Vitalism and the Scientific Image in Post-Enlightenment Life Science, 1800–2010*. Berlin: Springer (2013a) 1–15.
Nyord, R. 'Analogy and Metaphor in Ancient Medicine and the Ancient Egyptian Conceptualisation of Heat and the Body.' In *The Comparable Body – Analogy and Metaphor in Ancient Mesopotamian, Egyptian, and Greco-Roman Medicine*, ed. J. Wee. Leiden and Boston: Brill (2017) 12–42.
Paglia, C. *Sexual Personae: Art and Decadence from Nefertiti to Emily Dickinson*. New Haven and London: Yale University Press (1990).
Petridou, G., and C. Thumiger. 'Introduction.' In *Homo Patiens. Approaches to the Patient in the Ancient World*, ed. G. Petridou and C. Thumiger. Leiden: Brill (2015) 1–22.
Pitman, V. *The Nature of the Whole. Holism in Ancient Greek and Indian Medicine*. Delhi: Motilal Banarsidass (2006).
Port, A. 'History from Below, The History of Everyday Life and Microhistory.' In *International Encyclopedia of the Social and Behavioral Sciences*, vol. 11. Munich: Elsevier (2015) 108–13.
Pouillon, J. 'Plus c'est la même chose, plus ça change.' *Nouvelle Revue de Psychanalyse*, 15 (1977) 203–12.
Poynton, J. C. 'Holistic Thinking in Medicine: Pitfalls and Possibilities.' *Holistic Medicine*, 4.3 (1989) 137–44.
Renehan, R. 'The Meaning of ΣΩΜΑ in Homer: a Study in Methodology.' *CSCA* 12 (1981) 269–81.
Rosenberg, C. E. 'Holism in Twentieth-Century Medicine.' In *Greater than the Parts: Holism in Biomedicine 1920–50*, ed. C. Lawrence and G. Weisz. Oxford: Oxford University Press (1998) 335–55.
Schliesser, E. (ed.) *Sympathy: A History*. Oxford Scholarship Online (2015).
Settis, S. 'Nécessité des ruines: les enjeux du classique.' *European Review of History*, 18 (2011) 717–40.
Silk, M. S., I. Gildenhard and R. Barrow. *The Classical Tradition. Art, Literature, Thought*. London: Wiley Blackwell (2014).
Slingerland, E. *Mind and Body in Early China: Beyond Orientalism and the Myth of Holism*. Oxford: Oxford University Press (2019).
Smith, J. E. H. *Divine Machines: Leibniz and the Sciences of Life*. Princeton: Princeton University Press (2011).
Smith, K. 'From Dividual and Individual Selves to Porous Subjects.' *The Australian Journal of Anthropology*, 23 (2012) 50–64.
Snell, B. *Die Entdeckung des Geistes*. Hamburg: Claaszen & Govert Verlag (1946).
Sober, E. 'Holism, Individualism, and the Units of Selection.' *Proceedings of the Biennial Meeting of the Philosophy of Science Association*, (1980) 93–121.
Strathern, M. *The Gender of the Gift: Problems with Women and Problems with Society in Melanesia*. Berkeley: University of California Press (1988).

Sturdy, S. 'Hippocrates and the State Medicine: George Newman Outlines the Founding Policy of the Ministry of Health.' In *Greater than the Parts: Holism in Biomedicine 1920–50*, ed. C. Lawrence and G. Weisz. Oxford: Oxford University Press (1998) 112–34.

Tallon Russell, H. *Irigaray and Kierkegaard: On the Construction of the Self.* Macon: Mercer University Press (2009).

Taub, L. 'Physiological Analogies and Metaphors in Explanations of the Earth and the Cosmos.' In *Blood, Sweat, and Tears: The Changing Concepts of Physiology from Antiquity into Early Modern Europe*, ed. M. Horstmanshoff, H. King and C. Zittel. *Intersections 25*. Leiden and Boston: Brill (2012) 41–63.

Temkin, O. *Hippocrates in a World of Pagans and Christians*. Baltimore: Johns Hopkins University Press (1991).

Thumiger, C. 'Metatheatre in Modern and Ancient Fiction.' *Materiali e Discussioni per l'Analisi dei Testi Classici*, 63 (2009) 9–58.

Waisse, S., M. T. Cera Galvão do Amaral and A. M. Alfonso-Goldfarb. 'Roots of French Vitalism: Bordeu and Barthez, between Paris and Montpellier.' *Hist. Cienc. Saude-Manguinhos*, 18.3 (2011) 625–40.

Wee, J. Z. (ed.) *The Comparable Body – Analogy and Metaphor in Ancient Mesopotamian, Egyptian, and Greco-Roman Medicine*. Leiden and Boston: Brill (2017).

Williams, E. A. 'Hippocrates and the Montpellier Vitalists in the French Medical Enlightenment.' In *Reinventing Hippocrates*, ed. D. Cantor. London: Ashgate (2001) 157–77.

Williams, E. A. 'Of Two Lives One? Jean-Charles-Marguerite-Guillaume Grimaud and the Question of Holism in Vitalist Medicine.' *Science in Context*, 21.4 (2008) 593–613.

Wohl, V. 'Afterword.' In *Cosmos in the Ancient World*, ed. S. P. Hornky. Cambridge: Cambridge University Press (2019) 295–303.

Wolfe, C. T. 'Introduction: Vitalism without Metaphysics? Medical Vitalism in the Enlightenment.' *Science in Context*, 21.4 (2008a) 461–63.

Wolfe, C. T. 'Models of Organic Organization in Montpellier Vitalism.' *Early Science and Medicine*, 22 (2017) 229–52.

Wolfe, C. T. *La philosophie de la biologie avant la biologie: une histoire du vitalisme*. Paris: Garnier (2019).

Wolfe, C. T. 'Il Problema del Tutto e delle Parti. Il Caso del Vitalismo di Montpellier.' In *Morfologie del Rapporto Parti-tutto*, ed. G. D'Anna, E. Massimilla, F. Piro, M. Sanna and F. Toto. Milan: Mimesis (2019) 257–70.

Wolfe, C. T., and M. Terada. 'The Animal Economy as Object and Program in Montpellier Vitalism.' *Science in Context*, 21.4 (2008) 537–79.

Zimmermann, F. *The Jungle and the Aroma of Meats*. Motilala Banarsidass: Delhi (1992) (originally published as *La jungle et le fumet des viandes. Un thème écologique dans la médecine hindoue*, Paris 1982).

Zimmermann, F. *Généalogie des médecines douces: de l'Inde à l'Occident*. Paris: Les Presses universitaires de France (1995).

Primary Texts: Editions and Translations Used

Iohannis Cantacuzeni Refutationes Duae Prochori Cydonii et Disputatio cum Paulo Patriarcha Latino Epistulis Septem Tradita. Ed. F. Tinnefeld and E. Voordeckers. Corpus Christianorum. Series Graeca 16. Turnhout: Brepols (1987) 175–239.

CHAPTER 2

Holism, Sympathy, and the Living Being in Ancient Greek Medicine and Philosophy

Brooke Holmes

Abstract

This paper takes up ancient holism as a significant problem in ancient Greek medicine and philosophy that has to be approached with a critical awareness of modern receptions of ancient Greek medicine and science as naively vitalist, and of ancient Greece, more broadly, as the site of a pure, unified form of life. I argue that viewing questions of part and whole within the living being from the perspective of sympathy (*sumpatheia*) can help us articulate the major conceptual axes operative within ancient holism as a problem. I begin by situating the inquiry into ancient holism both in relationship to a history of scholarship on ancient Greek medicine and science that has focused on cultural and historical difference, and in relationship to the contested status of ancient, or premodern, 'life' within continental philosophy. I then turn to the two major axes that I argue help to structure the conceptual field of sympathy as it develops from the late fourth and early third century BCE in learned medicine and philosophical psychology. I focus on the development of sympathy in the Stoics, the Epicureans, and Galen, while also considering the theorization of living beings in the Hippocratics, Plato, and Aristotle. The first axis moves from 'part-to-part' sympathy to 'part-to-whole' sympathy; the second from the sympathy of body and soul to a sympathy that encompasses all the parts of the living thing. Following these axes helps us identify, in turn, persistent questions about the material structure of the body that allows for the communication of affections between its parts but also its coordinated work as a living whole. It also focuses attention on what guarantees the unity of the whole over and above that structure. Through tracking sympathy as both the occurrence of co-affection between the parts of a living thing and the relationship enabling that occurrence, we can gain insight into the theorization of a living being as a dynamic and complex but unified whole in the centuries after Aristotle.

The subject of 'ancient holism' is uniquely positioned at the juncture of historicist inquiries into ancient Greek science, medicine, and philosophy and

 | DOI:10.1163/9789004443143_004

modern ideas about the nature of 'life' in Greek antiquity. On the one hand, the problems of part and whole demonstrably concern a wide range of ancient Greek and Roman writers who are working with the living body as both a philosophical puzzle and a clinical challenge. The rise of interest in the living body as a whole greater than the sum of its parts is especially visible in the fourth century BCE with Aristotle's conceptualization of the 'organic body' and the emergence of 'untaught nature' as a principle governing life in the Hippocratic text *Epidemics VI*. On the other hand, the 'wholeness' of the living body, either as a theoretical construct in ancient texts or, more broadly, as a lived experience attributed to the ancient Greeks, is by no means a neutral property from the perspective of modernity's relationship to an antiquity deemed classical. In inquiring into 'ancient holism,' we stand in the wake of a complex interplay between vitalism, Romanticism, Philhellenism, racial science, and biopolitics from the late eighteenth century to the present. The inquiry, therefore, cannot be mistaken for one of historical interest alone. For this reason, the question of ancient holism must be considered through a perspective mindful of the modern reception of classical antiquity and, more specifically, the reception history of ancient Greek medical and philosophical theories of life and living bodies.

In this paper, I argue that we can chart a robust relationship between the theorisation of the living being as a whole greater than the sum of its parts in ancient Greek medical and philosophical texts from the fifth century BCE onwards and the multi-faceted concept of sympathy (*sumpatheia*). By using sympathy as a lens to view ancient holism, we can identify two intersecting axes that help to structure the field within which various views of the living being in terms of parts and whole are articulated. The first of these axes runs between, on the one hand, the transfer of a disease (*nosos*, *nosēma*) or an affection (*pathos*, *pathēma*) from one part of the living thing to another part ('part-to-part' sympathy); and, on the other hand, the communication of a disease or an affection from one part to the whole body or the whole living thing ('part-to-whole' sympathy). The second axis runs between a concept of the living thing as a whole comprising two parts – in particular, body and soul, whose interaction produces 'psychosomatic' sympathy – and a concept of the living thing as a unified whole comprising many parts that work together. I refer to the sympathy deployed to support this concept of the living thing as 'vital' sympathy.

These two axes, which run through the conceptual field of *sumpatheia*, help us chart, in turn, a number of important problems across different texts and between different ancient philosophical and medical schools and sects. In elaborating these axes in the second and third sections of the paper, we will come across two problems in particular. First, what is the structure that enables the transfer of an affection from either one part to another part or a part to the whole? The answer to this question usually goes in one of two directions. It focuses either on the minimal means of contact (a connecting vessel, bodies in contact, a material continuum) or on an underlying relationship that enables the parts not only to exchange affections but to work together to achieve a specific outcome: life, or a particular form of life (plant or animal, or the life of a particular kind, such as a beaver or a human being).[1] The second question concerns what it is that is required for this working relationship. One strong candidate, especially after Aristotle, is soul. But soul turns out to raise problems of its own for a holistic account of the living body, as we will see in thinking about vital sympathy in Galen.

Each of these questions, and the problems and solutions they raise, rewards far more attention than I give it here. My aim within the scope of this chapter is circumscribed: to draw selectively on a range of ancient Greek medical and philosophical texts to give a schematic overview of how, from the late fourth and early third centuries BCE into the first centuries CE, attempts to understand living things in terms of parts and whole increasingly turn to the conceptual field of sympathy. I would argue further that by facilitating the conceptualization of the living being as a whole comprising different parts, sympathy becomes a hinge between holistic accounts of the living being and attempts in philosophy, natural history, and political theory to think about the larger wholes within which the living being pursues its life: Nature, or the cosmos.

This last claim is one whose defense I must defer at present.[2] I nevertheless mention it here to indicate the broad scope and significant stakes of ancient sympathy and, by extension, the question of holism in Graeco-Roman antiquity. The significance of these stakes, in my view, concerns not only our understanding of ancient Greek life science but also the relationship between the present (modern or contemporary) and the 'classical' past. The problem of ancient holism matters to this relationship in two major ways. First, there is a strong vitalist or romantic component to the valuation of ancient Greece inherent within the formation of modern classicism as it has been developed within the context of European literature, philosophy, and science. Second, the

1 On holism and continuum theories, see Coughlin in this volume.

2 I defend this claim in Holmes (forthcoming b), which also develops a much more detailed account of 'sympathy within,' that is, sympathy as a concept deployed to explain the flourishing and suffering of the living being. On sympathy within, see also Holmes (2012b); (2013); (2014a); (2014b); (2015). On sympathy in Pliny's *Natural History*: Holmes (2017). On cosmic sympathy in the Stoics, see Holmes (2019b).

Greeks continue to attract attention within a complex of modern and contemporary lines of thought about life that harbour under the labels 'vitalism' and 'biopolitics.' In short, 'the (ancient) Greeks' and 'life' are deeply entangled for us in ways that demand further attention. If I do not give this entanglement adequate attention here, I nevertheless point to it for the reason that I outlined at the outset: namely, that an inquiry into ancient holism needs to be situated in light of modern and contemporary investments in both 'the Greeks' and 'life.'[3] Before turning to the axes of ancient sympathy, then, I take a few pages to situate this historical inquiry in relationship to developments in the study of ancient Greek science and medicine over the past few decades, to classical reception studies, and to recent disciplinary and transdisciplinary conversations around the history and philosophy of 'life' and 'life science.'

1 Continuity and Discontinuity in the History of Ancient Greek Science and Medicine

The last half-century of work within the history of Graeco-Roman medicine and life science can be understood as a collective resistance to the demons of presentism. In resisting the rip tide of 'Whiggish' history and the mid-century triumphalist narratives of ancient Greek science and medicine culminating in the achievements of their Western heirs, historians in these fields, influenced by the ground-breaking work of G. E. R. Lloyd and broader critiques of presentism within the history of science, anthropological methods, and the philosophy of science, have reworked the frameworks within which we stage a 'return' to antiquity.[4]

It is difficult to overstate the significance of these ongoing currents of research. Most important, they have converged to disrupt, time and again, assumptions about the continuity between the past and the present. 'The issue,' as Heinrich von Staden has written, 'is not 'presentism' nor whether or not there are significant conceptual, methodological, and other continuities between ancient and modern science. There *are* …'. Rather, he goes on, 'the issue is the distorting consequences entailed by the historiographic habit of brightly foregrounding elements of legitimate continuity, with which we tend to be culturally more at home, while relegating discontinuities to a shadowy, obscure

3 For more sustained discussion, see Holmes (2019a), on *bios* and biopolitics; Holmes (forthcoming a), on 'the Greeks' and 'the ancients' in Georges Canguilhem's theorization of vitalism as a philosophical-historical phenomenon.

4 See esp. Lloyd (1979); (1983); (1987).

background at best.'[5] Such a 'historiographic habit,' von Staden argues, is powerfully conditioned by 'two mutually reinforcing collective experiences: the modern reception of ancient Greece as the fountainhead of our culture and, second, modern Western scientific culture as our lodestar.'[6]

Von Staden's article appeared within a pivotal cluster of essays edited by the Assyriologist and historian of science Francesca Rochberg and published in 1992 in *Isis* (the other contributors were Martin Bernal, G. E. R. Lloyd, and David Pingree). The essays together critically reexamined historiographies invested in ancient Greece as the origin of Western science and philosophy, in part by examining the ways in which these historiographies have been shaped by nineteenth-century Philhellenism's troubling fixation on the purity of Greek origins, negotiated overtly or covertly through contemporaneous racial science, and in part by focusing on the neglected contributions of the ancient Near East and Egypt to ancient Greek medicine and science as well as the intrinsic value of these traditions. Such a project of 'decolonizing' the history of ancient science and medicine, as Rochberg described it in her introduction to the essays, is far from complete.[7]

The conceptual field of 'holism' within ancient Greek medicine and biology poses particular challenges to our engagements with it in the present because of the role played by vitality and wholeness within the Romantic idealization of classical Greece and the fetishization of the Greek body at the crossroads of vitalism and classicism in German National Socialism.[8] If, in turning our attention to ancient holism as a concept resonant with contemporary concerns and the reception of ancient Greek medicine, we are shifting attention back to continuities, we need to reflect on the conditions under which we make claims for what von Staden calls 'legitimate continuity' and, more broadly, for the value of ancient holism in the present.

At the same time, the very terms under which holism qualifies as an exciting topic, at least in contemporary biology as well as within the interdisciplinary fields in the humanities and social sciences called 'critical life studies' and

5 Von Staden (1992) 584. On the problem of continuity or 'continuism,' see also Rochberg (1992) 552, though Rochberg also seeks a path that refuses a hard line on incommensurability and historical difference in order to consider how a tradition may function transhistorically. See further Rochberg (2016).

6 Von Staden (1992) 584.

7 Rochberg (1992) 549.

8 See further Holmes (2019a). On Nazi 'biocracy,' see Esposito (2008) 110–45 (without considering the Greeks); on the idealization of the Graeco-Roman past in National Socialism, see McCoskey (2012) 167–99; Chapoutot (2016).

'biopolitics,' should perhaps exclude classical antiquity from consideration.[9] For if historians of ancient medicine and biology have turned their backs on the present in recent decades, historians of later periods (to say nothing of medical and scientific practitioners) have been all the more ready to turn their backs on the ancients. Biology, despite its Greek name, is an invention of the early nineteenth century.[10] Its object, 'life,' literally does not exist prior to this moment, but rather only 'living beings, which were viewed through a grid of knowledge constituted by natural history.'[11] That, at any rate, is the hard line taken by Michel Foucault in *The Order of Things*, published in French in 1966. It has received far less challenge, especially from classicists and scholars of other premodern periods, than the analogous claim that Foucault made for sexuality as an invention of the nineteenth century in the first volume of the *History of Sexuality*, published twelve years later.[12] Foucault was not the first or the last to draw a line before and after modern biology. But together with the new historicisms and social histories of truth that his work has been associated with, he certainly made any movement from a loosely defined modern 'now' to an ancient 'then' in the realm of biology and the philosophy of medicine that much less smooth. In any event, the Graeco-Roman 'life sciences' have always been among the best candidates for arguments about the obsolescence of classical antiquity.[13]

Nevertheless, at the philosophical edges of the life sciences, which is to say, in the vicinity of questions about what life is and how best to care for it, the

9 For 'critical life studies,' see Weinstein and Colebrook (2017); on biopolitics, Holmes (2019a).

10 Two books, both employing the language of 'biology' and both published in 1802, are usually cited as foundational: Gottfried Reinhold Treviranus, *Biologie, oder, Philosophie der lebenden Natur für Naturforscher und Aerzte* (Göttingen, 1802) and Jean-Baptiste Lamarck, *Recherches sur l'organisation des corps vivants* (Paris, 1802). Kant's Third Critique, with its heuristic approach to teleology, also often functions as a decisive point of rupture between ancient and modern in the historiography of the life sciences: see Bianchi (2017).

11 Foucault (1970) 139. Canguilhem adopts this position at Canguilhem (1989) 546.

12 Foucault (1978). On the reception of Foucault's claims about sexuality in Graeco-Roman antiquity, see Holmes 2012a: 76–125.

13 Historians of ancient medicine have long been aware that the field's two monumental nineteenth-century editions – Littré's Hippocrates and Kühn's Galen – appeared at a moment when their primary audience was shifting decisively away from practicing physicians. Kühn was himself not simply a physician but the head of one of Europe's most important medical schools in Leipzig. See esp. Nutton (2002), noting that the interest among physicians in Galen was due a strong eclectic streak in early nineteenth-century German academic medicine that sought to bring together new discoveries with ancient insights, rather than to a monolithic 'premodern' or obsolescent Galenism. Littré had initially trained as a physician before turning to classical philology as a means of livelihood.

ancients, and especially the Greeks, refuse to die. Indeed, Foucault himself turned from the nineteenth century to Graeco-Roman antiquity in the second and third volumes of the *History of Sexuality*, producing a series of questions that continue to trouble the sprawling field of work on biopolitics, biopower, and the history of life.[14] The stubborn persistence of these questions within modern and contemporary conceptualizations of life demands further interrogation both from those whose focus is on modernity and the present, who scarcely reckon with this spectral antiquity, and from those whose primary aim is to make sense in the present of the ancient 'life sciences.' For ghosts have a way of disturbing the present and the stories it tells of the past. Nor can any sense be made of the classical past without tackling again, as part of – and in the light of – the recent work of disrupting narratives of continuity flagged by von Staden, the very problem of *what counts* as continuity from antiquity to the present in a history of life. We have lived for some time now with the appeal of emphasizing difference when we look at ancient Greek medical and scientific texts. But are we so sure about what stays the same?

I think not. And so there is good reason to take seriously the possibilities of an encounter at this juncture between the history of science, within which antiquity has been increasingly marginalized as irrelevant to the history of science proper (and the history of biology more specifically), and the flourishing subfield of reception studies within classics, which has remained mostly focused on literature, art, and historiography, despite a growing interest in ancient philosophy, science, and medicine (and interest in reception from historians of ancient philosophy, science, and medicine).[15] On the one hand, there are compelling resonances between the work 'the ancients' do within the history and philosophy of the life sciences and the tenacity of 'the ancients' in other domains, from visual art to political theory to the history of mathematics. These resonances point to the tangled reception histories of classical antiquity across different landscapes over many centuries.

On the other hand, the question of what the Greeks have to do with histories and philosophies of life, the body, nature, and the organism also requires

14 The ubiquitous but misleading distinction that Giorgio Agamben makes between *bios* and *zōē* has done much to keep the Greeks in play: see Agamben (1998), which I have critiqued in Holmes (2019a). See also Dubreuil (2006); Finlayson (2010); Brill (2019).

15 Interest in the specific encounter between reception studies and ancient medicine has been increasing more quickly in recent years, but I would point to Helen King's reading of the case of the daughter of Leonidas (1998, 54–74) as an example of the kind of work I am attempting here. And of course, much work on the reception of ancient Greek medicine and science has been done within the disciplinary parameters of the history of medicine and science.

attention to the specific nature of these reception histories and, more broadly, the relationship between history and philosophy within medicine and the life sciences, with their ever-more-privileged claims on truth. The sciences' snowballing claim on truth and legitimation means that the history of medicine and the life sciences, to the extent it is approached as a history extending into ancient Greece, bears an especially fraught relationship to stories of origin, the constitution of a Western 'we,' and the formulation of philosophical problems in the present, as we saw at the outset. Over the past fifty years, historicism and cultural studies have dismantled the overly confident stories of inheritance and continuity that have been told about ancient Greek science and medicine and modernity. The resources of reception studies can help us develop strategies now for handling the aspects of those ancient traditions that we find resonant with problems in the present.

In this chapter, I take up sympathy as a site for thinking about holism as one such resonant aspect of ancient Greek science, medicine, and philosophy. I continue to honor the spirit of work on ancient medical and philosophical texts that draws out their historical and cultural specificity as a defense against facile claims of continuity. But my interest is not so much in blocking the idea of resonance. The aim, rather, is to draw out holism as a conceptual problem in antiquity and, in so doing, to hold at bay the persistent modern idea of Greece as a site of lost wholeness or a more fully integrated life. We should be wary, too, of simplified contrasts between a fuzzily mystical antiquity and modern science with its hard-headed materialism. The different holistic tendencies in antiquity are developed in the face of ancient materialism, especially atomism, as a real threat. Moreover, as we will see, as far as living things are concerned, the Epicureans develop their own ideas of holism and psychophysical sympathy.

In short, in sympathy we see the acknowledgement of the problem posed by holism in the prefix *sun-*, which reminds us that this whole is not a mereological atom but a being-in-parts. In *sym*-pathy, we see, too, the promise of a reintegration of parts in an affection experienced by the whole. I therefore turn now to chart what I identified earlier as the two major axes within sympathetic thinking around parts and wholes: between part-to-part transmission and part-to-whole transmission, and between an ensouled body comprising many parts and the specific partnership of body and soul.

2 Part-to-Part, Part-to-Whole

It is worth starting by recognizing the historical-philological challenge involved in charting the conceptual scope of sympathy and its interaction with forms of ancient holism. The language of sympathy (*sumpatheia*, *sumpaskhō*, *sumpathēs*) only starts to appear in the fourth century BCE; even then, it is relatively rare. Its use grows in the Hellenistic period, becoming even more widespread in the first centuries AD across a range of discourses concerned with natures, human or otherwise, as well as with a trans-individual Nature, usually aligned with a providential care for human beings and other living things. These discourses encompass medicine, psychology and ethics, natural history, cosmology, astrology, astronomy, the genre of 'problem' literature, learned magic, pharmacology, and historiography.

The rise of sympathy in the post-classical period means that later writers regularly read sympathy back into classical-era authors who do not use the term. The phenomenon is especially evident in Galen's engagement with 'Hippocrates' – that is, with texts that he sees as genuine works of Hippocrates. In his Hippocratic commentaries, Galen at times attributes to Hippocrates a concept of part-to-part sympathy that is integral to his own understanding of disease's movement between 'affected parts' and shared by other Imperial-era physicians.[16] He also, like a number of early modern philosophers and physicians, takes up a maxim on sympathy from the text *On Nutriment*, almost certainly Hellenistic but often ascribed to Hippocrates, as paradigmatic of a Hippocratic philosophy of nature, holistic in spirit and dutifully upheld by Galen himself in the face of atomistic materialism.[17] Similarly, the late second- and early third-century CE philosopher Alexander of Aphrodisias, the most famous and committed of Aristotle's ancient commentators, does not dispute the reality of sympathy when he attacks the Stoic theory of total mixture. Rather, he accounts for it in the terms of Aristotle's system.[18]

Already in antiquity, then, sympathy poses problems of reception not so different from those posed by ancient holism in modernity. On the one hand, the arc of sympathy's development in post-classical antiquity, and especially its significant role as a technical or quasi-technical term across different discourses, leads ancient authors to read earlier texts in a way that modern scholars see as obviously anachronistic. On the other hand, in early writings on the physical or

16 Holmes (2012b). See also Holmes (2014b). Siegel (1968) 360–82 gives Galen too much credit in developing a concept of translocal sympathy.

17 [Hp.] *Alim.* 23 (IX.106 L. = 143,1–3 Joly): σύρροια μία, σύμπνοια μία, συμπαθέα πάντα· κατὰ μὲν οὐλομελίην πάντα, κατὰ μέρος δὲ τὰ ἐν ἑκάστῳ μέρει μέρεα πρὸς τὸ ἔργον ('One flowing together, one breathing together, all thing in sympathy; all the limbs are in a whole, and the parts in each part, each in a particular way, in line with the function'). For Galen's appropriation, see esp. Gal. *Nat. Fac.* 1.12–1.13 (II.26–44 K. = 119,25–133,10 Helmreich) with Vegetti (1999); Holmes (2014a); (2015), discussed further below, p. 75. See also De Lacy (1979) on the significance of continuity in Galen's understanding of the body, esp. 361–63.

18 Alex. Aphr. *Mixt.* 223,32–33 Bruns (= *SVF* 2.441).

the organic body, especially the Hippocratic texts and the Aristotelian corpus, we can see emerging theories of living beings and the world around them that will come to be defined in relationship to *sumpatheia*.

I take seriously the absence of the language of sympathy in these early texts. For I would argue that, when it does appear, such language, and the noun *sumpatheia* in particular, marks a transition from observing that two things are affected together to positing an underlying relationship or shared zone of interaction, which is what allows the transmission of affect from one body to another. At the same time, for my purposes here, I spend a lot of time with these classical-era texts in charting what I have been calling the two axes of sympathy. For these texts shed light on how different models of sympathy took shape along tracks that at times run in parallel and at times cross. They can help us see, too, how *sumpatheia* came to name different relationships of part and whole in the living thing. In moving between earlier and later texts, I will note explicitly when the language of sympathy comes into play.

Let us at this point, then, turn to these two axes. The first moves from part-to-part sympathy to part-to-whole sympathy. With part-to-part sympathy, we are already within some kind of larger whole: hence the language of 'parts.' But insofar as I am primarily concerned in this chapter with living things, the 'whole' in question is in a sense already and unproblematically given in advance as the person conventionally identified by a proper name, or a kind of animal, or, for the medical writers, the body, understood as co-extensive with the person. That is not to say that the question of what guarantees the person or body to be a whole is not subject to elaboration and debate. On the contrary, this question will receive considerable attention from both physicians and philosophers. Rather, the possibility of assuming a whole in advance means that in part-to-part sympathy the nature of the whole can be minimally important to the conditions that allow an affection to be transmitted from one part to another. What is emphasized, rather, is the connection between the parts themselves, sometimes to the point that they constitute a community within the body as a whole.

In the tradition of learned medical writing that is organized around the physical body as an object of expert knowledge, a form of part-to-part sympathy is already evident in the writings of the Hippocratic Corpus. Indeed, from one perspective, part-to-part sympathy is rampant in the Hippocratic writings because they virtually all share a commitment to constituent fluids or humours that in some way transmit damage from one part of the body to another. The author of the treatise *On Affections*, for example, describes sciatica in terms of blood corrupted by bile or phlegm that travels through the body, causing pain in whatever part of the body (e.g. the leg) it stops in.[19] The movement of affections throughout the body lies behind the programmatic claim of the Hippocratic author of *On Places in a Human Being* that 'all the parts (*merea*) of the body, on becoming ill, immediately produce disease in another part.'[20]

Yet it is also possible to detect a shift of emphasis between the two texts that will become increasingly relevant in later medical writing. While it is true that sciatica starts in one part (the hip, coccyx, or buttock) and moves to another (the leg), the author of *On Affections* zeroes in on the fluid itself (corrupted blood), with less attention to the affected part. By contrast, the author *On Places in a Human Being* specifically highlights the movement of the disease from one part or 'member' of the body to another. This focus on the affected part looks forward to Galen's most extensive text on part-to-part sympathy, *On the Affected Parts*. The heart, for example, might suffer sympathetically with the liver, or with the lungs, or with the pericardium, or with the opening of the stomach. The voice can be lost, through sympathy, if the intercostal muscles are damaged.[21]

More important still, Galen now describes affections of this kind in terms of sympathy (*sumpatheia*). Galen himself makes it clear that the term is one he shares with other physicians in this period. Although we are hampered by gaps in the evidence, it does seem likely that a more systematic discourse around 'affected parts' (*peponthotes topoi*; *loci affecti*) and affections transmitted 'by sympathy' developed in the first centuries CE; Galen seems to associate it with the early second-century CE physician Archigenes in particular.[22] It is true that Theophrastus, writing in the late fourth and early third century BCE, uses 'sympathy' to describe an affection shared between 'nerves' and 'vessels.'[23] But it is

19 [Hp.] *Aff.* 29 (VI.240–42 L.).

20 [Hp.] *Loc.* 1 (VI.276 L.= Craik 36, 9–10).

21 Heart with liver, lungs, pericardium, opening of the stomach: Gal. *Praes. Puls.* 4.2 (IX.394 K.), 4.4 (IX.399 K.); *Loc. Aff.* 5.1 (VIII.299 K.); *Caus. Sympt.* 1.7.7 (VII.136–38 K.). The voice affected by damage to the intercostal muscles: *Loc. Aff.* 1.6 (VIII.49 K.).

22 On the formation of a medico-doxographical tradition on 'the affected parts,' see van der Eijk (1998), esp. 349–53; van der Eijk (1999) 321–23. See also King (2018) 14, emphasizing 'locative diagnosis' as characteristic of Imperial-era medicine, broadly informed by the anatomical developments in Ptolemaic Alexandria. On Archigenes and affected parts, see Gal. *Loc. Aff.* 2.1 (VIII.136–37 K.)

23 Thphr. *On Fatigue* 10.75–76 Sollenberger: συμπάθειαν τῶν νεύρων καὶ φλεβῶν. The apparently early fragment from Erasistratus on epilepsy (fr. 293 Garofalo), which uses the standard language of sympathy to describe a translocal traffic in affections, is classed as spurious by Garofalo. The doxographical context makes it difficult to know if these are Erasistratus' *ipsissima verba*.

hard to know what to make of this early occurrence. What we can say is that part-to-part sympathy becomes especially visible in Roman Imperial-era medical writing addressed to the migration of disease or affection within the body, particularly with a shift of attention from the movement of fluids, as in the Hippocratic Corpus, to places or parts invested with specific functionality.[24] An increasingly robust discourse of affections that migrate among parts seems to have helped generate 'sympathy' as a technical term in learned medicine.

But whether we are looking at *On Affections* or *On Places in a Human Being* or at Galen's writings, we see the transmission of a disease or affection from one part to another very often explained in terms of a vessel that connects them. These vessels are generic in the Hippocratic texts. By Galen's time, they have been divided into veins, arteries, and nerves, following the work of Praxagoras of Cos in the fourth century BCE and Herophilus of Chalcedon in the next century. But regardless of what specific form or function they are given, vessels regularly serve, from the Hippocratic Corpus to Galen and beyond, as the concrete network that enables parts to transmit disease to one another across distances within the body. The capacity of vessels to put even parts at a remove from one another in communication creates a specific kind of part-to-part sympathy that I call 'translocal sympathy.' The vessels can even be said to allow the body to 'communicate with itself,' as the author of *On Places in a Human Being* puts it.[25] With this last statement, we can see part-to-part communication being reframed in terms of the larger whole, the body. But before turning our gaze towards the whole, I would like to point briefly to another way in which parts may be seen to enter into a relationship with one another in the Hippocratic Corpus, a means of connection that moves beyond a concrete point of contact (the vessel) into a more abstract zone of interaction.

The first of these alternative means of relation is the positing of a kind of 'community' or 'kinship' among parts. The author of the Hippocratic text *Epidemics II*, describing a subset of critical signs – that is, signs that indicate turning points in the drama of disease (recovery, relapse, imminent death) – offers the following cases: the breasts shrivel in women who are about to miscarry; a chronic cough disappears after a testicle swells. 'The testicle that has swollen because of the cough,' the author goes on, 'is a reminder of the community (*koinōniē*) between the chest, breasts, genitals, and the voice.'[26] The

---

24 For the contrast between parts as way-stations for humours and parts as defined primarily by function, see Byl (1971); Ioannidi (1983); Gundert (1992), all emphasizing the importance of Aristotle to the discourse of functionality in relationship to parts. See also Holmes (2014b).

25 [Hp.] *Loc.* 9 (VI.292 L. = 48,13–14 Craik). See below, p. 62.

26 [Hp.] *Epid. II* 1.6 (V.76 L.).

symptoms here – the shriveled breasts, the swollen testicle – recall a web of relationships within the (sexed) body with which the expert reader is presumed to be familiar. In another passage, this time from the Hippocratic *Diseases of Women II*, the author explains that the breasts swell following a uterine affection because of the parts' *homoethniē*, their being-of-the-same-kind.[27]

In both these examples, the *koinōniē* or *homoethniē* of the breasts and the uterus creates a micro-community within the body premised on a kind of affinity that sets the stage for the sharing of affections. The authors assume a tightknit (sub)-group within the body, without the body being cast itself as an integrated and unified community. At the same time, in identifying 'commonality' or 'kinship' as the grounds for shared affections, they point to a more robust sense of what must be held in common for a part to share an affection with another part beyond a concrete vessel running from one point to another. It is fascinating that when, centuries later, Galen tries to interpret the 'community' of chest, breasts, genitals, and voice in his commentary on *Epidemics II*, he pivots back to translocal sympathy, trying to find a vessel that explains the connection between what look on the surface to be scattered symptoms.[28] His quest to find the connecting vessel may reflect the consolidation of a concept of part-to-part – and, more specifically, translocal – sympathy in medicine tethered to anatomically identifiable paths within the body.[29]

Over the course of the fourth century BCE, we can see that inquiries into the nature of a living body become increasingly interested in attributing 'community' to *all* the parts of the body as members of a single whole. We already saw this turn from specific parts of the body in communication with one another to *all* the parts in communication with one another within the body as a totality

27 [Hp.] *Mul. II* 174 (VIII.354 L.). The word only appears again at [Hp.] *Loc.* 1 (VI.278 L. = 36,33 Craik), discussed below, but the adjective *homoethnēs* appears in Herodotus (1.91) and Aristotle (*Rh.* 2.6, 1384a11). The use of *ethnos* was very broad in classical Greek, applicable to 'any class of beings shar[ing] a common identification' – Homer uses it of swarms of bees and flocks of birds – as well as to communities 'in which membership is thought to be ascribed through birth' (Hall 1997, 35). Elsewhere in fifth-century medical writing, *ethnos* is used of a group of people living together, often under the same climactic and environmental conditions: see e.g. [Hp.] *Aer.* 12 (II.52 L. = 219,12 Jouanna), 13 (II.56 L. = 222,11 Jouanna), 17 (II.66 L. = 230,6 Jouanna); *Vict.* II 37 (VI.528 L. = 158,5 Joly-Byl).

28 See Holmes (2012b).

29 Galen does posit other means for the transfer of sympathetic affections in *On the Affected Parts*, including transmission by vapours. But although vaporous transmission is vaguer than vascular transmission, it still moves beyond the claim of kinship to posit a transmitting body. The community of the breasts and the uterus became a *locus classicus* for sympathy: see e.g. Sor. *Gyn.* 1.15 (10,27–28 Ilberg) *tis … phusikē sumpatheia*. But for Galen, even here there is a need for a vessel connecting the two: Holmes (2012b) 55–57.

in *On Places in a Human Being*. This text offers one of the most programmatic accounts in the Hippocratic Corpus of the body as an integrated whole, modelled on the circle insofar as every part is both beginning and end.[30] Indeed, it will go on to a flourishing afterlife in early modern medicine and philosophy as a paradigm of a Hippocratic holism, sometimes aligned with sympathy.[31]

The body communicating with itself, however, is only one of two models of the body understood as a whole in the introduction to *On Places in a Human Being*. Having posed the figure of the circle, the author sententiously begins another line of thought: 'the body is the same as itself and is composed of the same things, though not in uniform disposition, in its small parts and its large; in parts above and parts below.' He goes on: 'If you take the smallest part of the body and injure it, the whole body (*pan to sōma*) will feel the injury, whatever sort it may be, for this reason: that the smallest part of the body has all the things that the biggest part has.'[32] Whatever the smallest part suffers, good or bad, is passed on along a chain of parts which are related to each other through a kind of kinship. The word here is again *homoethniē*, as in *Diseases of Women II*. The author goes on to attribute the body's experience of pain and pleasure to the *ethnos*, the 'clan,' of 'the smallest.' He explains again that 'the smallest (part)' has all the parts (*pant' … ta merea*), which then announce their experiences to their relatives. It is admittedly difficult to understand exactly what the smallest parts are here and what it is they contain.[33] But it seems clear enough that, on the author's account, the *whole* body's experience of the pain of even the smallest *part* is attributed to a kind of sympathy (*avant la lettre*) along kinship lines among tiny parts distributed throughout the body.

In both the circle model and the model of 'sympathy' among tiny parts, we move from the part to a sense of a larger whole because two conditions are met. First, there is a concrete structure in place that enables affections to

30 [Hp.] *Loc.* 1 (VI.276 L. = 36,1–3 Craik). On the circle, see also [Hp.] *Vict.* I 19 (VI.492–94 L. = 138,28–29 Joly-Byl); [Hp.] *Nat. Oss.* 11 (IX.182 L. = 149,14–18 Duminil) for the use of the circle to describe a single vessel from which all others branch off.

31 See Lonie (1981) 138–39 for Friedrich Hoffmann's extensive use of the treatise and this passage in particular, and 138 n. 71 for its appearance in other eighteenth-century medical texts; Wolfe and Terada (2008) 551 n. 16 for Herman Boerhaave's (1668–1738) citation of the text's image of the body as a circle, glossed by Boerhaave as showing '[sc. the body's] parts are indeed so entwined and tied up with others that the single parts are dependent on the whole.'

32 [Hp.] *Loc.* 1 (VI.278 L. = 36,26–38,3 Craik).

33 Vegetti (1965) 202–3 has argued for the influence of Anaxagoras' ideas on a mixture in which all the seeds are present. But Democritus' account of perception is also resonant: see Solmsen (1968) 544–45, 552–53 on a relationship with the account in Plato's *Timaeus*, which is similar to that in *On Places in a Human Being*.

be transmitted not only from one place to another but throughout the entire body. In the case of fluxes of diseased matter, it is the distribution of vessels throughout the body – detailed by the author at some length – that licenses the programmatic statement that the body is a circle without beginning or end: the body, as we saw earlier, is in communication with itself.[34] In the case of pain and pleasure, the distribution of these small parts within kinship networks throughout the body makes it possible for what happens to one small part to be transmitted to the body as a whole. Second, this structure has to facilitate the transmission of disease or damage from part to part in the first place. The vessels can do this because they communicate with one another, allowing diseased matter to pass from one place to another. The smallest parts, by contrast, seem bound together only by kinship, which is sufficient for their experiences to be passed along the chain until they are properly experiences of the whole body.

From one perspective, both models yield an idea of difference *within* a larger community that will be crucial to the conceptual field of sympathy.[35] The very language of sympathy is predicated, after all, on the idea of different parts. Otherwise, the affections (*pathē*) would just belong to the body as a whole, rather than being communicated. Yet such language also puts those parts into some kind of a community and perhaps even one that can be called a whole.

From another perspective, the models frame the body as a whole in quite different ways. In the case of fluxes of diseased matter, the migration of disease via connecting vessels happens throughout the body because of an extensive vascular network. What the author is in fact describing is the amplification of translocal sympathy. The result is not exactly part-to-whole sympathy. But we can say that the author of *On Places in a Human Being* does not take the body in its totality for granted as the backdrop for the sharing of affections among parts, as in the passages I cited earlier from *On Affections*, *Epidemics II*, and *Diseases of Women II*. Rather, it is the network of intercommunicating vessels that licenses the author's comparison of the body to a circle, a figure of wholeness over and above the parts.

34 [Hp.] *Loc.* 9 (VI.292 L. = 48,13-14 Craik) τὸ σῶμα κοινωνέον αὐτὸ ἑωυτῷ. The verb *koinōneō* is used elsewhere to speak of vessels that 'communicate' with one another, especially in the surgical treatises: see e.g. [Hp.] *Artic.* 13 (IV.118 L. = 134,8 Kühlewein), 45 (IV.190 L. = 172,3 Kühlewein), 49 (IV.216 L. =184,13 Kühlewein); *Fract.* 9 (III.450 L. = 62,4 Kühlewein); *Prorrh. II* 38 (IX.68 L.). At *Epid.* VI, 3.23 (V.304 L. = 76,4–5 Manetti-Roselli) and *Hum.* 20 (V.500 L.), we find references to *hai koinōniai* with the sense of sympathetic affections.

35 The difference in this account of pain and pleasure seems twofold: between discrete (but 'related') parts and between different types of parts that create chains of kinship within the larger whole.

Pain and pleasure look more straightforwardly like cases of 'part-to-whole' sympathy. We begin with a very small part and we end up at the whole body feeling pleasure or pain. The scalar shift from small part to whole body gives specificity to the initial claim that the body is uniform and continuous while also comprising many different, tiny parts that are continuous *with one another* on account of their kinship and extend throughout the body, even more ubiquitous than the vessels. These kinship relations magnify the experience of one part so that it becomes an experience of the whole. The felt experience of pain or pleasure as an experience of the body, rather than of a part, distinguishes this model from a model of circular flux, where the humours' freedom of movement is in contrast to the fixedness of the disease in a given place at a given time.

The idea of the pain of a part being experienced by the body, or the living thing, as a whole recurs in other medical and philosophical texts. In the discussion of the mechanics of *aisthēsis* in Plato's *Timaeus*, for example, where *aisthēsis* refers above all to pain and pleasure, Timaeus gives a detailed account of how some impacts to the body are passed on from one small part to another – the 'chain' model resembles that in *On Places in a Human Being* as well as the atomist model described by Lucretius – and eventually are transformed into an affection of 'the whole living thing.' But for Timaeus, the transformation of an affection into pain or pleasure requires that the chain of affects reaches what he calls *to phronimon*.[36] With this term he is clearly referring to some part of the soul, though there is controversy about which part. But before looking at the involvement of the soul or a psychic part in sensing, I would like to point to part-to-whole sympathy as exemplified by pain as an occurrence that could be used by Plato himself as proof of a unified whole.

In Book 5 of Plato's *Republic*, Socrates proposes that in the ideal city, the citizens are united in their pleasures and pains, as is true of an individual human being. If the finger is wounded, 'the entire community stretching through the body to the soul in one system of control senses it, and this entire community suffers in pain together with the affected finger, as a whole.'[37] The passage falls over itself in emphasizing the sense of a community (*koinōnia*) encompassing the body and soul together as a whole, a community that feels with each of its parts and is confirmed, in turn, *as* a whole through shared pain. The language of 'sharing in pain' (*sunēlgēsēn*) thus works, like the language of sympathy, to affirm both the whole and the part in the same word. The part in this case is obviously different from the particle in the *Timaeus* that is first moved, and

36 Pl. *Tim.* 64b.

37 Pl. *Resp.* 5, 462d.

Plato's language seems to allow, presumably under the pressure of the analogy, that the finger is sentient (as the individual citizen is). But what matters is Plato's emphasis on pain as an experience that involves the body-soul compound, the *whole animal*, as an entire community. The experience of shared pain in a human community thus points to the unified fabric binding its members together.

If we turn now to the Stoics, we can see how the pain of the finger felt by the whole comes to serve as paradigmatic of sympathy in a context where sympathy is being taken explicitly as the index of a unified body. In a critical account of Stoic theology, Sextus Empiricus reports that the Stoics had a taxonomy of bodies that proceeds along three stages from the loosest of aggregates to unified bodies (*hēnōmena sōmata*).[38] The first category of bodies encompasses flocks, choruses, and armies – in other words, loose groupings composed of separate (*diestōta*) elements that may nevertheless be organized around a common purpose. The next category includes bodies whose elements are joined together (*sunaptomena*), like ships or cables. In both these types of bodies, Sextus reports, the parts do not 'sympathize' with one another. So even if an entire army, save a single soldier, dies, the lone survivor does not suffer anything 'by transmission' (*kata diadosin*) – because an army is not a unified body.[39] By contrast, unified bodies have a kind of sympathy (*tis sumpatheia*) between the parts. The example the Stoics give in support of this claim is that 'if a finger is cut, the whole body shares in the pain.'[40] The unified body thus declares itself by exhibiting sympathy, and the classic case of sympathy is the pain of the finger, shared by the whole.

On Sextus' account, however, the cut finger is only one part of an argument that aims to prove the unity of the cosmos as a whole on the basis of its manifest sympathies: the effects of lunar cycles on the growth and diminution of animals both on land and at sea; the tides; changes to the atmosphere in accordance with the risings and settings of the stars. He says, too, that this argument, in turn, formed part of Stoic arguments for the existence and nature of god as the immanent mind of the cosmos unifying its parts.[41] What is interesting here is the resurgence of part-to-part sympathy (e.g. between the moon and sea creatures). Nevertheless, for the Stoics, these particular sympathies are

---

38 S. E. *Adv. Math.* 9.78; see also 1.102.

39 S. E. *Adv. Math.* 9.80. On the army as an example used by Plato to show what contemporary mereology would call 'the innocence of composition,' see Pl. *Theaet.* 204b10–e10, with Harte (2002) 41–47, esp. 45.

40 S. E. *Adv. Math.* 9.80.

41 S. E. *Adv. Math.* 9.79.

marshalled as evidence of an underlying unity or wholeness. This unity is their primary concern.

Like we saw with the vessels in the medical writers, the Stoics posit a concrete medium of connectivity between the parts: namely, *pneuma*, which creates a continuum between all the parts of the unified body.[42] *Pneuma* does not only put parts in contact across distances within a unified body. It also succeeds in creating a whole out of these parts because it imbues the unified body with a more robust sense of structure, as was intimated by earlier notions of a kinship between parts.

In the case of the living animal body, the capacity to unify the body is ascribed to the soul. Having returned to the soul as in some way implicated in the experience or identity of the animal as a whole, I would like to turn now to my second axis of sympathy. My aim in this final section will be to show how the axis we have just traced, which moves from material connectivity (and part-to-part sympathy) to a more robust sense of community or commonality (and part-to-whole sympathy), interacts with an axis that moves from an emphasis on many parts, as in most of the texts we have looked at so far, to a focus on two parts in particular, body and soul.

3 The Partnership of Body and Soul, the Community of Parts

In the account of sensation-perception in the *Timaeus*, Plato, as we saw, uses a model of what I have called 'chain sympathy' to describe the transmission of an affect from a part to the living being as a whole. In *On Places in a Human Being*, the Hippocratic author seems to imagine that the transition from part to whole occurs because of the spatial distribution of all the small parts that come to participate in the affection. In Plato, however, it is clear that this transition reflects a consequential leap from a chain of particles passing on the affection to one another to a single privileged part that turns an unfelt affection (*pathos*) into an experience of the whole animal. The leap is so consequential that Timaeus elsewhere describes it in terms of the *two* parts on either side of the divide: the body and the soul.[43]

In the *Philebus*, body and soul take on these binary roles in an even more defined way, especially in the 'violent' affections of pain and pleasure with which the dialogue is primarily concerned. Plato here again classifies affections into those that produce sensing and those that do not, and he says that what makes

42 On *pneuma* and the continuum, see Coughlin and Rocca in this volume.

43 See e.g. Pl. *Tim.* 43c.

the first class of affections different from the second is simply that their motions reach the soul, rather than being first 'extinguished' in the body.[44] It is only if the body and the soul experience one common affection (*heni pathei … koinē*) and are moved in common, Socrates says, that the affection is called *aisthēsis* (34a3–5). In the *Philebus*, then, sensing is defined as something common to the body and the soul, and sensing, in turn, defines the common ground between them. The partnership of body and soul, crucially, does not erase the difference between them: each partner participates in sensation in its own way (*idion*, 33d).[45] Nevertheless, if sensation preserves a boundary between the body and the soul, it also defines the community that they make together as parts of a single whole by manifesting the communication of a movement from *sōma* to *psuchē*.

The discussion in the *Philebus* of what is 'common to body and soul' has a long afterlife in accounts of the soul in the ancient Greek philosophical tradition. Even more than Plato, Aristotle looks to sensation as a privileged domain for the community of *sōma* and *psuchē*. On the first page of the treatise *On the Senses*, which stands at the head of Aristotle's writings on the soul in the *Parva Naturalia*, he classifies virtually every aspect of human life as 'common to body and soul' because it participates in sensation, including being awake, desire, and pleasure and pain.[46] But where Aristotle parts ways with Plato, at least in the *De Anima*, is in refusing an understanding of the body-soul relationship in sensation-perception in terms of translocal 'sympathy.' In the *Philebus* or the *Timaeus*, an affect or movement crosses a boundary into the soul, where it registers as felt experience. By contrast, Aristotle denies that motion can belong to the soul, at least 'in itself.'[47] The alternative account developed by Aristotle in the *De Anima* is too complicated to trace out here. Suffice to say that Aristotle

---

44 The criterion for *aisthēsis* in this case has to do with intensity rather than the part of the body affected: only strong movements will travel all the way to the soul. Plato addresses the role of 'violence' as a factor in pain and pleasure at *Tim.* 64c–65b; the strength and violence of the movements is also at stake in the account at 43c.

45 On the difference of the body and the soul, see e.g. Pl. *Phlb.* 36b8–9, 41b11–d2.

46 Arist. *Sens.* 1, 436b1–3. For the expression 'common to body and soul,' see also *De an.* 3.10, 433b19–21; *Part. an.* 1.3, 643a35, with Balme (1992) 116; *Somn. vig.* 1, 454a7–11. On continuities between the *Parva Naturalia* and the *De Anima*, see Johansen (2006); Morel (2006). Many readers have noted that Aristotle's use of the phrase probably looks back explicitly to the *Philebus*: see Menn (2002) 100; Johansen (2006) 146–47; Carpenter (2010b): 29; Boeri (2018) 161–63. Menn (2002) 85–90 argues that Aristotle has in mind not only Plato's views but his own, earlier views on perception and motions in the soul, especially in *Physics* 7; see also Boeri (2018) 161–63.

47 Arist. *De an.* 1.3, 406a2. For what Aristotle means by motion 'in itself', see Shields (2016) 116–34.

seems committed in the treatise to resisting a model in which soul and body interact as discrete parts.

Yet it is precisely the *interaction* of body and soul that comes center stage in two of the most influential psychophysical theories to develop after Aristotle, Stoic and Epicurean.[48] Both Hellenistic schools were deeply committed to the corporeality of the soul as part of their broader commitments to physicalism.[49] In each case, their arguments for the soul's corporeality turn on such interaction, described in terms of the 'sympathizing' (*sumpaskhō*) or 'sympathy' (*sumpatheia*) of the body and the soul. For this reason, I suggest that we see the language of (psychosomatic) sympathy coming to redefine what was described by Plato and Aristotle in terms of 'common to body and soul' – and redefining it, moreover, as manifest evidence of the soul's corporeality.

Let us begin with an argument attributed by the late fourth-century CE Christian Platonist Nemesius of Emesa to Cleanthes (ca. late-fourth to late-third century BCE), the second head of the Stoic school after its founding by Zeno (333–264 BCE). The argument aims to demonstrate the corporeality of the soul by appealing to the sharing of affections between the body and the soul – that is, the sympathizing of one with the other. Cleanthes begins the argument with a strategic version of the well-known Stoic claim that only bodies can act on bodies:[50] 'only a body can sympathize with another body.' To sympathize assumes causal interaction. Cleanthes then offers, as his next premise, the observation that the soul 'sympathizes' with the body if it is sick or cut, while the body 'sympathizes' with the soul when it is ashamed or afraid: it turns red and pale respectively. From these two premises he concludes that the soul is a body.[51] Cleanthes thus argues for the corporeality of the soul on the basis of what he describes as the evident 'sympathizing' of the body and the soul. The observation of part-to-part psychosomatic sympathy establishes corporeality as the common ground of both parts. But if Cleanthes' argument establishes

48 Gill (2006) addresses these theories precisely as exemplars of psychophysical holism without addressing sympathy.

49 The question of whether the soul is corporeal or incorporeal became a fixture of the doxographical tradition: see Mansfeld (1990) 3065–85.

50 Cic. *Ac.* 1.39 (LS 45A); S. E. *Adv. Math.* 8.263 (LS 45B). The passage from Nemesius appears as LS 45C.

51 Nem. *Nat. Hom.* 2 (21,6–9 Morani) οὐδὲν ἀσώματον συμπάσχει σώματι οὐδὲ ἀσωμάτῳ σῶμα, συμπάσχει δὲ ἡ ψυχὴ τῷ σώματι νοσοῦντι καὶ τεμνομένῳ καὶ τὸ σῶμα τῇ ψυχῇ· αἰσχυνομένης γοῦν ἐρυθρὸν γίνεται καὶ φοβουμένης ὠχρόν· σῶμα ἄρα ἡ ψυχή ('No incorporeal sympathizes with a body, and no body with an incorporeal, but one body sympathizes with another body. Now the soul sympathizes with the body when it is sick and being cut, and the body with the soul; thus when the soul feels shame and fear, the body turns red and pale respectively. Therefore, the soul is a body').

the corporeality of the soul, it assumes much more besides. He describes sympathy in a way that implicitly casts the body and the soul as separable entities, each of which has affections of its own that can be shared with the other: the body gets sick or is cut; the soul is ashamed or afraid.[52]

Given the deep association between Epicureanism and materialism in the reception of both philosophical traditions, it will come as no surprise that Epicurus (341–270 BCE) also argued that the *psuchē* is corporeal. Perhaps more surprisingly, the Epicureans also relied on an argument from sympathy to prove that the body and the soul hold corporeality in common. Like the Stoics, the Epicureans claim that only bodies can affect bodies. If the soul were incorporeal, Epicurus says at the end of the psychology in the *Letter to Herodotus*, it would not be able to act on and be acted on.[53] But it is so manifestly an agent and a patient that it must be corporeal.

Epicurus does not explicitly lay out a formal argument from sympathy in the *Letter* in defense of the soul's corporeality.[54] But if we turn to Book 3 of Lucretius' *De Rerum Natura*, we see psychosomatic sympathizing being explicitly appropriated for a physicalist argument about the soul. Lucretius begins his demonstration that the soul is a body by first pointing to the soul's capacity to rouse the body from sleep and steer it in locomotion.[55] Such interaction, he declares, is possible only through touch; and touch, in turn, is possible only between bodies – a version of the claim that only bodies can affect bodies, which Lucretius had already introduced in the first book of the poem.[56] Lucretius then proceeds to offer another class of evidence for the interaction of body and soul, this time showing not that the soul acts on the body but that the body acts on the soul. 'You see,' he writes, 'that mind suffers along with the body and shares our feeling (*consentire*) in the body.' That the mind is thrown into a tumult when the body is struck by weapons or blows, Lucretius concludes, proves definitively that its nature is corporeal.[57]

There is one clear difference between Cleanthes' presentation of the mutual sympathy of the body and the soul and that given in Lucretius. Lucretius does not foreground the emotions in describing the soul's action on the body. He

52 See Gal. *PHP* 5.2.3–7 (V.432–433 K. = 294,33–296,17 De Lacy), on the analogy between diseases of the soul and those of the body in Chrysippus and Posidonius.

53 Epic. *Ep. Hdt.* 67.

54 Sedley (1998) 119 speculates that the soul's corporeality would have occupied all of Book 9 of *On Nature*.

55 Lucr. *DRN* 3.162–67.

56 Lucr. *DRN* 1.304, 1.443–44.

57 *ergo corpoream naturam animi esse necessest, / corporeis quoniam telis ictuque laborat* (Lucr. *DRN* 3.175–76). Cf. 3.463–525, 819–29.

instead uses the example of locomotion to establish this part of the argument for mutual interaction.[58] But Lucretius' apparent reticence about the emotions is easily explained. Right before introducing his proof for the corporeality of the soul, he had used the emotions to prove a different kind of interaction. He argues that there are two parts of the soul that interact with one another: the mind (*mens, animus*) and the irrational, sensing soul (*anima*).[59] Lucretius adopts the case of fear in order to establish that the whole spirit (*anima*) shares in the feeling (*consentire*, 3.153) of the mind, detailing its many effects: sweating, pallor, loss of voice, faltering speech, and so on. But if Lucretius exploits the effects of fear to establish that the spirit and the mind are conjoined, this claim does not preclude him from also recognizing the conjunction of the soul and the body. In fact, he goes on to take the dramatic symptoms of fear as evidence not only that the mind and spirit are linked, but also that as soon as the spirit is struck by the mind's power, it 'straightaway strikes and drives forward the body.'[60] Fear therefore proves the interaction of parts of the soul. But it also proves the interaction of a unified soul and the body, as Lucretius makes clear in transitioning from his argument about the interaction of the parts of the soul to his argument about the composite soul's interaction with the body: 'this same reasoning teaches that the nature of the *animus* and the *anima* is corporeal.'[61]

Lucretius thus uses sympathy to establish a twofold conclusion. First, there are two, interacting parts of the soul, the *animus* or *mens* and the *anima*, which together comprise a unified nature; second, we can see that this bipartite, but unified, soul is corporeal from its interaction with the body. His twofold argument from sympathy is more complicated than the one we find attributed to Cleanthes (and, in fact, the Stoics would not want to establish parts of the soul). Lucretius nevertheless confirms how psychosomatic sympathy could be used by Hellenistic philosophers as evidence that the soul is *a* body, precisely because it acts and is acted upon within its partnership with *the* body. Indeed, later Platonist and Aristotelian commentators explicitly aim to refute

58 For locomotion as common to body and soul: Arist. *De an.* 3.10, 433b19–21.

59 He is presumably following Epicurus, but there is no argument for 'parts' of the soul in Epicurus' *Letter to Herodotus* (Kerferd 1971). Other sources do report that Epicurus did identify a rational and an irrational part: see Aët. 4.4.6; the scholiast to D. L. 10.66 (= fr. 311 Usener). See also Diogenes of Oenoanda fr. 37.1. Sedley (1998) 68–72 takes Lucretius' decision to locate the rational part of the soul in the chest as evidence of what he calls Lucretius' 'fundamentalism' because it shows no awareness of debates around cardiocentrism sparked by the Alexandrian anatomists.

60 Lucr. *DRN* 3.160. Cf. the account of locomotion at Lucr. *DRN* 4.881–91.

61 Lucr. *DRN* 3.161.

what we might call the argument from (psychosomatic) sympathy to defend the soul's incorporeality.

I suggest that we understand the argument from (psychosomatic) sympathy as a version of what I earlier classified as 'part-to-part' sympathy. In part-to-part sympathy, we can recall, what tends to be foregrounded is the concrete means by which one part transfers an affection to another, usually a vessel. Less attention is paid to the conditions of kinship or similarity that enable the formation of a community between the parts or the larger whole that can make sense of their relationship. The targeted use of sympathy in the arguments of Cleanthes and Lucretius similarly posits a minimal means of contact between soul and body: namely, shared corporeality. But they do not specify what makes the interaction of soul and body different from the interaction of any two bodies.

Another way to put this would be to say that corporeality alone does not make for much commonality (*koinōnia*). It is precisely the failure to specify the *koinōnia* of body and soul for which Aristotle faults his predecessors, including Plato, in the first book of the *De Anima*. It is not the case, he complains, that any old body can work with any old soul, as is assumed by theories of metempsychosis. Indeed, the problem with his predecessors is that they yoked soul to body without giving any thought to the partnership, *koinōnia*, that makes it possible for one to act and the other to be affected, and for one to move and the other to be moved.[62]

Aristotle's phrasing here aligns everything the soul does with its capacity to act on the body. But he is also emphasizing that the body must have a particular form and shape to be moved by its soul. His complaint about his predecessors' lack of attention to the partnership of the soul and the body brings into relief the *way* in which a soul acts on a body – namely, in the way that 'a craft makes use of its tools.'[63] The tool analogy looks forward to how important the ideas of function and purpose will be when Aristotle gives his own positive account of the soul and the soul-body compound in Book 2. The emphasis on function is marshalled by Aristotle there to give an account of the body and the soul as a unified whole.

62 Arist. *De an.* 1.3, 407b15–19. Aristotle describes the process by which a desire initiates motion as 'among the functions common to body and soul' at *De an.* 3.10, 433b19–21. For the relation of soul and body in locomotion, see the discussion of *De Motu Animalium* 10 at Nussbaum (1978) 143–64.

63 Arist. *De an.* 1.3, 407b26; see also 2.1, 412b1,12. For *technē* as a model for the soul that enables both an instrumentalist understanding of the soul-body relationship and hylomorphism (that is, not interactionism), see Menn (2002); see also Morel (2006) 133–38 on the *Parva Naturalia*.

Despite their disagreements with Aristotle, neither the Stoics nor the Epicureans give up on this idea of the body and the soul as a unified whole. Both schools agree that shared corporeality is insufficient for the body and the soul to make a life together: more commonality is needed. Each school accordingly develops an account of the living thing, and especially a sentient being, as a unity. In each case, moreover, the language of sympathy is deployed to describe not only individual occurrences of an affection shared by the body and the soul but also their underlying, permanent relationship, that is, their shared life. Let us take a very brief look at how, for both Epicureans and Stoics, sympathy cues a form of psychophysical holism that ascribes unity and wholeness to the community of body and soul.

The Stoics, as we have seen, are deeply committed to the category of the unified body. The cause of unity in any unified body is its *pneuma*, which the Stoics, at least from Chrysippus onwards, claim stands in a relationship of 'total blending' (*krasis di' holōn*) with the matter that it permeates. In total blending, the constituent parts are fully co-extensive with one another without losing their own properties.[64] By means of total blending, *pneuma* can be present everywhere in the body while retaining its special capacity to impart unity.[65] What total blending entails, as we saw in the example of the cut finger, is that the parts of a body exist in sympathy with one another or, as Chrysippus seems to have put it in speaking about the cosmos as a whole, a body is 'sympathetic with itself.'[66]

It is worth emphasizing that a unified body need not be sentient. Much as they rank categories of bodies, the Stoics also rank unified bodies depending on the particular 'tension' (*tonos*) of their *pneuma* in a scale that ascends from rocks, unified only by a minimal cohesion (*hexis*); to plants, unified by nature (*phusis*); to animals, whose unity is due to soul (*psuchē*). Yet the soul's mixture with the body functions as a privileged example of total blending, and total blending, in turn, accounts for the shared life of body and soul beyond the corporeality they hold in common.

64 See Alex. *Mixt.* 217,26–32 Bruns (= LS 48C; *SVF* 2.473), where total blending is contrasted with juxtaposition (an aggregate) and fusion, in which the constituent elements are destroyed (or present only potentially) in the mixture.

65 It seems that not every instance of total blending creates a unified body (the infamous example is a drop of wine in the sea), but Alexander says that accounting for the *unity* of the world is the aim of the theory of mixture: Alex. Aphr. *Mixt.* 216,4–6 Bruns (= LS48C; *SVF* 2.473). At *Mixt.* 227,5–10 Bruns, Alexander insists that 'the unification and sympathy of everything' depend on the theory of mixture.

66 Alex. Aphr. *Mixt.* 216,14–17 Bruns (= LS48C; *SVF* 2.473) ἡνῶσθαι μὲν ὑποτίθεται τὴν σύμπασαν οὐσίαν, πνεύματός τινος διὰ πάσης αὐτῆς διήκοντος, ὑφ᾽ οὗ συνέχεταί τε καὶ συμμένει καὶ σύμπαθές ἐστιν αὑτῷ τὸ πᾶν; cf. *Mixt.* 223,6–9 Bruns.

We can see this more robust sense of psychosomatic sympathy quite clearly in Hierocles' *Elements of Ethics*, probably written in the mid-second century CE. Hierocles is especially interested in proving that animals perceive themselves continuously from the moment of birth to the end of their lives.[67] The first premise in the argument is one that we have already encountered as the conclusion to the argument from psychosomatic sympathy: the soul and the body are both bodies and therefore capable of interacting. Hierocles, noting that this premise has been proven elsewhere, says he will not bother to demonstrate it here. He next introduces the doctrine of total blending in order to specify the *relationship* of the soul and the body: 'the soul is not enclosed in the body as in a bucket, like liquids surrounded by jars, but is wondrously blended and wholly intermingled, so that not even the least part of the mixture fails to have a share in either of them.'[68] Due to the total blending of the body and the soul, 'what has to do with sympathy (*ta tēs sumpatheias*) is complete for both.' For, Hierocles goes on, each one is sympathetic (*sumpathes*) with the other. Neither is the soul unaware of the body's troubles, nor is the body deaf to the soul's.[69] Here, then, we see psychosomatic sympathy used to claim not simply that the body and the soul share in corporeality, as in the argument ascribed to Cleanthes. Body and soul are *totally* blended. As a result, 'what has to do with sympathy is complete for both.' The common ground required to account for the sympathy of body and soul is far more extensive than shared corporeality.

If we turn back to the Epicureans, we find a similarly robust sense of sympathy as more than an occurrence of transferred affections, but as the condition of the shared life – and shared death – of body and soul. Again, it may be surprising that the Epicureans have their own strong concept of sympathy as a condition of life, given how closely the concept has traditionally been associated with the Stoics. But in fact, Epicurus's *Letter to Herodotus* is one of the earliest

---

67 Hier. *Elem. eth.* col. 1.38–39.

68 Hier. *Elem. eth.* col. 4.3–8. Trans. Ramelli/Konstan. That we are within the theory of total blending is clear from Hierocles' reference to fire passing through iron: Hier. *Elem. eth.* col. 4.8–9. Cf. Alex. *Mixt.* 218,1–2 Bruns.

69 ταύτῃ καὶ τὰ τῆς συμπαθίας ἐστὶν ἀμφοῖν κατακορῆ. θάτερον γὰρ τῷ ἑτέρῳ συμπαθὲς καὶ οὔτε τῶν σωματικῶν παθῶν ἀνήκοος ἡ ψυχὴ οὔτε αὖ τέλεον ἐκκεκώφηται πρὸς τὰ τῆς ψυχῆς δεινὰ τὸ σῶμα. (Hier. *Elem. eth.* col. 4.10–13). Trans. Ramelli/Konstan. The adjective *katakorēs* can mean 'deep' or 'intense' but also 'complete' as a modifier of 'harmony' (*sumphōnia*) (LSJ I 4), and it is this last sense that is probably in play here. Hierocles' examples are familiar: the impact of the body's troubles on the soul's capacities (delirium, for example, caused by an inflammation in a vital part); the bodily effects of the emotions (knocking of teeth, trembling of legs, changes of colour). But he now ascribes them to the body and soul being 'mixed together in the way we have said': Hier. *Elem. eth.* col. 4.20–22.

attestations that we have for the noun 'sympathy' (*sumpatheia*).[70] Epicurus there emphasizes that sensation-perception is a joint project of the soul and the rest of the compound, made possible by the soul's closeness with the aggregate and its 'sympathy' with it.[71] Although the account here is compressed and at times obscure, it is clear that it is because the soul is a certain kind of body, spread throughout the rest of the body, that it (or a part of it) is 'sympathetic' (*sumpathes*) with the aggregate. Its sympathy with the aggregate, together with its spatial juxtaposition with the rest of the atoms in the compound, enables sensation as an occurrence (*sumptōma*) of the entire compound. Epicurus thus seems to have adopted the term 'sympathy' to capture the fundamental interdependence and continuous communication that defines the soul-body relationship. That relationship is most fully expressed in the defining and, in fact, enabling activity of their shared life: sensation-perception.

We can see the significance of the robust sympathy of the soul and the body even more clearly in Book 3 of Lucretius. Epicureans are committed not only to the shared life of the soul and the body but to their shared death. The soul's mortality was fundamental to Epicurean arguments that, in Lucretius' famous phrase, 'death is nothing to us' (3.830). It is Lucretius' interest in demonstrating the mortality of the soul and, more specifically, its dependence on the body for life that gives sympathy such an important role to play in Book 3 as a witness to the relationship of the soul and the body, beyond what we have already seen of its role in Lucretius as a sign of the soul's corporeality. After Lucretius' discussion of the nature of the soul and its relationship to the body, he turns to a suite of arguments running for more than four hundred lines and designed to prove that the soul is not just mortal but inextricably bound to the body, born together with it and dying with it.[72] I single out two of these arguments to show

70 Outside of the discussion of sensation-perception, Epicurus uses *sumpatheia* four times (*Ep. Hdt.* 48, 50, 52, 53) in his account of the relationship between the emanations that cause perception and the objects generating them.

71 *Ep. Hdt.* 65 οὐ γὰρ αὐτὸ ἐν ἑαυτῷ ταύτην ἐκέκτητο τὴν δύναμιν, ἀλλ' ἑτέρῳ ἅμα συγγεγενημένῳ αὑτῷ παρεσκεύαζεν, ὃ διὰ τῆς συντελεσθείσης περὶ αὐτὸ δυνάμεως κατὰ τὴν κίνησιν σύμπτωμα αἰσθητικὸν εὐθὺς ἀποτελοῦν ἑαυτῷ ἀπεδίδου **κατὰ τὴν ὁμούρησιν καὶ συμπάθειαν** καὶ ἐκείνῳ, καθάπερ εἶπον ('For it (sc. the body) never possessed this power in itself, but used to afford opportunity for it to another existence, brought into being at the same time with itself; and this existence, owing to the power now consummated within itself as a result of motion, used spontaneously to produce for itself the capacity of sensation and then to communicate it to the body as well, in virtue of its juxtaposition and sympathy, as I have already said,' trans. Bailey, slightly modified). On *homourēsis* as the 'vicinity' of body and soul, see also *Ep. Pyth.* 106 and fr. 7 of *On Nature*, with Németh (2017) 51–52.

72 Lucr. *DRN* 3.425–829. Lucretius formally frames these arguments with a *nunc age* at 3.417, and they run right up to the famous conclusion at 3.830.

the Epicureans' conception of sympathy as the foundation of the shared life and death of body and soul.

In the first argument, Lucretius, like Hierocles, acknowledges that the body is not simply a vessel for the soul. He had in fact used the vessel argument earlier to emphasize the soul's dependence on the body.[73] But shortly afterward, he admits that the relationship of water to a container fails to capture the intimacy and complexity of the relationship of the body and the soul, 'since the body does cling closely to it.'[74] If Hierocles, in rejecting the image of the body as a vessel, proposes Stoic mixture as the physical basis for a total interpenetration of body and soul, Lucretius will point to the 'weaving together' of soul atoms and body atoms in order to illustrate the grounds for their interdependence. The deep commonality of body and soul also leads Lucretius, like Aristotle, to reject the argument for metempsychosis. For souls, he argues, could never slip into bodies that are already made: 'for they will not be able to conjoin themselves closely with these, nor could communication be established through sympathy (*consensu*).'[75] These passages drive home that, for Lucretius, sympathy proves not only that the soul is a body. It proves, too, that it is a particular *kind* of atomic compound, one capable of being 'sympathetic' with the (rest of the) body, as we saw in the *Letter to Herodotus*.

I have spent considerable time on psychosomatic sympathy because, as we started to see at the end of the last section, soul, in one form or another, comes to play such an important role in bringing about the unity of the living thing. The unity that soul makes possible encompasses body and soul, of course. But it may also ensure that the many parts that make up a living thing, from its most elemental parts to its most complex organs, are a unified whole rather than a mere heap or aggregate. In mapping the conceptual landscape of holism through the lens of sympathy, I therefore close by gesturing towards this more populous community of parts in the living animal. We started to see earlier that part-to-part sympathy can spark reflection on how sympathy is enabled not simply by a conduit but by the parts' inclusion in a larger whole.

73 Lucr. *DRN* 3.434–35.

74 Lucr. *DRN* 3.557. See also 3.324–27.

75 Lucr. *DRN* 3.738–40. The meaning of *consensus* at 3.740 (which appears only here) has been misunderstood. Lachmann emended the mss. reading *consensu* to *consensus*, a correction that Kenney claims is called for 'by the sense: the interconnexions are not brought about by *consensus*, but cause it; the genitive is that of definition' (2014, 170). See also Bailey (1962) 1117–18: 'it is true that logically *contagia* should come first and *consensus* be its result (i.e. *contage consensus fiet* would be the natural way of putting it).' Ernout's 'datif de but' (1926, 112) seems not to have convinced anyone. But Lucretius is using *consensus* here to name the underlying condition that enables occurrences of sympathy.

The integration of the body's many and heterogeneous parts into a unity lies at the heart of Aristotle's teleology, which credits soul with this unifying work. Aristotelian teleology will shape instances of what I have been calling 'vital' sympathy in the later tradition.

From Aristotle's teleological perspective, (nearly) every part of a living thing exists for the sake of something.[76] More specifically, Aristotle holds that each part exists for the sake of the function(s) or activities to which it is 'naturally adapted.' As Aristotle famously writes in the introduction to *Parts of Animals*, 'every instrument (*organon*) is for the sake of something, and each bodily part is for the sake of something, and what they are for the sake of is an activity (*praxis*).'[77] But each part and its activity cannot be understood in isolation. Rather, it has to be evaluated in terms of the living thing as a whole and the activity proper to it as a particular kind of living thing.[78] Just as every part of the body is for the sake of some activity, he continues on in *Parts of Animals*, 'it is plain that the body, too, as a whole is composed for the sake of a certain complete activity.' It is 'for the sake of the soul,' he says, that the body has come to be in a certain way. In other words, not only the parts of the body but also and most importantly the manifold activities of that body and its parts are unified by a common purpose. The purpose in question is achieving, and then maintaining, a fully-fledged existence as a living thing engaged in a particular form of life (*bios*).

Aristotle's teleology has an enormous impact on the account of the living body that Galen develops across his vast corpus. But Galen is also an avowed Platonist and, as a result, committed to a transcendent Demiurge. This commitment leaves him with the problem of how to make sense of the 'mindfulness' of immanent teleology, especially within the physiological or vegetal body: 'who [the Demiurge] is and how he resides in the body of a living creature is one of the most problematic and insoluble of questions,' he writes in *On Problematical Movements*.[79] In his attempt to answer this question, Galen turned again and again to what he took to be Hippocrates' own maxim on the sympathy of all the body's parts in *On Nutriment*: 'One flowing together, one breathing together, all things in sympathy; all the limbs are in a whole, and

76 For synthetic accounts of Aristotle's teleology, see Johnson (2005); Leunissen (2010). Aristotle left some parts without a function, leaving an opening for Galen's claim that only he has given a complete teleological account of the human body: see van der Eijk (2010).

77 Arist. *Part an.* 1.5, 645b14–21. Trans. Balme.

78 For Aristotle, a part cannot be a substance because it is not unified: Arist. *Metaph.* Z 16, 1040b5–10.

79 Gal. *DMD* 4.8 (136,22–23 Nutton).

the parts in each part, each in a particular way, in line with the function.'[80] The maxim looms large within Galen's account of a Hippocratic philosophy of nature. Galen aims to show, among other things, the primacy of Hippocrates vis-à-vis the Stoics, although nearly all modern scholars would reverse the line of influence and date the Hippocratic text to the third century BCE or later. Galen's deployment of the 'Hippocratic' maxim is flexible and complicated. For the purposes of sketching 'vital sympathy,' I emphasize two points.

First, this ostensibly Hippocratic, avowedly holistic sympathy is not the same as the translocal sympathy that Galen tries to identify in his commentaries on Hippocratic texts. It is likely because *sumpatheia* had a relatively narrow technical sense related to translocal sympathy that when Galen wants to invoke this more philosophically expansive, holistic, 'Hippocratic' sympathy, he does not use the noun *sumpatheia* and instead cites the passage from *On Nutriment*, usually in an abbreviated form. The contexts in which he cites the passage, moreover, tend to be programmatic and adversarial, with the Epicureans, Asclepiades of Bithynia and Erasistratus of Ceos – all mechanists of one kind or another in Galen's view – as targets. In an especially memorable attack in *On the Natural Faculties*, where Galen sides with continuum theorists against the atomists, he accuses Asclepiades of claiming that 'nothing is naturally sympathetic (*sumpathes ... phusei*) with anything else, all substance being divided and broken up into inharmonious elements and absurd 'particles.''[81] Asclepiades' fatal flaw thus comes down to the denial of sympathy.

On the Natural Faculties is one of the most important texts for Galen's development of a 'vital' sympathy aligned with Hippocrates' legacy. But I want instead to close with his use of the maxim from *On Nutriment* in his magnum opus on what he sees self-consciously as Aristotelian teleology, *On the Usefulness of Parts*, which he composed over ten years.[82] In the preface to the work, Galen turns, predictably, to Hippocrates as his tutelary deity and invokes the passage from *On Nutriment*: 'taken as a whole, all the parts in sympathy, but taken severally, the parts in each part cooperate for its effect.'[83] Many people, he goes on, get confused about the saying, because it is too concise and too archaic in its style. Galen therefore steps up with a paraphrase: 'all the parts

80 [Hp.] *Alim.* 23 (IX.106 L. = 143,1–3 Joly): σύρροια μία, σύμπνοια μία, συμπαθέα πάντα· κατὰ μὲν οὐλομελίην πάντα, κατὰ μέρος δὲ τὰ ἐν ἑκάστῳ μέρει μέρεα πρὸς τὸ ἔργον.

81 Gal. *Nat. Fac.* 1.13 (II.39 K. = 129,7–9 Helmreich).

82 On Galen's engagement with *Parts of Animals*, see Moraux (1985). See also van der Eijk (2010), esp. 264–65 on the influence of Aristotle on Galen and his familiarity with Aristotle's corpus.

83 Gal. *UP* 1.8 (III.17 K. = 1.12.24–25 Helmreich): κατὰ μὲν οὐλομελίην πάντα συμπαθέα, κατὰ μέρος δὲ τὰ ἐν ἑκάστῳ μέρει μέρεα πρὸς τὸ ἔργον.

of the body are in sympathy with one another, that is to say, all cooperate in producing one work.'[84] His citation and his paraphrase, which drop the first part of the maxim, strategically amplify the teleological cues that are already present in the passage (including an intricate triple play on the word for 'part,' *meros*, in the original Greek and the use of *ergon*, Aristotle's preferred word for function). In so doing, Galen binds 'Hippocratic' sympathy to Aristotle's teleological account of the unity of a living thing.[85]

We therefore find ourselves back along the axis running from part-to-part sympathy to part-to-whole sympathy. I had earlier suggested in connection with *On Places in a Human Being* that specific claims of part-to-whole sympathy, whose paradigmatic example is the pain of a single part felt by the whole, should be read together with cases where part-to-part sympathy is being redefined as a general principle governing all the parts, whose interrelation invites further attention to the larger whole to which they belong and, increasingly, an overt holism grounded in the unity of the living thing. Certainly in the preface to *On the Usefulness of Parts*, Galen is thinking about the (organic) body as a totality in which each part has a function in relationship to others and to the life of the whole.

At the same time, Galen is less confident than Aristotle, or the Stoics for that matter, that soul is capable of creating this unity. He parts ways with them, first, in his Platonic commitment to a tripartite soul, whose parts he maps very concretely onto the anatomical body. Yet he parts ways with them, too, in his worries about the relationship of our rational, sentient soul to the vegetal part of the animal that he often refers to as nature, *phusis*.[86] What undermines the possibility of a single unitary soul, for Galen, is the fact that 'the soul that manages us has no knowledge of the parts that obey its urges.'[87] He marvels at the fact that children can speak without any understanding of how the muscles involved produce the sounds or, for that matter, the work done by the nerves.[88]

84 Gal. *UP* 1.8 (III.18 K. = 1.13.7–9 Helmreich); cf. 1.9 (III.24 K. = 1.17.13–15 Helmreich).

85 Cf. Alex. Aphr. *De An.* 100,1–4 Bruns. Here the argument for total 'part-to-part' sympathy is negative – Alexander is trying to refute encephalocentric arguments based on localized symptoms; but the passage suggests that Galen was not the only reader of Aristotle in the first centuries CE who saw the organic body in terms of (total) part-to-part sympathy.

86 He credits the *psuchē/phusis* distinction to the Stoics, but see von Staden (2000) 105–16, esp. 110–11, arguing that Galen is more likely inspired by the contrast between soul and nature in the Hellenistic anatomists.

87 Gal. *Foet. Form.* 6.25 (V.697 K. = 100,28–29 Nickel).

88 Gal. *Foet. Form.* 6.23 (V.696 K. = 100,14–20 Nickel), 6.26 (V.697 K. = 100,30–102,9 Nickel). Galen makes this point in other treatises as well. See also Gal. *In Hipp. Epid. VI* 5.2 (259,6–261,14 Wenkebach-Pfaff); *Loc. Aff.* 6.6 (VIII.445 K.); *PHP* 5.5.1–8 (316,21–318,19 De Lacy), where Galen is interested in the child's natural inclinations towards pleasure or goodness.

Even as adults, we do not have any knowledge of the parts of our bodies or their activity before the study of anatomy. Yet our ignorance about anatomy does not prevent us from moving our arms or having a conversation. In practice, then, Galen's ambivalent relationship to holism seems to have less to do with either his Platonist commitments or his belief in the unity of the (vegetal) body celebrated in terms of a Hippocratic, 'vital' sympathy.[89] Rather, it arises from an idea that he could not shake: that we humans are creatures designed around a fundamental blindness to our own nature understood as our vital being.

4 Conclusion

The preceding discussion, however schematic, should make it clear that ancient Greek medical and philosophical authors pursued a robust inquiry into the nature of parts and wholes — 'mereology,' in the language of contemporary philosophy. Verity Harte has persuasively shown how the problem of structure becomes increasingly important to Plato as he grapples with the unity of wholes that are not 'mereological atoms,' that is, wholes with (proper) parts.[90] But Plato's understanding of structure is primarily mathematical, rather than biological. By contrast, Aristotle's paradigmatic substances are living things – 'unities and individuals par excellence'; they may be the *only* things that enjoy the 'dignity of substance.'[91] Aristotle's holism is predominantly vitalist. Whatever Aristotle's debts to biological and medical writings of the previous century, it is clear from texts in the Hippocratic Corpus, and also writers like Praxagoras of Cos and Diocles of Carystus, that theoretical medical writers were also starting to pursue an account of the living thing as a whole in the late fifth into the fourth centuries BCE, as they became more and more interested in relationships among the parts of the body not only in disease but also in health. We increasingly see, in different discourses, the living thing imagined

---

He takes up the problem again in his *On Problematical Movements*: see e.g. 4.5 (136,13–16 Nutton), 7.17 (159,6–10 Nutton), 8.17–18 (158,6–16 Nutton) with Nutton and Bos (2011) 286–87, 341.

89 I therefore read Galen's relationship to Stoic holism differently than does Gill (2010), esp. 16–17, who primarily contrasts Galen's tripartite soul with the unitary soul of the Stoics; but cf. Gill (2010) 103–24.

90 The mereological atom has one 'improper' part: itself. See Harte (2002), esp. 46–47, 122–34, 158–67, 267–81 on wholes as 'contentful structures' in Plato.

91 Frey (2007) 191 ('unities and individuals par excellence') with Arist. *Metaph.* Z 7, 1032a18–19. The only things worthy of 'the dignity of substance': Shields (2008) 129 (adopting the phrasing of W. D. Ross).

and theorized as a unity, and unity imagined and theorized in turn through the paradigm of the living thing.

These holistic or vitalist tendencies in ancient, especially late and post-classical medical and philosophical texts, are not unknown to scholars. But they have often been a cause of anxiety or overinvestment. Much of the work on Aristotle's biology over the past few decades has sought to redeem him as a disciplined philosopher of biology in the face of worries that his teleology is precisely too vitalist – that is, that it isolates life too much from the workings of the physical world, invoking mysterious substances or processes to account for it. Or, as we saw at the outset, these 'vitalist' tendencies are read as reflections of a more unified philosophical spirit, before the onset of modernity and its concomitant ruptures – temporal, psychological, spiritual – and racialized impurities.

I would argue that by focusing on the emergence of sympathy as a conceptual habit in learned medicine and philosophical psychology, especially from the late fourth century BCE on, we can reframe ancient holism in terms of a series of problems that arise from the increasingly complicated and increasingly vexed theorisation of living beings, especially sentient animals, as complex wholes. As I indicated in the beginning, I do not think that the growth of different discourses of sympathy vis-à-vis the living thing can be understood apart from discourses (such as that of sympathy-antipathy) that look to the larger whole in which the living thing lives. But my more limited purpose here has been to plot two axes that run through the conceptual field of sympathy *within* a living being as a way of getting clearer about how the problem of living things as wholes comprising many parts takes shape in different authors who, despite sometimes virulent disagreement, also share sympathy as a conceptual resource, even trading strategies for how to use it. What emerges is not a placidly holistic and paradigmatically premodern veneration of life. It is, rather, the efflorescence of 'life' as a problem for the project of human flourishing.

Bibliography

Agamben, G. *Homo Sacer: Sovereign Power and Bare Life*. Trans. D. Heller-Roazen. Stanford: Stanford University Press (1998).

Balme, D. M. Aristotle. *"De Partibus Animalium I" and "De Generatione Animalium I" (with passages from II.1–3)*. Reprinted with new material. Oxford: Clarendon Press (1992).

Bianchi, E. 'Aristotle's Organism, and Ours.' In *Contemporary Encounters with Ancient Metaphysics*, ed. A. J. Greenstine and R. J. Johnson. Edinburgh: Edinburgh University Press (2017) 138–57.

Boeri, M. D. 'Plato and Aristotle on What Is Common to Soul and Body: Some Remarks on a Complicated Issue'. In *Soul and Mind in Greek Thought: Psychological Issues in Plato and Aristotle*, ed. M. D. Boeri, Y. Y. Kanayama and J. Mittelman. Cham: Springer (2018) 153–76.

Brill, S. 'Aristotle's Meta-Zoology: Shared Life and Human Animality in the Politics.' In *Antiquities beyond Humanism*, ed. E. Bianchi, S. Brill and B. Holmes. Oxford: Oxford University Press (2019) 97–122.

Byl, S. 'Note sur la polysémie d'ΟΡΓΑΝΟΝ et les origins du finalisme.' *L'Antiquité Classique*, 40 (1971) 121–33.

Canguilhem, G. 'Vie.' *Encyclopedia Universalis*, 23 (1989) 530–46.

Carpenter, A. 'What Is Peculiar to Plato's and Aristotle's Psychologies? What Is Common to Them Both?' In *Aristotle and the Stoics Reading Plato*, ed. V. Harte, M. M. McCabe, R. W. Sharples and A. Sheppard. London: Institute of Classical Studies (2010) 21–44.

Chapoutot, J. *Greeks, Romans, Germans: How the Nazis Usurped Europe's Classical Past*. Trans. Richard R. Nybakken. Oakland: University of California Press (2016).

De Lacy, P. 'Galen's Concept of Continuity.' *GRBS*, 20 (1979) 355–69.

Esposito, R. *Bíos: Biopolitics and Philosophy*. Trans. Timothy Campbell. Minneapolis: University of Minnesota Press (2008).

Foucault, M. *The Order of Things: An Archaeology of the Human Sciences*. New York: Random House (1970).

Foucault, M. *The History of Sexuality. Vol. 1: An Introduction*. Trans. R. Hurley. New York: Random House (1978).

Frey, C. 'Organic Unity and the Matter of Man.' *Oxford Studies in Ancient Philosophy*, 32 (2007) 167–204.

Gill, C. 'Psychophysical Holism in Stoicism and Epicureanism.' In *Common to Body and Soul: Philosophical Approaches to Explaining Living Behaviour in Greco-Roman Antiquity*, ed. R. A. H. King. Berlin: De Gruyter (2006) 209–31.

Gill, C. *Naturalistic Psychology in Galen and Stoicism*. Oxford: Oxford University Press (2010).

Gundert, B. 'Parts and Their Roles in Hippocratic Medicine.' *Isis*, 83 (1992) 453–65.

Hall, J. *Ethnic Identity in Greek Antiquity*. Cambridge: Cambridge University Press (1997).

Harte, V. *Plato on Parts and Wholes: The Metaphysics of Structure*. Oxford: Oxford University Press (2002).

Holmes, B. *Gender: Antiquity and its Legacy*. London: I. B. Tauris (2012a).

Holmes, B. 'Sympathy between Hippocrates and Galen: The Case of Galen's Commentary on 'Epidemics', Book Two.' In *"Epidemics" in Context: Greek Commentaries on Hippocrates in the Arabic Tradition*, ed. P. E. Pormann. Berlin: De Gruyter (2012b) 49–70.

Holmes, B. 'Disturbing Connections: Sympathetic Affections, Mental Disorder, and Galen's Elusive Soul.' In *Mental Disorders in Classical Antiquity*, ed. W. V. Harris. Leiden: Brill (2013) 147–76.

Holmes, B. 'Galen on the Chances of Life.' In *Eikos: Probabilities, Hypotheticals, and Counterfactuals in Ancient Greek Thought*, ed. V. Wohl. Cambridge: Cambridge University Press (2014a) 230–50.

Holmes, B. 'Proto-Sympathy in the Hippocratic Corpus.' In *Hippocrate et les hippocratismes: médecine, religion, société: Actes du XIVe Colloque International Hippocratique*, ed. J. Jouanna and M. Zink. Paris: Académie des Inscriptions et Belles Lettres (2014b) 123–38.

Holmes, B. 'Galen on Sympathy.' In *Sympathy*, ed. E. Schliesser. Oxford Philosophical Concepts. New York: Oxford University Press (2015) 61–69.

Holmes, B. 'The Generous Text: Animal Intuition, Human Knowledge, and Written Transmission in Pliny's Books on Medicine.' In *Knowledge, Text, and Practice in Ancient Technical Texts*, ed. M. Formisano and P. J. van der Eijk. Cambridge: Cambridge University Press (2017) 231–51.

Holmes, B. 'Bios.' *Political Concepts: A Critical Lexicon* 5 (2019a). http://www.politicalconcepts.org/bios-brooke-holmes/. Last accessed 20 May 2020.

Holmes, B. 'On Stoic Sympathy: Cosmobiology and the Life of Nature.' In *Antiquities beyond Humanism*, ed. E. Bianchi, S. Brill and B. Holmes. Oxford: Oxford University Press (2019b) 239–70.

Holmes, B. 'Canguilhem and the Greeks: Vitalism between History and Philosophy.' In *Vitalism and Its Legacies in the Twentieth Century*, ed. C. Donohue and C. Wolfe. New York: Springer (forthcoming a).

Holmes, B. *The Tissue of the World: Sympathy, Life, and Nature in Greco-Roman Antiquity*. Chicago: University of Chicago Press (forthcoming b).

Ioannidi, H. 'Les notions de partie du corps et d'organe.' In *Formes de pensée dans la Collection hippocratique*, ed. F. Lasserre and P. Mudry. Geneva: Droz (1983) 327–33.

Johansen, T. K. 'What's New in the *De Sensu*? The Place of the *De Sensu* in Aristotle's Psychology.' In *Common to Body and Soul: Philosophical Approaches to Explaining Living Behaviour in Greco-Roman Antiquity*, ed. R. A. H. King. Berlin: De Gruyter (2006) 140–64.

Johnson, M. R. *Aristotle on Teleology*. Oxford: Oxford University Press (2005).

Kerferd, G. B. 'Epicurus' Doctrine of the Soul.' *Phronesis*, 16 (1971) 80–96.

King, D. *Experiencing Pain in Imperial Greek Culture*. Oxford: Oxford University Press (2018).

King, H. *Hippocrates' Woman: Reading the Female Body in Ancient Greece*. London: Routledge (1998).

King, R. A. H. (ed.) *Common to Body and Soul: Philosophical Approaches to Explaining Living Behaviour in Greco-Roman Antiquity*. Berlin: De Gruyter (2006).

Leunissen, M. *Explanation and Teleology in Aristotle's Science of Nature*. Cambridge: Cambridge University Press (2010).
Lloyd, G. E. R. *Magic, Reason, and Experience: Studies in the Origins and Development of Greek Science*. Cambridge: Cambridge University Press (1979).
Lloyd, G. E. R. *Science, Folklore, and Ideology: Studies in the Life Sciences in Ancient Greece*. Cambridge: Cambridge University Press (1983).
Lloyd, G. E. R. *The Revolutions of Wisdom: Studies in the Claims and Practice of Ancient Greek Science*. Berkeley: University of California Press (1987).
Lonie, I. M. 'Hippocrates the Iatromechanist.' *Medical History*, 25 (1981) 113–50.
Mansfeld, J. 'Doxography and Dialectic: The Sitz im Leben of the Placita.' *ANRW* II 36.4 (1990) 3056–29.
McCoskey, D. *Race: Antiquity and Its Legacy*. London: I. B. Tauris (2012).
Menn, S. 'Aristotle's Definition of Soul and the Programme of the *De Anima*.' *OSAP*, 22 (2002) 83–139.
Moraux, P. 'Galen and Aristotle's *De Partibus Animalium*.' In *Aristotle on Nature and Living Things: Philosophical and Historical Studies Presented to David M. Balme on his Seventieth Birthday*, ed. A. Gotthelf. Pittsburgh: Mathesis Publications (1985) 327–44.
Morel, P.-M. "Common to Body and Soul' in the *Parva Naturalia*.' In *Common to Body and Soul: Philosophical Approaches to Explaining Living Behaviour in Greco-Roman Antiquity*, ed. R. A. H. King. Berlin: De Gruyter (2006) 121–39.
Németh, A. *Epicurus on the Self*. New York: Routledge (2017).
Nussbaum, M. C. *Aristotle's "De Motu Animalium."* Princeton: Princeton University Press (1978).
Nutton, V. 'In Defense of Kühn.' *Bulletin of the Institute of Classical Studies* Supplement 77: The Unknown Galen. (2002) 1–7.
Ramelli, I. *Hierocles the Stoic: Elements of Ethics, Fragments and Excerpts*. Trans. D. Konstan. Atlanta: Society of Biblical Literature (2009).
Rochberg, F. 'Introduction: The Cultures of Ancient Science: Some Historical Reflections.' *Isis*, 83 (1992) 547–53.
Rochberg, F. *Before Nature: Cuneiform Knowledge and the History of Science*. Chicago: University of Chicago Press (2016).
Sedley, D. *Lucretius and the Transformation of Greek Wisdom*. Cambridge: Cambridge University Press (1998).
Shields, C. 'Substance and Life in Aristotle.' *Apeiron*, 41 (2008) 129–51.
Shields, C. *Aristotle, De Anima*. Oxford: Oxford University Press (2016).
Siegel, R. E. *Galen's System of Physiology and Medicine: An Analysis of His Doctrines and Observations on Bloodflow, Respiration, Tumors, and Internal Diseases*. Basel: Karger (1968).

Solmsen, F. 'Greek Philosophy and the Discovery of the Nerves.' In *Kleine Schriften*. Hildesheim: Olms (1968) 536–82 (originally published in *Museum Helveticum*, 18 (1961) 150–97).
van der Eijk, P. J. 'Quelques remarques sur la méthode doxographique de Caelius Aurélien.' In *Maladie et maladies dans les textes latines antiques et médiévaux*, ed. C. Deroux. Brussels: Latomus, Revue d'études latines (1998) 342–53.
van der Eijk, P. J. 'The Anonymus Parisinus and the Doctrines of 'the Ancients'.' In *Ancient Histories of Medicine: Essays in Medical Doxography and Historiography in Classical Antiquity*, ed. P. J. van der Eijk. Leiden: Brill (1999) 295–331.
van der Eijk, P. J. "Aristotle! What a Thing for You to Say!' Galen's Engagement with Aristotle and Aristotelians.' In *Galen and the World of Knowledge*, ed. C. Gill, T. Whitmarsh and J. Wilkins. Cambridge: Cambridge University Press (2010) 261–81.
Vegetti, M. 'Il *De locis in homine* fra Anassagora ed Ippocrate.' *Istituto Lombardo (Rend. Lett.)*, 99 (1965) 193–213.
Vegetti, M. 'Historiographical Strategies in Galen's Physiology (*De usu partium, De naturalibus facultatibus*).' In *Ancient Histories of Medicine: Essays in Medical Doxography and Historiography in Classical Antiquity*, ed. P. J. van der Eijk. Leiden: Brill (1999) 383–95.
von Staden, H. 'Affinities and Elisions: Helen and Hellenocentrism.' *Isis*, 83 (1992) 578–95.
von Staden, H. 'Body, Soul, and Nerves: Epicurus, Herophilus, Erasistratus, the Stoics, and Galen.' In *Psyche and Soma: Physicians and Metaphysicians on the Mind-Body Problem from Antiquity to the Enlightenment*, ed. J. P. Wright and P. Potter. Oxford: Oxford University Press (2000) 79–116.
Weinstein, J., and C. Colebrook (eds.) *Posthumous Life: Theorizing beyond the Posthuman*. New York: Columbia University Press (2017).
Wolfe, C. T., and M. Terada. 'The Animal Economy as Object and Program in Montpellier Vitalism.' *Science in Context*, 21.4 (2008) 537–79.

Primary Texts: Editions and Translations Used

Alexander of Aphrodisias. *Alexandri Aphrodisiensis praeter Commentaria Scripta Minora*. Ed. I. Bruns. Berlin: De Gruyter (1961).
Epicurus. *Epicurea*. Ed. H. Usener. Leipzig: Teubner (1887).
Epicurus. *Epicurus, the Extant Remains*. Ed. C. W. Bailey. Oxford: Clarendon Press (1926).
Erasistratus. *Erasistrati Fragmenta*. Ed. I. Garofalo. Pisa: Giardini (1988).
Galen. *Claudii Galeni Opera Omnia*. 20 vols. Ed. C. Kühn. Leipzig: C. Cnobloch (1821–1833).

Galen. *Galeni Pergameni Scripta Minora*, 3 vols. Ed. I. Müller, J. Marquardt and G. Helmreich. Leipzig: Teubner (1884–1893).

Galen. *Galeni, In Hippocratis Epidemiarum Libros I et II*. Ed. E. Wenkebach and F. Pfaff. CMG V 10,1. Leipzig: Teubner (1934).

Galen. *Galeni, Über die Ausformung der Keimlinge*, Ed. D. Nickel. CMG V 3,3. Berlin: Akademie Verlag (2001).

Galen. *Galeni De Placitis Hippocratis et Platonis*. 3rd ed. 3 vols. Ed. P. De Lacy. CMG V 4,1,2. Berlin: Akademie Verlag (2005).

Galen. *Galen, On Problematical Movements*. Ed. V. Nutton, with G. Bos. Cambridge: Cambridge University Press (2011).

Hippocrates. *Hippocrate, Du régime des maladies aigués; Appendice; De l'aliment; De l'usage des liquides*. Ed. R. Joly. CUF t. 6.2. Paris: Les belles lettres (1972).

Hippocrates. *Hippocratis Opera Quae Feruntur Omnia*, 2 vols. Ed. H. Kühlewein Leipzig: (1894–1902).

Hippocrates. *Œuvres complètes d'Hippocrate*. 10 vols. Ed. É. Littré. Paris: Baillière (1839–1861).

Long, A. A., and D. N. Sedley. *The Hellenistic Philosophers*. 2 vols. Cambridge: Cambridge University Press (1987). = **LS**.

Lucretius. *Lucreti De Rerum Natura. Libri sex*. Ed. C. W. Bailey. Oxford: Clarendon Press (1962).

Lucretius. *Lucrèce*. Ed. A. Ernout. Paris: Les belles lettres (1947).

Lucretius. *Lucretius, De Rerum Natura, Book III*. Ed. E. J. Kenney. Cambridge: Cambridge University Press (2014).

Nemesius of Ephesus. *Nemesii Emeseni De Natura Hominis*. Ed. M. Morani. Leipzig: Teubner (1987).

Soranus. *Sorani Gynaeciorum libri IV, De Signis Fractuarum, De Fasciis, Vita Hippocratis secundum Soranum*. Ed. J. Ilberg. CMG 4. Leipzig: Teubner (1927).

Theophrastus. 'Theophrastus, *On Fatigue*'. Ed. M. G. Sollenberger. In *Theophrastus of Eresus, On Sweat; On Dizziness; and On Fatigue*, ed. W. W. Fortenbaugh, R. W. Sharples and M. G. Sollenberger. Leiden: Brill (2003) 253–323.

von Arnim, H. F. A. (ed.) *Stoicorum veterum fragmenta*. 4 vols. Leipzig: Teubner (1903–1924). = *SVF*.

CHAPTER 3

'Holism' in Cognitive Approaches to the Ancient Emotions

William Michael Short

Abstract

Emotional experience is at once bodily, mental, cultural and social. Methods for studying the emotions, especially those of historical societies, must therefore be equally multidisciplinary to avoid reducing affective experience to a single dimension. This chapter evaluates two kinds of approach to studying the ancient emotions drawing inspiration from the cognitive sciences: in particular, the Wierzbickian script-based and Lakovian metaphor-based methods. It argues that whereas the Wierzbickian approach falls short of an adequate cultural emotionology, an embodied semantics along cognitive-linguistic lines can enable emotion concepts to be studied in a way that is both emically sensitive and etically sound, as well as in their several dimensions simultaneously – thus affording a more holistic perspective on this aspect of ancient experience.

The study of human emotions is necessarily an interdisciplinary undertaking that must bring together many different perspectives simultaneously and avoid reducing its 'object' to a single dimension.[1] This is because emotional experience itself is inherently multifaceted, being at once bodily, mental, and social. Whatever basic theory one may subscribe to – whether we believe, for instance, that emotions derive from the autonomic physical responses that precede our intellectual awareness of those experiences (the James-Lange theory), or that physiological arousal and psychological awareness of emotions occur simultaneously (the Cannon-Bard theory), or again that raw feelings are experienced as emotions only after they have been coded in certain conceptual terms (the Schachter-Singer cognitive appraisal theory) – any adequate account has to acknowledge that emotions involve complex states of feeling, thinking, and behaving in constant interaction with the social and cultural

1 Barrett (2017); Ogarkova et al. (2009).

 | DOI:10.1163/9789004443143_005

environment, which includes language.[2] In other words, emotional experience is shaped both by our common human embodiment and by our global and local socio-cultural situatedness.[3] What's more, it is inherently temporal, insofar as emotions are conditioned by personal and collective memories and play out dynamically through time. Thus, scholarly investigation into the emotions must incorporate insights from neuroscience and biology, psychology, philosophy, and sociology, as well as from linguistics, history, and even literary studies. Their study must also include an anthropological point of view sensitive to the possible diversity of emotional experience across cultures as well its commonality.[4]

Developing an interdisciplinary emotionology along these lines would seem to emblematize the kind of 'holism' that forms the central theoretical concern of this volume. Therefore, in this chapter, I evaluate two methods of studying Roman emotions that have recently emerged from the cognitive sciences. (Though perhaps most prevalent, the kind of good old-fashioned philology that tries to describe emotion concepts by comparing explicit definitions of terms in ancient philosophical or technical authors to their actual linguistic behaviour and contextual usage – including their syntactic and collocational patterns, etymological histories, and semantic evolution through time – is touched on only in passing, as this method has been evaluated already elsewhere).[5] The first (and earlier) method I shall introduce is inspired by the 'cultural scripts' approach of Anna Wierzbicka and Cliff Goddard. The second incorporates elements of the contemporary theory of conceptual metaphor in cognitive linguistics, most associated with George Lakoff and Mark Johnson. I argue that whereas the Wierzbickian approach falls short of an adequate cultural emotionology, an embodied semantics along cognitive-linguistic lines appears capable of enabling ancient emotion concepts to be studied in a way that is both emically sensitive (i.e., that privileges 'the native's own view') and etically sound (expressed in scientifically validated and psychologically realistic terms). Most importantly, it provides a foundation for studying such concepts holistically in more than one sense – that is, as something simultaneously mental and bodily, as well as social and cultural through and through.

The multifacetedness of human emotional experience – the fact that it is in part determined by the particulars of human embodiment, in part conditioned

2 Levenson (2003). A survey of theories is given in Scherer and Ekman (1984).

3 On the debate between universalists and constructivists, see esp. Harré (1986) and Griffiths (1997).

4 Mesquita and Frijda (1992). The point is emphasized esp. by Goody (2002).

5 Most notably by Cairns (2008).

by our historical and cultural situatedness, and in part constructed through emergent social interactions – requires that emotionological research be equally multifaceted and multidisciplinary. This requirement is perhaps particularly marked in the case of historical societies, where scholarship is immediately confronted with challenges of sources and methods. As David Konstan notes, scholars have no direct access to living native informants from ancient Greece and Rome, and so cannot rely on methods like ethnographic interview or participant observation to investigate the emotional lives of members of these cultures.[6] Trying to characterize what ancient people 'really' felt on the inside is perhaps beside the point, but even the different aim of explaining the cognitive processes and conceptual structures that define the contents and contexts – in short, the meanings – of emotions in antiquity seems to require a kind of access that scholars of historical societies cannot possess. This means they must find alternative ways of reconstructing the ancient 'emotosphere' (to use Nick Herbert's handy coinage)[7] from different kinds of representational evidence: lexical data (vocabularies), literary narratives, expert (above all philosophical) definitions, and visual images.

Classical scholars have taken several different approaches.[8] Probably the most widespread approach is the philological one, which combines linguistic analysis with close reading of word usage in context, often in reference to the explicit definitions or characterizations of emotions that can be found in contemporary philosophical or other technical writers. Though in practice this approach takes a variety of forms and probably cannot be described as a single coherent methodology, studies can be classified under two general rubrics. In the more terminological type, analysis takes its impetus from an emotional category of English – say, *anger*, *fear*, or *jealousy* – and attempts to ascertain how the lexical resources of Greek or Latin map onto the situation of this language of reference. The thrust of this kind of broadly structuralist analysis can be onomasiological – asking what term or terms Greek or Latin speakers used in referring to the emotion in question, and what distinctions of meaning may be covered by these terms – or semasiological – asking what exact emotional experience may be captured by a given word or cluster of words.[9] In the more literary approach, focus is on how representations of a given emotion are constructed and deployed in particular genres or by particular authors. Such

6 Konstan (2003) 6.
7 Herbert (2004).
8 For a good introduction, see Cairns and Nelis (2017).
9 Good examples of this method are Fantham (1986) and Harris (2003).

studies interrogate the programmatic or thematic work that emotions do in imaginative contexts rather than try to characterize lived affective experiences.

I pass over the literary approach, which tends to concern itself with more narrowly local than broadly cultural characterizations of emotions. As others have pinpointed the shortcomings of terminological approaches, it is enough to highlight certain challenges of this methodology that arise from defining ancient emotion terms in relation to the categories of another language.[10] The problem is not in using modern categories as an initial heuristic – this may be productive and in fact necessary – but in treating equivalencies so established between concepts as definitional. This can amount merely to a kind of semantic 'flattening', when the meanings of ancient words are viewed as basically constrained by those of English lexemes – as when investigation of, for instance, *fastidium* is consumed in distinguishing different contextual senses of this word between 'disgust', 'dislike', or 'aversion', as if these constituted the limits of its possible value.[11] But remaining within an 'etic' frame of reference runs the risk of viewing one set of categories as objectively true (especially when these categories have been determined through scientific study) and thus of judging one society's conceptual resources by the standards of another. Defining native categories always in terms of 'our' (or 'science's') categories can introduce the bias of treating difference in and of itself as a kind of inadequacy.[12] Besides being ethnocentric, mapping native terminology to the semantic structures of another language can lead to hasty assumptions about the significance of concepts to a culture, if the salience of a category is taken to be directly proportional to the specificity and ramification of the semantic field relating to it.

(This can lead to situations akin to the famous case of Eskimo 'snow.' In one early paper, Whorf had claimed that the Inuit language, unlike English which must make due with just *snow*, possesses many terms that characterize subtle distinctions in the quality and circumstances of snowfall.[13] According to Whorf, Inuit speakers have no general concept of snow, but only highly specialized concepts – corresponding to things like 'heavy wet snow', 'light fluffy snow', 'snow mixed with rain', and so on – reflected in the language's ramified lexicon. This led to Whorf's conclusion that the robustness of Inuit speakers' available vocabulary of snow corresponds directly to their culture's extraordinary

10 In particular, see the critique in Sanders (2014).

11 Bettini and Short (2018) 8–10 discuss this problematic in general; Kaster (2005) 6–9, in relation to emotion terms. See also Hubscher-Davidson (2018).

12 This point is made by Enfield (1998).

13 Whorf (1940).

concern about snow. But further study revealed that the Inuit snow lexicon is hardly larger than English's, casting doubt on this kind of correlation).[14]

Often the terminological method amounts to definition by a kind of 'semantic triangulation', where the meaning of term is established through a process of approximation from neighbouring terms with the same field.[15] It may appear possible to determine the meaning of Latin *tristitia*, for instance, by distinguishing it from *dolor*, on the one hand, as an internal feeling of sorrow, and *luctus*, on the other, as its artificial external manifestation through socially-prescribed customs of mourning.[16] Within this system, *tristitia* can then be defined as the involuntary outward expression of sorrow, whose meaning thus covers the variety of contextual senses the word appears to have, ranging from 'sadness' understood in the broadest terms, over 'grief' due to bereavement, to simply 'melancholy' – and even to 'sternness' or 'severity' (through a kind of metonymical extension). The catalogue of glosses in this way substantiates and affirms the established general definition. However, whilst this methodology might be appropriate for constructing a translation dictionary (where the aim is to provide ready-to-hand approximate glosses for terms), for ethnographic description it appears inadequate. Rather than establishing what *tristitia* means to a Latin speaker, a definition for English speakers has been given. The value of the emotion concept within its proper linguistic and cultural context remains fuzzy ('the meaning of *tristitia* is somewhere between sadness, grief, melancholy …') By the same token, 'etic' definitions can be overly precise. When Cicero speaks of *aegritudo animi* he may be struggling to express a concept his language had no suitable word for, but this formulation cannot simply be explained as a Latin equivalent of 'depressive melancholy.'[17]

Focusing on explicit vocabularies may actually lead to overlooking categories that may be highly salient culturally but only marginally lexicalized. For instance, Latin has no straightforward way of expressing what in English would be called *jealousy*: the intense feeling of begrudging directed at someone who competes for, or already has won, the love or favour of another we would like to possess exclusively for ourselves.[18] Though *aemulus* (*aemula*) can be used in the sense of a 'rival' for the affection of a lover (cf. Ov., *Ars* 2.436, *si nulla subest aemula, languet amor*), *aemulatio* normally refers to positive feelings of competitive striving. *Invidia* is closer to something like self-righteous

14 For a debunking of the myth of Inuit's plethora of 'snow' terms, see Martin (1986).
15 For the idea of 'semantic triangulation', see Spinks (2016) 107–11.
16 Cf. the analysis of Bartlett (1996) 123–50.
17 I am referring to the conclusions of Toohey (2004) 46–48.
18 Cf. Baumgart (1990) 106–9; Grzywacz (1937).

contempt. *Zelotypia* is borrowed from Greek (in its earliest uses, it appears still unlatinized). Cicero's *rivalitas* captures the concept metaphorically: it derives from *rivus* and thus means, literally, the state of sharing (and fighting over) the same 'stream.' Does this mean that Latin speakers had no native concept of a lover's jealousy? Obviously not. Latin literature provides ample evidence of this concept from the earliest period. One thinks immediately of Lysidamus and his jealous wife in Plautus's *Casina* or of Daedalis in *Captivi*. Horace famously invoked this sentiment in his consolation to Tibullus – *Albi, ne doleas plus nimio memor / inmitis Glycerae neu miserabilis / decantes eleos, cur tibi iunior / laesa praeniteat fide*, 'Do not overly fret, Albius, remembering cruel Glycera, nor sing piteous elegies why a younger man outshines you now that faith has been broken!' (*Od.*, 1.33.1–4) – and much of Latin elegy is taken up in thematizing this concept.[19]

While philological approaches have delivered import insights into ancient emotional experience, a window has been left open for new methodologies that go beyond the circle of language, as it were, to try to encompass more than just the words that people use in characterizing these experiences. Recently, two approaches drawing on developments in the cognitive sciences have emerged within Classical Studies, moving away from more literary and lexicon-based approaches and towards a more 'holistic' perspective. 'Holistic' in this case is polyvalent: it characterizes not only an overall intellectual attitude, which seeks to incorporate insights from different scholarly traditions, but also a specific theoretical orientation, which views meaning as an emergent property of human beings' conceptualizing faculties and sense-making capacities as well as of cultural embeddedness – which may include world knowledge and, to a greater or lesser degree, bodily understanding – rather than as residing 'in' words themselves.

The first is inspired by the research programme of Anna Wierzbicka and Cliff Goddard, who have argued that most of the content of human cultural systems can be described in terms of 'scripts' – mental representations that define the normative 'recipe' of thoughts, attitudes and behaviours making up a concept – expressed through a 'natural semantic metalanguage' that consists of a small number of universally valid conceptual primitives. The second is aligned with the contemporary theory of metaphor in cognitive linguistics, which has been developed above all by George Lakoff and Mark Johnson.[20] This theory proposes that abstract concepts of all kinds derive, at a very basic level

19 On jealousy in Latin elegy, see Caston (2012).
20 Lakoff and Johnson (1980); Lakoff (1987); Johnson (1987); see also Kövecses (2005) and (2006).

of cognitive organization, from gestalt experiential structures ('image schemas') through metaphorical extension.[21] In being closely tied to the psychological theories of their underlying models (Ulrich Neisser's constructivism, or Jean Piaget's and Jerome Bruner's interactionism), these approaches, more than trying to define the meanings of words in the vocabulary of Greek or Latin *per se*, instead aim at characterizing the structure and content of the mental categories trafficked in by Greek and Latin speakers, and that therefore underpin language use and can account for the range of senses typically exhibited by words.

Although both belong to what can be referred to as the 'cognitive science of the emotions',[22] the Wierzbickian script-based and Lakovian metaphor-based approaches to the emotions come from quite different traditions within the cognitive interdiscipline and presuppose quite different views of cognition. In adapting concepts from early artificial intelligence research and cognitive psychology (in particular Shank and Abelson's 'script theory' of memory encoding), Wierzbicka's approach falls squarely within the theoretical and conceptual framework of the so-called 'first wave' of cognitive sciences, which treat the mind and the body as wholly distinct and separable and view cognition largely in information-processing terms.[23] Indeed, on the classical Cartesian theory of cognition, human thought consists in the syntactical manipulation of implementation-independent abstract symbol systems that mentally 're-present' the structures of an objectively existing physical world to the mind. In this view, that is, the mind receives input from a world that is structurally predetermined, translates this input into a language-like symbolic code that it can manipulate in algorithmic ways, and then issues commands to the body to execute in the environment as a function of the input.[24] In this computational-representational view of cognition, mental processes (e.g., reasoning, decision-making, and problem solving) 'just happen' to be realized by the human brain and 'just happen' to take place in the human body. Just as easily, thought – as an abstract symbol system – could be implemented by some other computational-representational 'hardware' having nothing to do with our bodily nature (for instance, as a mechanical or digital computer).[25] This information-processing model of cognition can be illustrated as in Figure 3.1:

21 See esp. Gibbs and Colston (1995); Feldman (2006). On the close relationship between Gestalt and cognitive linguistics, see Thumiger in Chapter 1 above, 37–8.

22 Oatley and Johnson-Laird (2014); cf. also Maiese (2010).

23 See esp. Rowlands (2010); Boden (2008); and Gallagher (2005).

24 As in Fodorian 'Mentalese': Fodor (1975).

25 Neumann (1958) is a classical statement of the position.

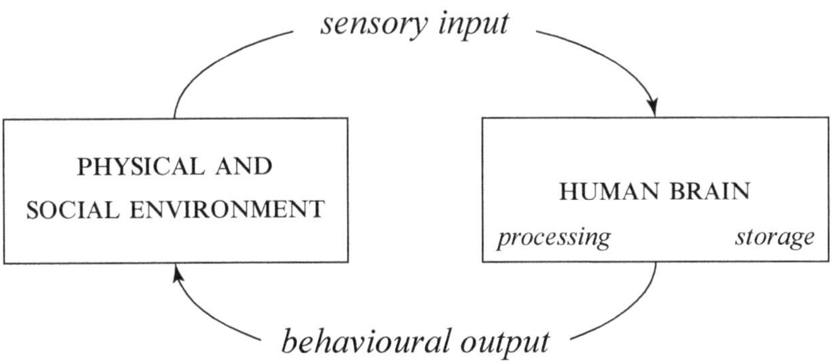

FIGURE 3.1 Information processing model of cognition

In Wierzbicka's approach, definitions of emotion concepts thus consist in descriptions of the algorithm-like mental structures which the speakers of a language utilize (unconsciously) as a basis for their interpretation of feelings and upon which they model their emotions and their relations with other people. As Wierzbicka (1992b, 552) explains: 'A definition of the kind proposed … embodies a hypothesis about a language-specific psychological script, unconsciously used by speakers of a given language in interpreting their own and other people's emotional experience.' Scripts are intersubjectively shared and define what people normally expect to think, feel, and say in respect to a given experience. They are stated in what Goddard and Wierzbicka call a 'natural semantic metalanguage', which provides a lexicon consisting of perhaps several dozen supposedly human-universal semantic primitives.[26] To be explanatory of emotion concepts, this vocabulary is limited to words which are, as Wierzbicka asserts, 'intuitively understandable' (that is, not belonging to the jargon of psychology or other expert disciplines, but to conventional, everyday language) and which are not themselves names of specific emotions.[27] The metalanguage thus includes generic terms like 'feel' and a set of basic non-emotion concepts, such as 'want', 'say', 'think', 'know', 'good', 'bad', and so on, which are claimed to be plausible candidates for irreducible and cross-linguistically valid conceptual building blocks. Scripts follow a standard lexico-grammatical frame and possess a basic grammar and rules of combination.

For example, the English emotion concept *surprise* is defined by Wierzbicka in terms of the following short script:

26 See esp. Goddard and Wierzbicka (1994).
27 Wierzbicka (1992b) 541.

SURPRISE
X feels something
sometimes a person thinks something like this:
something happened now
I didn't think before now: this will happen
if I thought about this I would have said: this will not happen
because of this, this person feels something
X feels like this

that sets out a sort of prototypical scenario of what someone experiences when *surprise*'d. According to the script, *surprise* is defined above all by the cognitive process of recognizing some event and becoming aware that this event was not part of one's prior expectations of what would happen, along with the affective response that this recognition brings about in a person. Thus, the script specifies an input (perception of an event, the 'trigger situation'), a series of mental states typically induced by this input (recognition, introspection, reflection), and an output, which consists in the occurrence of the feeling state labelled *surprise*. The key element for definitional purposes is the series of specific mental states a person passes through along the way to becoming surprised: that is, which unconscious thoughts precede, and directly cause, *surprise*.[28]

Because the metalanguage used in the definition of scripts is built up out of supposedly universal semantic primitives (established through cross-linguistic analysis), the more 'holistic' claim can be made, therefore, that scripts provide an objective framework for comparing concepts between cultures.[29] Differences between cultures in respect to the understanding of the 'same' concept can be identified, and explained, where their scripts for this concept diverge. For instance, the Malay concept of *terkejut* differs from English *surprise* insofar as its script entails a kind of mental paralysis resulting directly from the recognition of an unexpected event. Whereas in *surprise* the outcome is merely a certain affective experience ('because of this, this person feels something'), with *terkejut* there is the added consequence that 'this person couldn't think about anything' – which accounts for its more negative evaluation by Malay speakers. The script for Latin (*ad*)*miratio* – probably this language's closest equivalent to the 'surprise' concept, which is expressed through a metonymy from visual perception, as in *mirari* and *inopinari*, or through spatial

28 In this sense, scripts are similar to Fillmorean frames; however, scripts are unitary algorithmic mental structures, whereas frames may incorporate representations of all kinds, in addition to behavioural 'recipes': Fillmore (1982); Barsalou (1992); Barsalou and Hale (1993).

29 Goddard (2004); Wierzbicka (1994).

metaphor, as in *superoccupo* and *obrepo* – might differ again. As this concept is often associated with the combined feeling of astonishment and pleasure that accompanies perception of the sublime (especially relating to divinity), it would probably have an instead strongly positive evaluative dimension, or at any rate need to recognize this concept's entanglement with religion.[30]

As an illustration of the script-based approach, consider Robert Kaster's analysis of Latin *invidia*. Even if he does not always present scripts in the same schematic form as Wierzbicka and prefers to define emotion concepts in terms of stereotyped 'scenarios', the method is largely the same. Kaster distinguishes two types of *invidia*, which differ on the basis of whether someone's judgement about the pain they feel in contemplating another's good occurs in reference to some principle of what is 'right.' The first type of *invidia* – comparable to the Greek concept *nemesis* – is defined as 'the pain I feel from contemplating someone else's good, which is either rightfully someone else's, or affronts some general societal principle.'[31] The second type of *invidia* – comparable to Greek *phthonos* – is instead a feeling of pain 'just because you have some good, or because it is specifically *your* good.' We can therefore characterize *invidia* as embodying two different scripts:

INVIDIA 1
X feels something
sometimes a person thinks something like this:
I feel bad
I feel this way because person Y has something good
I know that the good belongs rightfully to person Z
because of this, this person feels something
X feels like this

INVIDIA 2
X feels something
sometimes a person thinks something like this:
I feel bad
I feel this way because I have something good
The good is mine
I do not want person Y to have the good
because of this, this person feels something
X feels like this

30 York (1993).
31 Kaster (2005) 87.

Making a distinction along these lines points up an obvious problem in casually translating *invidia* by English *envy*, as *envy* does not appear to cover the pain someone feels when another enjoys a good in defiance of accepted societal principles (which might be captured better by *righteous indignation*). In this sense, as Kaster concludes, Latin *invidia* and English *envy* are only partially overlapping categories whose scripts may reveal interesting cultural differences in conceptualization.

The Lakovian metaphor-based approach belongs, by contrast, to the 'second wave' cognitive sciences, which views the character of human cognition, and the structure of human conceptual systems, as inextricable from human bodily nature. 'Embodiment' is the principle that thought and language are in fact fundamentally dependent on the nature of the human brain and grounded in character of human bodily interaction with the social and physical environment.[32] Instead of viewing meanings as defined by 'necessary and sufficient conditions' expressed in purely symbolic (propositional, language-like) formats that are entirely independent of any sensory modality, as in traditional philosophical and linguistic semantics, an embodied semantics emphasizes how human categorization and conceptualization are deeply constrained by the way we encounter the world, and thus that the natural dimensions of concepts are given by properties defined by our sensory and motor capacities and embedded situational (ad-hoc) motives and purposes.[33] In particular, the theory of conceptual metaphor proposes that many (or indeed most) abstract elements of our conceptual system are delivered metaphorically by concepts from more readily comprehensible physical and spatial domains.[34] That is, abstract concepts – including our emotion concepts – are embodied to the degree that they piggyback, via metaphorical mappings, on more concrete spatio-physical concepts that emerge from our bodily interaction with the world, and make sense to us by virtue of their grounding in sensorimotor experiences that are directly meaningful.

Consider, for example, that in many languages the emotion called *anger* in English is conceptualized as HEATED FLUID IN A CONTAINER. In English, this conceptualization is captured in scores of idiomatic phrases such as *blow one's stack*, *lip one's lid*, and *let off steam*, where the notion of emotional intensity is mapped to that of the liquid's temperature, and anger's effects on the body to the pressurization of the liquid. Indeed, as Zoltán Kövecsecs argues, this metaphor delivers English's perhaps most conventionalized and most structurally

---

32 Barrett (2011); Clark (1999).

33 Cf. Barsalou (1983); Fillmore (1985); Lakoff (1987); Johnson (1987).

34 Lakoff (1993) and (1987); Johnson (1987); Lakoff and Johnson (1980).

articulated conceptualization of anger, providing a model for understanding – through various images associated with the heating of fluid in a pressurized container – not only anger's direct effects on the body but also its causes, its effects, and the potential outcomes for the angry person and those around him or her if anger is not somehow dealt with.[35] Andrew Riggsby has shown that a version of this metaphor also appears in Latin, as indicated by expressions such as:[36]

1) *iracundaque mens facile efferuescit in ira / … nec capere irarum fluctus in pectore possunt*, 'An irascible mind easily bubbles over in anger … nor can they contain the waves of anger in their chest' (Lucr., *RN*. 3.295, 298);
2) *exarsit iracundia ac stomacho*, 'He blazed forth in anger and irritation' (Cic., *Ver*. 2.2.48);
3) *talibus Allecto dictis exarsit in iras*, 'At such words Allecto blazed forth into anger' (Verg., *Aen*. 7.445);
4) *mortis fraternae feruidus ira*, 'Seething with anger at his brother's death' (Verg., *Aen*. 9.736);
5) *Quinctius quidem adeo exarsit ira*, 'Quinctius so blazed forth in anger …' (Liv., *AUC* 35.31.13);
6) *ignes ipse suos nutrit*, 'He (sc. Tereus) fuels the fires of his passion' (Ov., *Met*. 6.491–2);
7) *ardet et iram / non capit … / … exaestuat ira*, 'She (sc. Procne) burns and cannot contain her anger … boils over with anger' (610–11, 623);
8) *ira se profert et in faciem exit, quantoque maior, hoc efferuescit manifestius*, 'Anger brings itself forth and exits onto the face, and the greater it is, the more obviously it bubbles forth' (Sen., *De ira*. 1.1.5);
9) *rabida uocis eruptio colla distendet … impetus, rupturus se nisi eruperit!*, 'A furious eruption of sound distends the neck … a pressure that would burst itself unless it found an outburst' (2.35.3–5);
10) *aquariolus … ita ira extumuit, ita exarsit furore*, 'The philanderer … so swelled up with anger, so blazed forth in rage …' (Apul., *Apol*. 78).

It is the fact that such mappings involve the transfer of an organized system of knowledge from concrete physical experience (namely, how fluids behave in heated, pressurized conditions) to abstract emotional experience (namely, anger) that allows English and Latin speakers to think, and thus talk, coherently about an aspect of human life that may be difficult to comprehend in and of itself. Moreover, talking about anger in metaphorical terms of hot fluid is immediately meaningful to speakers of these languages, since the metaphor

35 Kövecses (1995).
36 Riggsby (2015).

is grounded in the apparently universal human experience of feeling hot and pressurized when angry.[37]

As another example, take Latin speakers' conceptualization of FEAR as captured by Latin *horror*. The etymology of this word from *horreo* 'stand erect; bristle' indicates this conceptualization centrally includes the idea of hair standing on end. As suggested by expressions like *mihi frigidus horror / membra quatit*, 'Cold fear shakes my limbs' (Verg., *Aen.* 3.29–30), *mihi gelidus horror ac tremor somnum excutit*, 'Cold fear and shaking knocks the sleep out of me' (Sen., *Tro.* 457) and *me luridus occupat horror*, 'Pale fear overwhelms me' (Ov., *Met.* 14.198), fear is additionally conceived by Latin speakers as cold, shivering, and paleness. *Horror* is also something that 'seizes' (*percapere*), 'strikes' (*excutere*), or 'penetrates' (*pervadere*) the body. These images are not simply fancy ways of talking about FEAR, however, nor are they selected at random. Instead, they are (part of) Latin speakers' absolutely regular and ordinary vocabulary of fear. Moreover, the metaphor itself constitutes the understanding that Latin speakers have of fear: for speakers of Latin, fear is – not simply 'is like' – cold, shivering, and paleness.[38] What again makes sense of these metaphors is their grounding in concrete physical experience: very specifically, the autonomic bodily responses – especially sharp fluctuations in body temperature, along with perspiration, shivering or shuddering, pallor, and piloerection – that characterize, and systematically correlate to, the lived experience of fear in human beings universally.

Even such a rapid sketch of the theoretical underpinnings of these two approaches will allow us to make a distinction between them from an anthropological perspective. I believe their theoretical commitments bear directly on their suitability to the study of ancient culture. I have already distinguished the Wierzbickian approach from the Lakovian approach on the basis of its adherence to a view of cognition rooted in Cartesian dualism. Given this volume's rooting in traditions of 'holism' – where the mind-body debate has been a central concern[39] – my critique of Wierzbicka's approach in terms of its commitment to this dualism was not incidental. Rather, this approach's rootedness in a view of the mind as basically separate from the body has important

37 Experimental studies have shown that the occurrence of anger coincides with objectively measurable increases in skin temperature and blood pressure: e.g., Ekman et al. (1983); Levenson et al. (1990); Levenson et al. (1991). In this way, (part of) the physiology of anger itself affords a ready metaphorical image for conceptualizing such experiences in the abstract.

38 Cairns (2013) suggests exactly this grounding for Greek's metaphors of fear in terms of 'shuddering.'

39 See the Introduction above (5–7), as well as Singer (156–73) in this volume.

ramifications for its anthropological usefulness, and, within this book's perspective, would appear to diminish its overall utility for studying the emotions – though scripts themselves have been offered as a more 'holistic' alternative to philology. In fact, in defining emotion concepts in terms of scripts formulated in a metalanguage whose elements – no matter how much they have been verified as candidates for universal semantic primitives – ultimately corresponds to English concepts, the Wierzbickian approach exhibits two major challenges from this point of view.

Very much like the semantic elements that play such a constitutive role in the componential feature analysis of the New Ethnography – elements like [MAN], [WOMAN], [CHILD], [YOUNG], [OLD], and so on that are used to build up the semantic profiles of words – Wierzbickian semantic primitives can only appear to be culture-neutral, when in fact they must presuppose a worldview: that of English speakers.[40] It may seem self-evident that every culture would have the basic categories that make up the building blocks of componential analysis (or a Wierzbickian emotion script). After all, everywhere there are men and women and children who are young or old – and indeed that the words of their languages could be analysed in these terms. Translation is largely possible between languages because they share some degree of conceptual compatibility. But we cannot take this for granted. Even a cursory examination of the ethnographic literature (Margaret Mead's studies of the Manus people of Melanesia, for instance) reveals that cultures may possess a very different understanding of what constitutes 'young' and 'old' or not possess simple binary descriptors like this.[41] In fact, the Manus have a social structure that is highly stratified generationally, so that belonging to a particular age-set is the determinant social category rather than some appurtenance to general category of 'the young' or 'the elderly.' Moreover, if recent anthropology has taught us anything, that is that even concepts so seemingly basic and natural as [MALE] and [FEMALE] attain their meanings within *cultural* contexts (as Judith Butler has emphasized for the ostensibly universal categories of sex).[42]

Though claimed to refer to universal, objective properties of human conceptual systems, Wierzbicka's 'primitives' thus correspond already to culturally embedded concepts. In this sense, the analysis of emotion scripts appears to pursue emic descriptions through a set of allegedly etic categories that are in fact emic categories! Umpteenth example of the imposition of the analyst's own set of conceptual categories on the subject of anthropological investigation.

---

40 See esp. Schneider (1965).
41 Cf. Arnett (2016); Eisenstadt (2013); Benedict (1937).
42 Butler (2004).

Only in this case the '-centrism' may be especially pernicious, because in the script-based approach the description of culture-specific categories occurs through atomic semantic components claimed to have universal validity, but whose human-level grounding has not been established (and probably cannot be, as the method always proceeds through language).[43]

Equally problematic is the question of the mental status of emotion scripts. The claim is that emotion scripts provide speakers of a given language with a template or recipe for thinking and behaving that is 'unconsciously used ... in interpreting their own and other people's emotional experience.'[44] Such scripts are therefore meant to *actually exist* and exist as such in people's minds (just as the 'scripts' written by artificial intelligence researchers for robots or computers do). But even if we accept that emotion scripts are descriptively adequate for understanding emotional experience, what mental status do we attribute to them in the human mind? How could their existence ever be proven? It hardly needs to be said that probably no one of us experiences emotions as a sequence of discrete feelings and metacognitions in some reproducible and easily expressible propositional format. Indeed, recent research suggests that we interpret others' emotions not by referring lived experiences to some stereotyped mental template (represented mentally in whatever format), but through a kind of affective 'simulation.'[45] From this point of view, emotion scripts seem to be the ultimate in etic constructs.

By contrast, a metaphorical approach along cognitive linguistic lines enables us to develop robust emic analyses sensitive to how concepts are understood 'in the native's own terms.' By illustrating how human-universal structures and processes of conceptualization (i.e., body-based metaphor) give rise to idiosyncratic systems of understanding, conceptual metaphor theory, in my view, provides exactly the sort of language-independent, 'etic' framework of analysis that can enable an 'emic' accounting of ancient conceptual systems, especially when combined with a culturally-comparative perspective, since this helps highlight how different constellations of metaphors may converge on the 'same' concepts in different languages. Comparing Latin's metaphors with those from other languages reveals that metaphorical conceptualization is in fact highly variable across cultures. Though they may share certain experience-based conceptualizations, different languages, through their metaphors, highlight and emphasize different aspects of experience. Such differences stand out most

43 The 'non-validity' argument has been set out most forcefully by Cattelain (1995) and Riemer (2006).

44 Wierzbicka (1992b) 552.

45 Damasio (2003); Levi (2008); Weinrich (2014).

especially in what cognitive linguists refer to as the 'range of the target': that is, the narrower or wider set of source domains that the speakers of a language utilize in conveying a given concept. Very often, through juxtaposition it is possible to discern the main conceptual foci of different metaphor systems – what dimension of a concept a system's metaphors are largely aimed at defining – and these foci can be seen to characterize cultural themes.

Take Latin's metaphorical construal of ANGER again. Evidence suggests that in addition to the 'HOT FLUID' metaphor it shares with English (and many other languages besides), Latin possesses several other metaphorical ways of expressing anger.[46] For instance, to become angry is, literally, to 'fall into anger' (*in iram incidere*) or to 'turn towards madness' (*in rabiem vertere*) or to 'arrive at madness' (*in insaniam pervenire*). In these expressions, anger is represented both in terms of another psychological experience – insanity – and in terms of spatial movement: namely, as a location to which the angry person 'goes.' Anger can also be construed metaphorically as a kind of rigid, brittle structure that one 'breaks' or 'beats down', as in formulations like *odium iramque frequentissime frangat*, 'Often it (sc. laughter) dispels hatred and anger' or *iram contundit* (Mart. Cap. 6.2). Or anger can be construed a kind of wild animal needing to be tamed, as in Quintilian's *lenire iram* (*IO*. 3.8.12). Or anger can be construed in terms drawn from the stadium, as a kind of chariot, as in Juvenal's *pone irae frena* (8.88) and Lucan's *frenos furentibus ira laxat* (7.125). In this metaphor, the speed of the chariot corresponds to the degree of anger a person feels. Another frequent metaphor depicts anger as a bodily fluid that is 'vomited out' onto someone, as in Terence's *ego iram hanc in eos evomem omnem* (*Ad.* 3.4). The extension of *stomachor*'s literal reference (it has to do with the stomach, *stomachus*) to have the meaning of 'anger' very likely depends on the same image. In the Vulgate, anger is represented also in terms of sharpness (*acuit iram*: Sap. 5: 21).

The set of Latin metaphors can be compared with the range of metaphors in English, illustrated by Figure 3.2.[47]

This illustration shows that whilst certain metaphors grounded in human-universal bodily experiences may be shared between Latin and English, English also makes available to its speakers several metaphors that are mostly, or entirely, lacking in Latin. Three in particular stand out: the 'NATURAL FORCE', 'FUNCTIONING MACHINE', and 'SOCIAL SUPERIOR' metaphors. What can account for this difference? Obviously, the specific images of English's 'MACHINE' metaphor, in which the angry person is construed as a mechanical or electronic

46 Cf. the catalogue of anger metaphors in Harris (2009) 68–69.

47 Cf. Constantinou (2014).

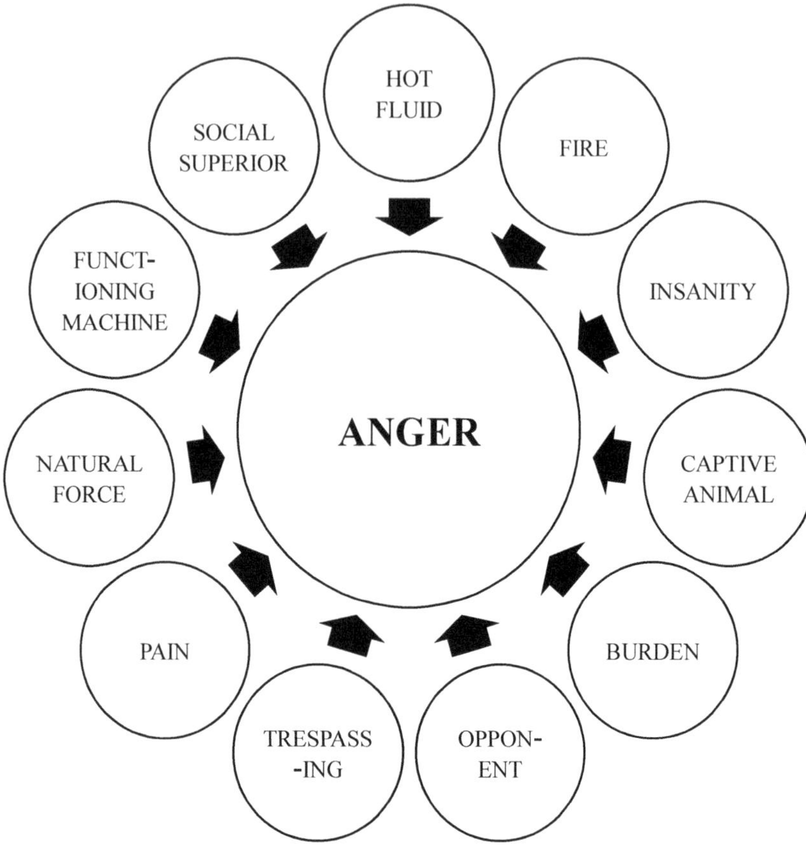

FIGURE 3.2 Metaphors of anger in English

device (as in *He went off like an alarm, He's really geared up, His pistons were pumping*) derive from technologies unknown to ancient societies, and so its absence from Latin may be a matter of historical contingency.[48] Yet an historical explanation is not necessarily the only one. Even if alarms and engines could not have afforded imagery to metaphorical conceptualization, nevertheless Latin speakers might have relied on technological metaphor in this instance, as they did in others: e.g., in their use of the tracing arm the drafting compass (*centrum*) as a metaphor for any central position, or of the carpenter's square (*norma*) as a metaphor for any 'rule' or 'precept.' Furthermore, the absence of any 'NATURAL FORCE' metaphor for anger from Latin – represented in English by expressions like *a stormy meeting* – cannot be explained on historical grounds. Its absence is all the more surprising as Latin speakers did not

48 For examples and discussion, see Kövecses (1987).

hesitate, contrariwise, to utilize personifying metaphors to characterize natural forces like the weather (as, e.g., when Vergil describes a storm as 'suddenly raging with anger': *tempestas sine mora furit*, *Aen.* 5.694). Similarly, although something like English's 'SOCIAL SUPERIOR' metaphor[49] appears to have suggested itself to Latin speakers in relation to other abstract psychological concepts, such images are not normally applied to anger.

The different make-up of Latin's and English's respective metaphor systems vis-à-vis ANGER can probably instead be related to broader cultural patterns of conceptualization. What emerges most immediately from the imagery of the English metaphors is a view of anger as imposed on someone from the outside and against their will.[50] This is certainly entailed by the NATURAL FORCE and SOCIAL SUPERIOR metaphors: in both cases, anger is understood as something that originates externally to a person and whose power a person is helpless to resist. At the same time, the MACHINE metaphor implies that an angry person's feelings (and behaviours) occur mechanistically – as it were, in automated, pre-programmed ways – and which thus cannot be avoided. Overall, the view of anger engendered by these images is that an angry person is not in control.[51] By contrast, Latin's privileging of a spatial metaphorics and especially of images of 'HOT FLUID' in conceptualizing anger imparts an ontology to this concept that emphasizes the internal origins of anger, and a directionality of affect that moves from the angry person outward towards the world. (By 'ontology' I mean that the metaphor delivers the structure and content of understanding: in being mapped to the conceptualization of anger, images of 'HOT FLUID' directly constitute an inferential pattern that Latin speakers rely on in thinking and reasoning about this dimension of experience). Even if Latin's anger-as-a-wild-animal metaphor is similar to the English metaphor in engendering a view of anger as a dangerous outside force working on a person, it is hardly common and may in fact derive from the image of the angry person as a bull in Greek literature from Aeschylus onward.[52]

In this respect, consider as well the network of metaphors of converging on Latin speakers' conceptualization of FEAR, as expressed by *metus*, *pavor*, *timor*, *formido* and so on. Evidence indicates that FEAR was not only construed metaphorically in terms of the body's autonomic responses (cold, shaking, horripilation). It could be conceived also as a kind of slowness, as in Plautine *timore torpeo* ('I am sluggish in fear': *Truc.* 824), or as a kind of muteness or silence, as

49 Kövecses (2005).
50 Cf. Soriano (2003).
51 Carmelo Pérez Rull (2002).
52 Cf. Anderson (2014) 325.

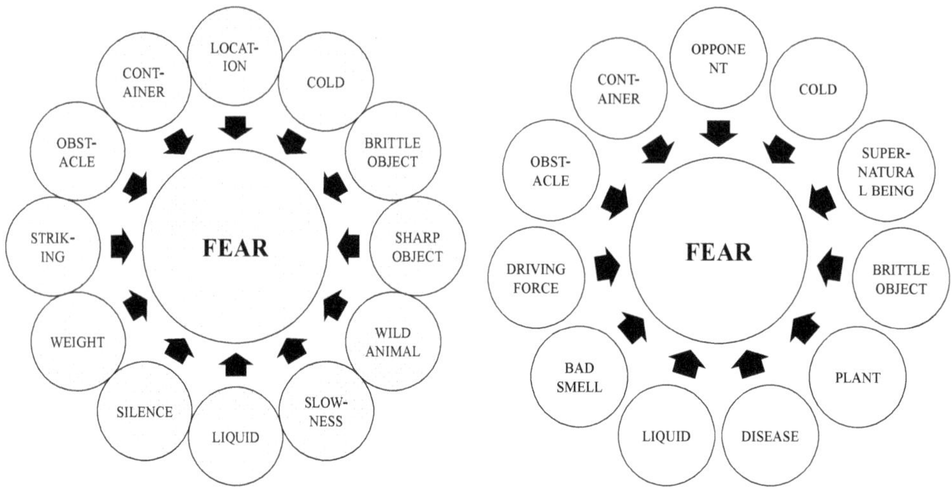

FIGURE 3.3 Systems of metaphors of fear in Latin and English

in Terence's *animus timore obstipuit*, 'the spirit became mute with fear' (*Ad.* 612) or even as a kind of weapon that strikes someone, as in Livy's *alicui pavorem incutere* (*AUC* 27.42). *Metus* is very often conceived metaphorically as a weight or burden on someone, as illustrated by expressions like *metum alicui adimere* (Ter., *Heaut.* 2.3.100), *metu exonerare* (Liv., *AUC* 2.2), *removere metum* and *metum levare alicui* (Cic., *TD* 2.59). In other words, the system of metaphor that characterizes FEAR in Latin can be illustrated as in Figure 3.3, where it is also juxtaposed to the corresponding system of metaphors in English.

Again, certain overlaps in conceptualization are noticeable. For instance, the two languages share, the 'OBSTACLE' and 'CONTAINER' metaphors (whose highly schematic imagery suggest they operate at a very low level of conceptualization) as well as the more imagistically rich 'BRITTLE OBJECT' metaphor (cf. Cic., *Off.* 1.68, *frangi metu* with expressions like *crumble in fear*). They also share the 'COLD' metaphor, as we might expect from its clear physiological grounding. But the two systems demonstrate telling divergences, as well. English possesses several metaphors that Latin does not: e.g., the 'OPPONENT', 'SEED', 'DISEASE', and 'BAD SMELL' metaphors.[53] Meanwhile, Latin has several metaphors – such as the 'SLOWNESS', 'SILENCE', and 'WEIGHT' metaphors – which do not appear to be present in English (or are very attenuated in this language). What is striking about these divergences is that they are again patterned in terms of their 'main meaning focus.' English's metaphors again imply

53 Details in Kövecses (2003) 23–24.

that fear has external causality. In each image, FEAR is something that originates externally to the person and either acts upon them from outside (OPPONENT, BAD SMELL) or enters from outside, as it were (DISEASE, SEED). By contrast, Latin's metaphors once more largely ontologize FEAR as something 'inside' a person, or at any rate *not* originating from outside. It is not that this image is absent from Latin (the 'WILD ANIMAL' and 'STRIKING' metaphors clearly construe FEAR as coming from *outside* a person and – what's more – hostilely), but the point is that the major portion of Latin's metaphorization of FEAR focuses, through its specific imagery, on an entirely different aspect of this experience than English's metaphors.

I believe that what can be anthropologically revealing about this kind of analysis is the way that specific inferential structures may emerge across different systems of metaphorical conceptualization. What I mean is that internally to Latin's system of metaphors of FEAR, the cluster of images constellating around this concept consistently entail the notion that fear is something 'inside' affecting the experiencer that is directed outward (differently from English, where fear tends to be metaphorized as something affecting the experiencer from 'outside', directed inward). This entailment shared by the different metaphorical images constituting the concept of FEAR characterizes an overall ontology of emotional experience. As it happens, this ontology turns out to be recapitulated by the images of Latin's ANGER metaphors – not only by the 'HOT FLUID' metaphor, which imagines anger as a fluid inside the angry person's body, but also in the 'VOMITING', 'INSANITY', and 'BRITTLENESS' metaphors, which again entail an 'inwardness' of emotion. The whole cluster of metaphors of ANGER in Latin, that is, portrays a picture of emotion as again somehow 'in' the experiencer, just as its metaphors of FEAR do. By contrast, across English's systems of metaphor for these concepts, the inferential structure is that FEAR and ANGER are things that come from 'outside', again characterizing a (different) overall ontology of emotional experience.

When a consistent entailment pattern emerges not only from *within* a particular metaphor system, but also from *across* several metaphor systems all within a single domain, it stands to reason that this patterning corresponds to the conceptualization of the domain (in this case, emotion) as a whole. Whereas the metaphorical imagery capturing emotion concepts in English tends to emphasize the *external* origin of affective experience, the images that Latin speakers rely on in understanding emotion concepts as a category instead emphasize its *internal* origin. Of course, it is well known that in ancient (especially Stoic) philosophy a common theory of the emotions construed affective experience in expressly 'motional' terms, so that the emotions were understood as what Margaret Graver called 'affective movements' (especially 'outpourings').[54] In this theory, emotions are represented explicitly as originating internally to the person and moving outward. (Hence the use in classical Latin of the verb *emoveo* to express the effects of emotions – as in Seneca's *mens emota* (*Polyb.* 37.5), and, at a later period, of *emotio* as a covering term for this domain). But the same theory manifests itself implicitly also in the metaphors that constituted Latin speakers' conventionalized ways of speaking about emotion. In this sense, whilst the notion of 'affective movement' may belong to the context of expert philosophical theorizing, it also appears to underpin a 'folk' understanding of the emotions in Roman culture as well.

I have argued that the different theoretical commitments of the Wierzbickian script-based approach and the Lakovian metaphor-based approach afford different opportunities for studying the emotions of ancient cultures. As I see it, the Lakovian approach affords a more productive means of studying ancient emotions emically. It also permits a more 'holistic' perspective to be taken on the ancient emotions, in at least two senses. The Wierzbickian approach views concepts as algorithm-like cognitive procedures correlating environmental stimuli to mental states. The scripts a culture provides to its members operate almost as mathematical functions: They take a certain input (the perception of some conditions in the environment) and generate a certain output (a feeling). The body is thus largely written out of the equation, leaving the emotions as colourless and idealized. The Lakovian approach views emotion categories, like all categories, as constituted through systems of conceptual mappings from more concrete (and so more readily comprehensible) domains of experience, which jointly deliver the logic of metaphorically defined concepts. Rather than viewing the body as simply a platform for implementing the output of a wholly independent cognitive system, the metaphor-based approach thus treats it as integral to conceptualization. Besides acknowledging the fully both bodily and mental nature of emotional understanding, this can also allow us to view culture as a whole. By showing that understanding in both 'expert' theoretical and everyday 'folk' contexts is scaffolded on a common core of metaphors, this approach presents culture as a unified system of signs, meanings, and texts.

The metaphorical approach to ancient emotion concepts thus presents itself as particularly relevant to the 'holism' conceived, in several senses, by this volume. More than the philological method – which tends to reduce emotional experience to the choice between some different vocabulary items – and even the script-based Wierzbickian framework – which reduces affectivity to a flat input-output symbolic processing loop – a Lakovian approach permits

54 Graver (2008) 30.

the characterization of emotions at different levels simultaneously. Indeed, it avoids the chief pitfall of a Wierzbickian semantics, of defining situated concepts in terms of 'primitives' masquerading as universal but always already culturally embedded. This is possible because, in cognitive linguistics, metaphors are said to be grounded directly in experience. In this theory, metaphorical mappings are not arbitrary and unconstrained, but experientially motivated, typically by their grounding in systematic correlations in phenomenal experience. In particular, concepts are defined 'image schematically', that is, in terms of gestalt skeletal cognitive structures that emerge directly from sensorimotor experience. Therefore, their metaphorical projections provide a solution to the problem of how linguistic expressions and other symbols acquire their meanings, since in this view all concepts (literal as well as metaphorically derived ones) are grounded, at some level, in structures of cognition that emerge from bodily experiences that are directly meaningful to human beings. Unlike the semantic primitives of Wierbickian scripts, which are themselves purely symbolic, the grounding structures of metaphors are experiential 'primitives' with cross-cultural validity, because they arise from basic human sensorimotor interactions with the world.

It is in this sense, at least, that I take the metaphor-based approach to be holistic: namely, that human conceptualization, and thus the inferential processes guiding semantic extension, depends in large part on cognitive structures – i.e., images schemas – that arise naturalistically from (indeed are analogues of) recurring perceptual and kinaesthetic experiences. Through unidirectional mappings of image schematic structure to domains not directly grounded in experience, literal (physico-spatial and bodily) understanding comes to be extended to abstract reasoning, including of the emotions. Because they emerge from, or are grounded in, repeated human bodily experiences (physical sensations, movements, and so on), image schemas – unlike the Fodorian representations (amodal abstract symbols) of Wierzbickian scripts – are thus directly meaningful representational structures. At the same time, because they are cognitive structures which capture and organize patterns in our experience, image schemas are inherently multimodal. The 'holism' of an embodied metaphorical approach therefore pertains to the fact that abstract (figurative) *as well as* concrete (literal) understanding is based on at least partial activations of the same sensorimotor areas of the brain, and that culture-specific forms of understanding are scaffolded metaphorically on aspects of human-universal experience.

The character of the embodied-cognitive approach to the emotions I have been advocating thus appears of a piece with the kind(s) of 'holism' discussed in the other chapters of this book. Even as this approach is 'holistic' in the sense of its being simultaneously both universalist and relativist, it is also holistic in the sense that at its heart is exactly the sort of challenge to the mind-body dualism that inflected certain aspects of ancient philosophical thinking.[55] Unlike the Wierzbickian approach – where emotion concepts apparently operate as symbolic functions that translate some propositional input ('a person thinks something like this') into some sort of emotional representation as output ('because of this, a person feels …'), the body being entirely written out – the image schemas which underpin embodied metaphorical understanding are in the first and last instance structures of bodily experience. Between sensorimotor cognition and emotional cognition there is no representational transduction: in the form of image schemas, the same patterns of neural excitement that deliver literal (perceptual and motor) understanding are recruited to deliver abstract (emotional) understanding, via figurative projection. Furthermore, image schemas are cognitive structures with fundamentally gestalt properties, whose 'sum is greater than their parts' – so that bodily experience emerges not as a patchwork of disjointed sensorimotor processes but as a coherent and unified source of imagery for conceptualization.

Bibliography

Anderson, W. *Essays on Roman Satire*. Princeton: Princeton University Press (2014).

Arnett, J. J. 'Life Stage Concepts Across History and Cultures.' *Human Development*, 59 (2016) 290–316.

Barrett, L. *Beyond the Brain: How the Body and the Environment Shape Cognition*. Princeton: Princeton University Press (2011).

Barrett, L. F. *How Emotions are Made: The Secret Life of the Brain*. Boston: Houghton Mifflin Harcourt (2017).

Barsalou, L. 'Frames, Concepts, and Conceptual Fields.' In *Frames, Fields, and Contrasts: New Essays in Semantic and Lexical Organization*, ed. A. Lehrer and E. F. Kittay. New York: Routledge (1992) 21–74.

Barsalou, L., and C. Hale. 'Components of Conceptual Representation.' In *Categories and Concepts*, ed. I. Van Mechelen, J. Hapton, R. Michalski, and P. Theuns. San Diego: Academic Press (1993) 97–144.

Bartlett, G. *Translations and Translation Principles in the Old English and Old High German Versions of Boethius's De Consolatione Philosophiae*. PhD dissertation, University of Minnesota (1996).

55 Cf. esp. Coughlin in this volume and Leith in this volume.

Baumgart, H. *Jealousy: Experiences and Solutions*. Chicago: University of Chicago Press (1990).

Benedict, R. *Patterns of Culture*. Boston: Houghton Mifflin (1937).

Bettini, M., and W. M. Short. 'Introduction.' In *The World through Roman Eyes*, ed. M. Bettini and W. M. Short. Cambridge: Cambridge University Press (2018) 11–17.

Boden, M. *Mind as Machine: A History of Cognitive Science*. Oxford: Oxford University Press (2008).

Butler, J. *Undoing Gender*. New York: Routledge (2004).

Cairns, D. 'Look both Ways: Studying Emotion in Ancient Greek.' *Critical Quarterly*, 50.4 (2008) 43–62.

Cairns, D. 'A Short History of Shudders.' In *Unveiling Emotions II—Emotions in Greece and Rome: Texts, Images, Material Culture*, ed. A. Chaniotis and P. Ducrey. Stuttgart: Franz Steiner (2013) 85–107.

Cairns, D., and D. Nelis (eds.). *Emotions in the Classical World: Methods, Approaches, and Directions*. Wiesbaden: Steiner (2017).

Carmelo Pérez Rull, J. 'The emotional control metaphors.' *Journal of English Studies*, 3 (2002) 179–92.

Caston, R. *The Elegiac Passion: Jealousy in Roman Love Elegy*. Oxford: Oxford University Press (2012).

Cattelain, E. J. 'Must a Universal Semantic Metalanguage be Composed of Primitives?' *Pragmatics and Cognition*, 3.1 (1995) 159–79.

Clark, A. 'An Embodied Cognitive Science?' *Trends in Cognitive Science*, 3 (1999) 345–51.

Constantinou, M. 'Conceptual Metaphors of Anger in Popularized Scientific Texts.' In *Linguistic Approaches to Emotion in Context*, ed. F. Baider and G. Cislaru. Amsterdam: John Benjamins (2014) 159–88.

Damasio, A. *Looking for Spinoza: Joy, Sorrow, and the Feeling Brain*. Boston: Houghton Mifflin Harcourt (2003).

Eisenstadt, S. *From Generation to Generation: Age Groups and Social Structure*. New York: Routledge (2013).

Ekman, P., R. Levenson and W. Friesen. 'Autonomic Nervous System Activity Distinguishes among Emotions.' *Science*, 221 (1983) 1209–10.

Enfield, N. *Linguacentrism in Culture and Thought*. Essen: LAUD (1998).

Fantham, E. 'ΖΗΛΟΤΥΠΙΑ: a Brief Excursion into Sex, Violence, and Literary History.' *Phoenix*, 36 (1986) 45–57.

Feldman, J. *From Molecule to Metaphor: A Neural Theory of Language*. Cambridge MA: MIT Press (2006).

Fillmore, C. J. 'Frame Semantics.' In *Linguistics in the Morning Calm, Selected Papers from the Seoul International Conference on Linguistics*. Hanshin: Linguistic Society of Korea (1982) 111–37.

Fodor, J. A. *The Language of Thought*. Cambridge MA: Harvard University Press (1975).

Gallagher, S. *How the Body Shapes the Mind*. Oxford: Oxford University Press (2005).

Gallese, V. 'Finding the Body in the Brain.' In *Goldman and His Critics*, ed. B. McLaughlin and H. Kornblith. New York: Blackwell (2016) 297–317.

Gibbs, R., and H. Colston. 'The Cognitive Psychological Reality of Image Schemas and Their Transformations.' *Cognitive Linguistics*, 6 (1995) 347–78.

Goddard, C. *Cross-Linguistic Semantics*. Amsterdam: John Benjamins (2004).

Goody, J. 'The Anthropology of the Senses and Sensations.' *La Ricerca Folklorica*, 45 (2002) 17–28.

Graver, M. *Stoicism and Emotion*. Chicago: University of Chicago Press (2008).

Griffiths, P. *What Emotions Really Are: The Problem of Psychological Categories*. Chicago: University of Chicago Press (1997).

Grzywacz, M. *'Eifersucht' in den romanischen Sprachen*. Bochum-Langendreer: H. Pöppinghaus (1937).

Harré, R. *The Social Construction of Emotions*. Oxford: Blackwell (1986).

Harris, W. 'The Rage of Women.' In *Ancient Anger: Perspectives from Homer to Galen*, ed. S. Braund and G. Most. Cambridge: Cambridge University Press (2003) 122–43.

Harris, W. *Restraining Rage: The Ideology of Anger Control in Classical Antiquity*. Cambridge MA: Harvard University Press (2009).

Herbert, N. *Elemental Mind*. New York: Plume (2004).

Hubscher-Davidson, S. *Translation and Emotion*. New York: Routledge (2018).

Johnson, M. *The Body in Mind*. Chicago: University of Chicago Press (1987).

Kaster, R. *Emotion, Restraint, and Community in Ancient Rome*. Oxford: Oxford University Press (2005).

Konstan, D. 'Translating Ancient Emotions.' *Acta Classica*, 46 (2003) 5–19.

Kövecses, Z. 'Anger: Its language, Conceptualization, and Physiology in the Light of Cross-Cultural Evidence.' In *Language and the Cognitive Construal of the World*, ed. R. MacLaury and J. Taylor. Berlin: De Gruyter (1995) 181–96.

Kövecses, Z. *Metaphor and Emotion*. Cambridge: Cambridge University Press (2003).

Kövecses, Z. *Metaphor in Culture: Universality and Variation*. Cambridge: Cambridge University Press (2005).

Kövecses, Z. *Language, Mind and Culture*. Oxford: Oxford University Press (2006).

Kövecses, Z., V. Szelid, N. Eszter, O. Blanco, E. Akkök and R. Szabó. 'Anger Metaphors across Languages: A Cognitive Linguistic Perspective.' In *Bilingual Figurative Language Processing*, ed. R. Heredia and A. Cieślicka. Cambridge: Cambridge University Press (2015) 341–67.

Lakoff, G. *Women, Fire and Dangerous Things: What Categories Reveal about the Mind*. Chicago: University of Chicago Press (1987).

Lakoff, G. 'The Contemporary Theory of Metaphor.' In *Metaphor and Thought*, ed. A. Ortony. Cambridge: Cambridge University Press (1993) 202–51.

Lakoff, G., and M. Johnson. *Metaphors We Live By*. Chicago: University of Chicago Press (1980).

Levenson, R. 'Blood, Sweat, and Fears.' *Annals of the New York Academy of Science*, 1000 (2003) 348–66.

Levenson, R., Ekman, P. and W. Friesen. 'Voluntary Facial Action Generates Emotion-Specific Autonomic Nervous System Activity.' *Psychophysiology*, 27 (1990) 363–84.

Levi, S. 'Affective Simulation, Imitation, and the Motor Mirror System.' *International Postgraduate Journal of Philosophy*, 1 (2008) 1–11.

Maiese, M. *Embodiment, Emotion, and Cognition*. New York: Springer (2010).

Martin, L. 'Eskimo Words for Snow.' *American Anthropologist* 88.2 (1986) 418–23.

Mesquita, B., and N. Frijda. 'Cultural Variations in Emotions: A Review.' *Psychological Bulletin*, 112.2 (1992) 179–204.

Oatley, K., and P. Johnson-Laird. 'Cognitive Approaches to Emotions.' *Trends in Cognitive Sciences*, 18.3 (2014) 134–40.

Ogarkova, A., P. Borgeaud and K. Scherer. 'Language and Culture in Emotion Research.' *Social Science Information*, 48.3 (2009) 339–57.

Riemer, N. 'Reductive Paraphrase and Meaning: A critique of Wierzbickian Semantics.' *Linguistics and Philosophy*, 29.3 (2006) 347–79.

Riggsby, A. 'Tyrants, Fire, and Dangerous Things.' In *Roman Reflections: Studies in Latin Philosophy*, ed. G. Williams and K. Volk. Oxford: Oxford University Press (2015) 111–28.

Rowlands, M. *The New Science of the Mind: From Extended Mind to Embodied Phenomenology*. Cambridge MA: MIT Press (2010).

Sanders, E. *Envy and Jealousy in Classical Athens*. Oxford: Oxford University Press (2014).

Scherer, K. R., and P. Ekman (eds.) *Approaches to Emotion*. Hillsdale NJ: Erlbaum (1984).

Schneider, D. 'American Kin Terms and Terms for Kinsmen: A Critique of Goodenough's Componential Analysis.' *American Anthropologist*, 67.5 (1965) 288–308.

Soriano, C. 'Some Anger Metaphors in Spanish and English. A Contrastive Review.' *International Journal of English Studies*, 3.2 (2003) 107–22.

Spinks, C. W. *Semiosis, Marginal Signs and Trickster: A Dagger of the Mind*. New York: Springer (2016).

Toohey, P. *Melancholy, Love and Time: Boundaries of the Self in Ancient Literature*. Ann Arbor: University of Michigan Press (2004).

Von Neumann, J. *The Computer and the Brain*. New Haven: Yale University Press (1958).

Whorf, B. L. 'Science and Linguistics.' *Technology Review*, 42.6 (1940) 229–31, 247–48.

Wierzbicka, A. *Semantics, Culture and Cognition: Universal Human Concepts in Culture-Specific Configurations*. Oxford: Oxford University Press (1992a).

Wierzbicka, A. 'Defining Emotion Concepts.' *Cognitive Science*, 16 (1992b) 539–81.

Wierzbicka, A. 'Cultural Scripts.' In *Language Contact and Language Conflict*, ed. M. Pütz. Amsterdam: John Benjamins (1994) 69–86.
Wierzbicka, A. *Semantics: Primes and universals*. Oxford: Oxford University Press (1996).
Wierzbicka, A. *Emotions Across Languages and Cultures: Diversity and Universals*. Cambridge: Cambridge University Press (1999).
Wierzbicka, A. 'Language and Cultural Scripts.' In *The Routledge Handbook of Language and Culture*, ed. F. Sharifian. New York: Routledge (2015) 339–56.
Wierzbicka, A., and C. Goddard (eds.) *Semantic and Lexical Universals – Theory and Empirical Findings*. Amsterdam: John Benjamins (1994).
Wierzbicka, A., and J. Harkins (eds.) *Emotions in Crosslinguistic Perspective*. Berlin: De Gruyter (2001).
York, M. 'Toward an Indo-European Vocabulary of the Sacred.' *Word*, 44.2 (1993) 235–54.

PART 2

Is Graeco-Roman Medicine Holistic?

CHAPTER 4

Hippocratic Holisms

Hynek Bartoš

Abstract

The aim of this essay is to identify three different pre-Platonic forms of holism: the 'therapeutic', the 'environmental', and the 'cosmic.' With the help of passages from the Hippocratic *On the Nature of Man*, *On Regimen*, and *On Sevens*, on the one hand, and from Plato, the earliest independent authority on the holistic nature of Hippocratic medicine, on the other, I make the case that all three forms of holism play significant roles in dietetic medicine, that they are complementary, and that aspects of them can even be combined into a single account.

Hippocratic medicine has been characterized as 'holistic' since antiquity. As early as Plato, a contemporary of Hippocrates and most of the Hippocratic authors, we find mention of this specific feature of Hippocrates' method. In a discussion in the *Phaedrus* about the best possible way in which one can acquire the art of rhetoric, Socrates suggests that the 'method of medicine is in a way the same as the method of rhetoric.' 'In both cases', he explains, 'we need to determine the nature of something – of the body in medicine, of the soul in rhetoric.' To Socrates' question as to whether it is possible to reach a serious understanding of the nature of the soul 'without understanding the nature of the whole (*tou holou*)' (*Phaedr.* 270c1–2), his interlocutor Phaedrus replies: 'if we're to listen to Hippocrates, Asclepius' descendant, we won't even understand the body if we don't follow that method' (270c3–5).

This passage has been 'the source of bitter dispute among scholars' since Galen's time,[1] especially with regard to two relatively independent questions that each have distinct consequences for readers of Plato and Hippocrates: (1) what, specifically, does 'the whole' mean in the passage; and (2) which Hippocratic text (or texts), if any, served as Plato's source. As for the first question, which is of special importance for understanding Plato's own account, at least four different readings of the 'whole' (*holon*) have been suggested.

1 Jouanna (1999) 59.

It can stand for (a) the whole soul (composed of three parts);[2] (b) the whole of the human body,[3] or the totality consisting of body and soul taken together;[4] (c) the whole environment,[5] including such things as seasonal cycles, winds, and other meteorological phenomena that immediately influence the condition of human body; or, finally, (d) the cosmic whole,[6] i.e. the whole world and its component parts.[7]

The second inquiry has played an important role in discussions of the so-called 'Hippocratic question.' For if one were to succeed in identifying a corresponding passage in an extant Hippocratic text, this would provide a strong argument in support of Hippocrates' authorship of that particular text. No less than four strong candidates have been advanced as Plato's source. First, Galen claimed to see in this passage a reference to the Hippocratic *On the Nature of Man*.[8] Second, É. Littré believed he had definitively demonstrated that Plato alluded to the Hippocratic *On Ancient Medicine*.[9] Third, and more recently, W. Smith has vehemently argued that *On Regimen* served as Plato's source.[10] And finally, J. Mansfeld suggests that this role was most likely played by *Airs, Waters, Places*.[11]

Despite all these suggestions, neither of our questions has received a satisfactory and conclusive answer. Nevertheless, the discussion about sources has not been unproductive and has had some important consequences for our understanding of the various meanings of holism in the pre-Platonic medical

2 Hackforth (1952), de Vries (1969), Jouanna (1977), Rowe (1986), Yunis (2011).

3 Hermias, *in Plat. Phaedr. Scholia*, 245, 5 (Couvreur).

4 Verdenius (1982).

5 Gill (2003), Ferrari (1987), (1980), Korobili and Stefou (in this volume, p. 208 n. 20).

6 Galen *HNH* I.48 (XV.105 K. = 55.14–16 Mewaldt), Littré (1839), Kucharski (1939), Joly (1961), Brisson (1989), Thivel (1991), Brisson (1992), Brown (2003).

7 It is also possible that Plato is purposefully ambiguous in the passage. Smith (1979, rev. 2002, 48) assumes that Plato intentionally left 'the whole' ambiguous because both 'man as a whole' and 'cosmos' are comprehended in Hippocratic science. Thein (2012, 139–40) suggests that the 'whole' at 270c2 may be intended by Socrates to be the totality that consists of a body and a soul taken together, whereas Phaedrus (inspired by certain Hippocratic teachings and remarking that even the body demands a holistic approach) would take it for the totality of the universe.

8 Galen, *HNH*, prooem. (XV.4–5 K. = 4.19–5.9 Mewaldt).

9 Littré (1839) 295–320.

10 Smith (1979) 44–60, rejected by Mansfeld (1980) and Lloyd (1991), reiterated in Smith (1999). For similar views, see also Hutchinson (1988) 23, Cooksey (2010) 46, van der Eijk (2004) 188.

11 Mansfeld (1980), see also Vegetti (1965, 44–46), who considers both *On Ancient Medicine* and *Airs, Waters, Places* to be the Hippocratic theory reflected by Plato.

tradition. It is no accident that the four works identified as the most likely candidates for Plato's source all belong to a relatively small group of medical texts that discuss the methodological foundations of dietetic medicine, an innovative medical approach to health that had an enormous impact on the philosophical discussions of the day.[12] The aim of the present paper is to show that the variety of interpretations of the *Phaedrus* passage that have been suggested reflect the variety of holistic approaches attested in the Hippocratic works that promote dietetic medicine. In the course of this essay, I distinguish three different forms of holism (I call them 'therapeutic', 'environmental', and 'cosmic')[13] and demonstrate that they are all interrelated, complementary, and can even be brought together and combined into a single account.

As for my sources, both *Airs, Waters, Places* and *On Ancient Medicine* attest some characteristic features of the therapeutic and environmental approaches that are typical of dietetic medicine in general. However, neither text employs the term *holon* for the whole of the human body or for the whole world.[14] Accordingly, I shall focus instead on the remaining two texts, *On Regimen* and *On the Nature of Man* (including *On Regimen in Health*),[15] both of which are explicit in their terminology as well as being representative of the dietetic

12 For example, both Plato (*Symp.* 188a4–5) and Aristotle (e.g. *Ph.* 246b4–6) define health in terms of *krasis*, i.e. they both acknowledge and make use of the key theoretical term of dietetic medicine which is attested only in the four treatises mentioned above (i.e. *On the Nature of Man, On Ancient Medicine, On Regimen*, and *Airs, Waters, Places*) and in no other Hippocratic text (with the exception of *Aph.* 5.62, IV.556 L.), which most likely draws on the account in *Vict.* 2.37). See Smith (1992) and Bartoš (forthcoming).

13 In terms of the classification suggested by Singer (in his contribution to this volume, pp. 155 and 176–78), my 'therapeutic' category roughly corresponds to his 'whole-body' holism, and especially to its second variation (b2), while my 'environmental' class overlaps with his 'one-with-the-cosmos' holism. My 'cosmic' version, by contrast, is not considered by Singer, although it is, I believe, a clearly distinct and highly significant version of the holistic approach which should be duly recognized. At the same time, his 'mind-body holism' is not included in my discussion because it is not explicitly attested in any Hippocratic text (cf. Singer, pp. 155–63). As for the suggestion by Craik (in this volume) that ancient Greek medicine is fundamentally 'holistic' in the sense that 'it views the human organism as a complete mental and somatic unity', I am in complete agreement with her conclusion that 'these ideas are not purely medical, but are rooted in Greek language and thought.' Nonetheless, it should be noted that most of her examples from Hippocratic texts are limited to what I call 'therapeutic' holism and what Singer calls 'whole-body' holism, which is also the case for the examples of 'humoralism' discussed by Nutton in this volume.

14 Cf. *VM* 14 (I.604.10 L.), and *Aër.* 23 (II.86.5–6 L.).

15 In agreement with Jouanna (2002), Craik (2015) and other contemporary authorities, I consider *On the Nature of Man* and *On Regimen in Health* to be one continuous account. Hence, for the sake of clarity, when referring to passages in *Nat. Hom.* 16–24 (according

tradition. In addition, given the fact that the 'cosmic' form of holism is very rare in general and is absent from *On the Nature of Man* in particular, I will complement my pair of texts with *On Sevens*, a rarely discussed but philosophically highly significant treatise that contains a remarkably well-elaborated view of the relationship between the human body and higher-level macrocosmic structures.[16]

1 Therapeutic Holism

I start with the suggestion that *holon* in the *Phaedrus* passage refers to the whole of the human body. Before I turn to the Hippocratic evidence, it will be useful to consider a passage from Plato's *Charmides* in which Socrates refers appreciatively to physicians who cure the 'whole body' of their patients:

> You have probably heard this about good doctors, that if you go to them with a pain in the eyes, they are likely to say that they cannot undertake to cure the eyes by themselves, but that it will be necessary to treat the head at the same time if things are also to go well with the eyes. And again it would be very foolish to suppose that one could ever treat the head by itself without treating the whole body (ἄνευ ὅλου τοῦ σώματος). In keeping with this principle, they plan a regime (διαίταις) for the whole body with the idea of treating and curing the part along with the whole (μετὰ τοῦ ὅλου τὸ μέρος).[17]

Socrates refers here to a specific medical method according to which the head (like any other body part) must be treated together with the whole body, a

to Jouanna's edition), I also indicate its equivalent in Littré's edition (*Nat. Hom.* 16–24 = *Salubr.* 1–9).

16 While there is a consensus among scholars that *On the Nature of Man* (including *Salubr.*) and *On Regimen* are pre-Platonic (cf. Jouanna 1999, and Craik 2015), there is less agreement on the dating of *On Sevens*. Earlier commentators and editors of the text suggested dating between the sixth century (Roscher 1913, Lommer 1938) and the first half of the fourth century BCE (West 1971), while Mansfeld (1971) argues for the first century CE and Jouanna (1999, 412–13) suggests that 'the rare passages preserved in Greek do not justify assigning an early date and associating it with the ancient core of the Hippocratic Collection.' Nonetheless, 'there is nothing to rule out a date in the fifth century BCE' (Craik 2015, 128). In any case, in the following discussion I focus only on those topics in *Hebd.* that have a parallel in the other two texts.

17 Plato, *Charmides* 156b3–c5 (trans. R. K. Sprague, modified). For more details on this passage and its context, see Korobili and Stefou (in this volume).

method with which he expects Charmides to be acquainted ('you have probably heard this').[18] The holistic method of the 'good physicians' in this account employs two levels of bodily organization and, accordingly, two different levels of mereological relationship: eyes (parts) with regard to the head (whole), and the head (as a part) together with the body (as a whole). It is noteworthy that the approach of the good physicians is described as therapeutic and that regimen (*diaitai*) is mentioned explicitly.

If we focus on *On Regimen* and *On the Nature of Man*, we can see that both authors take for granted that a healthy condition consists in a balanced mixture of the primary constituents and that this balance can also be described at the level of their qualities, i.e. hot, cold, dry, and wet. On both accounts, an imbalance between the qualities causes pathology (*Nat. Hom.* 2 'In the body there are many constituents, which, by heating, by cooling, by drying or by wetting one another contrary to nature, engender diseases'),[19] and the suggested therapy is in principle allopathic (*Nat. Hom.* 9 'One must know that diseases due to repletion are cured by evacuation, and those due to evacuation are cured by repletion').[20] There are four basic types of repletion/excess (of heat, cold, moisture, and dryness) and four general forms of dietetic treatment, namely warming, cooling, moistening, and drying.

As for the therapeutic means, the authors provide instructions concerning food and drink, various exercises – such as walking, running, wrestling, swinging the arms, and holding the breath – also bathing, emetics and clysters, sexual activities (e.g. *Nat. Hom.* 16–22 = *Salubr.* 1–7; *Vict.* 3.68, 3.73, 3.80, 3.84), and even activities explicitly connected with the soul, such as seeing, hearing, thinking, speaking, and singing (*Vict.* 2.61). All these dietetic procedures, the authors of both texts believe, contribute to the increase or decrease of the hot or cold, dry or moist in the body and can accordingly be used in the preservation or restoration of health by dietetic means.

18 It should be noted that the aim of Socrates is not to convince Charmides to cure his headache together with the whole body (as the quoted part of the passage seems to suggest) but rather to cure his soul together with the body, which is a method that Socrates ascribes a few lines later to a Thracian doctor who suggests that 'it is necessary first and foremost to cure the soul if the parts of the head and the rest of the body are to be healthy' (157a1–3). Neglect of this principle is 'the very reason why most diseases are beyond the Greek doctors' (156e3–6). As far as the evidence of the Hippocratic texts is concerned, this principle is indeed almost absent in the medical literature of the Classical era, although it is relatively common among Greek philosophers of the time (cf. Bartoš 2018 and 2015, 165–229).

19 *Nat. Hom.* 2, VI.36 L. = 168.6–8 Jouanna, trans. Jones.

20 *Nat. Hom.* 9, VI.52 L. = 188.3–6 Jouanna, trans. Jones.

Although the sources of pathological imbalance are occasionally localized to particular organs or bodily parts in these accounts, therapy is applied, as a rule, to the whole body, either internally or externally, or in both ways.[21] For instance, when the author of *On Regimen* notes 'disease in the region of the head', he recommends the sufferer take longer walks in the early morning and after dinner.[22] When he diagnoses fluxes in the head or in the bowels, or tumours growing in the flesh, the suggested therapy is the same: 'In such cases it is beneficial to reduce food by one-third and to take an emetic, to be followed by a gradual increase of food for five days, the normal diet being resumed in another five; another emetic should be followed by the same gradual increase.'[23] When a corruption of the human seed is indicated, and the excess of hot and dry identified as the cause, the author simply suggests that regimen must be directed towards cooling and moistening.[24] When there are indications that blood is arrested by dryness, no matter where the stoppage happens, the author advises that one should 'cool and moisten the body.'[25]

To sum up, there is little room for local therapy or isolated therapy directed at particular organs in the dietetic approach. Treating and curing 'the part along with the whole', as Plato's Socrates puts it, is a necessary condition of dietetic therapy given its specific therapeutic means and corresponding theoretical assumptions.

2 Environmental Holism

To introduce the environmental form of Hippocratic holism – which can also be called 'prognostic', 'meteorological',[26] or 'one-with-the-cosmos'[27] – we should

21 As for possible exceptions to this rule, one can mention, for instance, 'some trouble of the bladder' indicated by springs and cisterns seen in a dream, in the case of which the author recommends a thorough purge with diuretics (*Vict.* 4.90, VI.656 L. = 226.17–18 Joly-Byl). Similarly, when the author indicates a disease of the belly, he advises that the patient should be thoroughly purged with light, soft aperients (*Vict.* 4.90, VI.656 L. = 226.18–19 Joly-Byl). Another exception is found when he prescribes in chap. 32 for individuals of the third constitution that 'their exercise should be directed more to the exterior of the body (πρὸς τὰ ἔξω τοῦ σώματος) than to the inner parts (πρὸς τὰ εἴσω)' (*Vict.* 1.32, VI.508 L. = 148.25–27 Joly-Byl), and to those of the fourth constitution that 'they profit more if their exercise be directed to the internal parts of the body (εἴσω τοῦ σώματος)' (*Vict.* 1.32, VI.508–10 L. = 148.27–34 Joly-Byl).

22 *Vict.* 4.90 (VI.654 L. = 226.5–7 Joly-Byl).

23 *Vict.* 4.89 (VI.650 L. = 224.6–8 Joly-Byl), trans. Jones (modified).

24 *Vict.* 4.90 (VI.654 L. = 226.10–13 Joly-Byl).

25 *Vict.* 4.93 (VI.660 L. = 230.2–3 Joly-Byl).

26 Le Blay (2005) 253.

27 Singer (in this volume) 176–78. See also Thumiger (in the introduction) 6–8.

start with the lowest level, i.e. with the primary constituents of the human body. In Plato's reflection of the medical method in the *Phaedrus*, immediately after the passage quoted above Socrates formulates the recommended methodology as follows:

> First, we must consider whether the object regarding which we intend to become experts and capable of transmitting our expertise is simple or complex. Then, if it is simple, we must investigate its power ... If, on the other hand, it takes many forms, we must enumerate them all and, as we did in the simple case, investigate how each is naturally able to act upon what and how it has a natural disposition to be acted upon by what.[28]

Socrates introduces this formulation as something that 'both Hippocrates and true argument say about nature' and as the right way 'to think systematically about the nature of anything.' Phaedrus replies in agreement that 'proceeding by any other method would be like walking with the blind.'[29]

The authors of *On the Nature of Man* and *On Regimen* both aspire to define the nature of the human body and to identify its constituents (and the relation between them in respect to health). As such, their accounts provide representative illustrations of the use of the method in dietetic texts. I start with a passage from the second chapter of *On Regimen*, identified by Smith and others as the closest parallel to Socrates's formulation.[30] Here the Hippocratic author introduces his own methodology:

> I maintain that he who aspires to treat correctly of human regimen must first acquire knowledge and discernment (γνῶναι καὶ διαγνῶναι) of the nature of man in general – knowledge of its primary parts and discernment of the parts by which (ὑπὸ τίνων μερῶν) it is controlled. For if he be

28 Plato *Phaedr.* 270c10–d7, trans. Nehamas-Woodruff.

29 Plato *Phaedr.* 270c9–e1.

30 Cf. Smith (1979), 48 'This impressive outline of a science of medicine is, I contend, what Plato refers to in the *Phaedrus*. A closer comparison of what Plato says with what Hippocrates says clarifies Plato's reasons for using Hippocrates' work as he does in the context he does. Plato sees a parallel between Hippocrates' gnosis and diagnosis (which mean "know together" and "know separately"; I translated "know and distinguish") and his own collection and division. Hippocrates says that one must know the nature of man as a whole and must know the parts that control him and the *dynamis* of all aspects of the environment that affect man. Plato found this a useful parallel to his thoughts about scientific oratory: distinguish kinds of souls and how each acts or is acted on and classify speeches according to their *dynameis* in relation to particular souls (*Phaedrus* 271a–b). Plato left 'the whole' ambiguous because both "man as a whole" and "cosmos" are comprehended in the Hippocratic science.'

> ignorant of the primary constitution, he will be unable to gain knowledge of their [i.e. the primary parts'] effects; if he be ignorant of the controlling thing in the body, he will not be capable of administering to a patient suitable treatment.[31]

In response to these methodological demands, the author posits in chapter 3 that 'all animals, including man, consist of two parts, different in power but working together in their use, namely of fire and water.' These parts depend on one another ('each by itself suffices neither for itself nor for anything else') and are inseparable. Fire is qualified as the moving agent ('fire can move all things always') and water as the source of nourishment ('water can nourish all things always').[32] Apart from the capacities to move and nourish, each of the elements is further characterized in chapter 4 by the possession of two qualities (fire has the hot and the dry, water the cold and the moist), and while the polarity hot-cold seems to define the opposition between fire and water, the polarity wet-dry refers to communication between the elements ('mutually, too, fire has the moist from water, for in fire there is moisture, and water has the dry from fire, for there is dryness in water also').[33] As for the 'discernment' of the parts by which human nature is controlled, the author makes clear that each element 'in turn masters or is mastered to the greatest maximum or the least minimum possible.'[34] This account of elements thus satisfies the methodological requirements announced in chapter 2 and also provides theoretical support for the author's main therapeutic principle, according to which food (nutriment/water = cold+moist) and exercise (activity/fire = hot+dry) must be kept in balance: 'For food and exercise, while possessing opposite qualities, yet work together to produce health. For it is the nature of exercise to use up material, but of food and drink to make good deficiencies.'[35]

The author of *On the Nature of Man* starts with the announcement that he will not address topics related to human nature 'beyond its relation to medicine' and will not speak about air or fire or water or earth or 'anything else that is not an obvious constituent of man.'[36] 'I for my part will prove that what I declare to be the constituents of man are, according to both convention and nature, always alike the same … I will also bring evidence, and set forth the

31 *Vict.* 1.2 (VI.468 L. = 122.22–27 Joly-Byl), trans. Jones.
32 *Vict.* 1.3 (VI.472 L. = 126.5–10 Joly-Byl), trans. Jones.
33 *Vict.* 1.4 (VI.474 L. = 126.21–22 Joly-Byl), trans. Jones.
34 *Vict.* 1.3 (VI.472 L. = 126.10–11 Joly-Byl), trans. Jones (modified).
35 *Vict.* 1.2 (VI.468–70 L. = 124.6–7 Joly-Byl), trans. Jones.
36 *Nat. Hom.* 1 (VI.32 L. = 165.3–7 Jouanna), trans. Jones.

necessary causes why each constituent grows or decreases in the body.'[37] As for growth, he makes clear that 'generation will not take place if the combination of hot with cold and of dry with moist be not tempered and equal.'[38] The same four qualities also play a crucial role in his humoral theory. In chapter 4, he introduces four humours (bile, black bile, phlegm, and blood) as the constituents of human beings that are responsible for the health of the individual, and argues that they differ not only by sight but also according to touch: 'For they are not equally warm, nor cold, nor dry, nor moist. Since then they are so different from one another in form and in power, they cannot be one, if fire and water are not one.'[39] The assumption that a person 'enjoys the most perfect health when these humours are duly proportioned to one another in respect of compounding, power, and bulk, and when they are perfectly mingled'[40] also presupposes a balanced proportion of the primary qualities.

It should be highlighted that, despite their disagreement on the number and nature of the primary elements of the human body (fire and water, on the one hand, the four bodily humours, on the other), both authors can translate the powers of the elements into the language of the primary qualities (i.e. hot, cold, dry, and wet).[41] In their practical therapeutic instructions, in particular, both authors prefer to speak of the four qualities rather than of their peculiar primary elements.[42]

Apart from the primary elements of the human body and their actual combination in a particular patient's body, both authors enumerate a whole list of other variables that must be taken into consideration in dietetic diagnosis, all of which can be classified according to the same four qualities. In *On the Nature of Man* (chapter 9) the author claims:

37 *Nat. Hom.* 2 (VI.36 L. = 170.1–7 Jouanna), trans. Jones.
38 *Nat. Hom.* 3 (VI.38 L. = 170.11–14 Jouanna), trans. Jones.
39 *Nat. Hom.* 5 (VI.42 L. = 176.7–9 Jouanna), trans. Jones.
40 *Nat. Hom.* 4 (VI.40 L. = 172.15–174.2 Jouanna), trans. Jones.
41 Already Galen (*HNH* 13–14, XV.4–5 K. = 9.19–24 Mewaldt; cf. *Hipp. Elem.* 5.32, I.456–57 K. = 100.19–24 De Lacy) identifies the four qualities as essential to the original doctrine of Hippocrates.
42 It is remarkable that outside the theoretical account of book one, i.e. in the practical dietetic instructions of books 2–4, the author of *On Regimen* does not need to speak about fire and water as the elements of the human body (with the exception in *Vict.* 2.56, VI.566 L. = 178.16–22 Joly-Byl, and VI.570 L. = 180.23–25 Joly-Byl; see Bartoš 2015, 91–99). Nor does the author of *On the Nature of Man* mention the four humours in his dietetic chapter 9 or in his account of regimen in health (chap. 16–24 = *Salubr.* 1–9), although he occasionally mentions phlegm in the body and the bilious body in chap. 20 (= *Salubr.* 5).

> To know the whole matter, the physician must set himself against the established character of disease, of constitutions, of seasons and of ages; he must relax what is tense and make tense what is relaxed … This one should learn and change, and carry out treatment only after examination of the patient's constitution, age, physique, the season of the year and fashion of the disease, sometimes taking away and sometimes adding, as I have already said, and so making changes in drugging or in regimen to suit the several conditions of age, season, physique and disease.[43]

Later on, he summarizes what is involved in fixing regimen. One must, he says, 'pay attention to age, seasons, habit, land, and physique, and … counteract the prevailing heat or cold.' 'For in this way', the author concludes, 'will the best health be enjoyed.'[44] In *On Regimen*, the enumeration in chapter 2 of the various dietetic conditions or variables to which attention must be paid even culminates with a remark on stars and the whole cosmos:

> And it is necessary, as it appears, to discern the power of the various exercises, both natural exercises and artificial, to know which of them tends to increase flesh and which to lessen it; and not only this, but also to proportion exercise to bulk of food, to the constitution of the patient, to the age of the individual, to the season of the year, to the changes of the winds, to the situation of the region in which the patient resides, and to the constitution of the year. A man must observe the risings and settings of stars, that he may know how to watch for change and excess in food, drink, wind, and the whole universe (τοῦ ὅλου κόσμου), from which diseases exist among men.[45]

Seasons of the year are mentioned among the dietetic variables in both Hippocratic accounts. Both authors divide the year into four seasons and presuppose that each season is dominated by one or two qualities (*Vict.* 3.67, *Nat. Hom.* 7). When the author of *On Regimen* advises that one watch for 'the risings and settings of stars', he still speaks about seasonal changes, defined in his account by the stars and constellations ('Winter lasts from the setting of Pleiades to the spring equinox, spring from the equinox to the rising of the Pleiades, summer from the Pleiades to the rising of Arcturus, autumn from Arcturus to

43 *Nat. Hom.* 9 (VI.52 L. = 188.6–190.12 Jouanna), trans. Jones.
44 *Nat. Hom.* 17 = *Salubr.* 2 (VI.76 L. = 208.20 Jouanna).
45 *Vict.* 1.2 (VI.470 L. = 124.8–17 Joly-Byl), trans. Jones (modified).

the setting of the Pleiades').[46] Accordingly, when he summarizes his position that one has to watch for changes 'in the whole universe from which diseases exist among men', he refers to all the various changes in a patient's environment that directly influence his/her body in terms of hot, cold, dry, and wet.

One of the most notable features of the dietetic accounts is that the practices described assume the possibility of making a timely diagnosis of any possible imbalance in the body (caused by predictable external factors) and of taking preventative measures in terms of applying a regime with counterbalancing effects. The account in *Nat. Hom.* 16–24 (= *Salubr.* 1–9) is oriented entirely towards prevention and pays special attention to seasonal changes. For instance, since summer 'is hot and dry, and makes bodies burning and parched', the author recommends counteracting these conditions with a diet that makes the body 'cold and soft.'[47] He also advises that one should prepare for changes ('from spring to summer', 'from summer to winter') by 'opposing opposites.'[48] The author of *On Regimen* spells out his prophylactic concerns with particular precision in the concluding lines of his methodological introduction in chapter 2:

> But I have discovered these things, as well as the forecasting of an illness before the patient falls sick, based upon the direction in which is the excess. For diseases do not arise among men all at once; they gather themselves together gradually before appearing with a sudden spring. So I have discovered the symptoms shown in a patient before health is mastered by disease, and how these are to be replaced by a state of health.[49]

The dietetic approach requires knowledge of the effects of a variety of changes in the environment, and as for regular changes, such as those coming with the turning of the seasons, a dietician is advised to predict them and to apply a counterbalancing regimen before these changes attack. It is advised that one should learn about the nature of these changes (i.e. when they come and what effect they have on the human body), but not necessarily about the whole cosmos or about the nature of the heavenly bodies within it. These preventative environmental concerns are also attested in other Hippocratic accounts of dietetics (most explicitly in *Aër.*).[50] In this context, when the authors speak of

46 *Vict.* 3.68 (VI.594 L. = 194.23–196.2 Joly-Byl), trans. Jones.
47 *Nat. Hom.* 16 = *Salubr.* 1 (VI.72–74 L. = 206.11–16 Jouanna).
48 *Nat. Hom.* 16 = *Salubr.* 1 (VI.74 L. = 206.16–208.7 Jouanna).
49 *Vict.* 1.2 (VI.470 L. = 124.16 Joly-Byl), trans. Jones.
50 Cf. *Aër.* 2 (II.14 L. = 57.2–10 Heiberg), trans. Jones: 'For knowing the changes of the seasons, and the risings and settings of the stars, with the circumstances of each of these

the 'whole universe' (*Vict.* 1.2: τοῦ ὅλου κόσμου) or 'this universe' (*Nat. Hom.* 7: ἐν τῷδε τῷ κόσμῳ),[51] they may well speak about the environment alone, without having any elaborated cosmological models in mind.

3 Cosmic Holism

While the first two kinds of holism are deeply embedded in the principles of dietetic medicine and are, therefore, relatively common in the Hippocratic literature, the third one is rare, attested only in *On Regimen* and *On Sevens*, as far as I know.[52] In this 'cosmic' approach, sometimes also called 'philosophical',[53] analogies are drawn between the human body (and its parts) and the cosmos (and its parts). Despite the fact that, as we shall see shortly, these analogies rarely signify a direct influence of the macrocosmic parts on the relevant parts of the human body, the Hippocratic authors consider them highly relevant to dietetic diagnosis and prognosis.

The author of *On Regimen* employs the analogy between the macrocosm and the microcosm of the human body in two different contexts, namely in the embryological account in book one and in the account of dream diagnosis in

phenomena, he [i.e. a physician] will know beforehand the nature of the year that is coming. Through these considerations and by learning the times beforehand, he will have full knowledge of each particular case, will succeed best in securing health, and will achieve the greatest triumphs in the practice of this art. If it be thought that all this belongs to meteorology, he will find out, on second thought, that the contribution of astronomy to medicine is not a very small one but a very great one indeed. For with the seasons men's diseases, like their digestive organs, suffer change.'

51 *Nat. Hom.* 7 (VI.48–50 L. = 186.1–2 Jouanna), trans. Jones: 'For just as every year participates in every element, the hot, the cold, the dry and the moist – none in fact of these elements would last for a moment without all the things that exist in this universe (ἐν τῷδε τῷ κόσμῳ), but if one were to fail all would, for by reason of the same necessity all things are constructed and nourished by another – even so, if any of these congenital elements were to fail, the man could not live.' Cf. *Vict.* 1.3 (VI.474 L. = 126.16–19 Joly-Byl) for a similar argument.

52 Cf. Mansfeld (1980) 347: 'It is somewhat paradoxical that a consistently cosmological brand of medicine is to be found only in marginal treatises of the *Corpus* such as *Regimen* – and of course also outside the *Corpus*, as in the system of Philistion of Locri, whom Plato to an extent followed in the medical section of his own cosmological treatise, *Timaeus*.' See also Le Blay (2005) 252–53, who ascribes the same approach to the author of *Fleshes*, which begins its account with a brief description of the creation of the cosmos before turning to the formation of man from the very same elements and by means of similar formations. Nevertheless, it should be noted that unlike in *On Regimen* and *On Sevens*, there is nothing explicit about the micro-macrocosmic relations in *Fleshes*.

53 Le Blay (2005) 252–53.

book four. In the former, found towards the end of the embryological account (starting in chapter 6 and culminating in chapter 10), we read a summary of the role of fire in the process of embryogenesis:

> In a word, the fire arranged all things in the body by itself properly, in resemblance with the whole (ἀπομίμησιν τοῦ ὅλου), small things in relation to great things and great things in relation to small things. It made the largest cavity, a store-room for dry water and moist, to give to all and to take from all, having the power of the sea, providing food for creatures suited to it, bringing destruction to those not suited. And around it fire made a concretion of cold and moist water, a passage for cold and warm breath, in resemblance with the earth (ἀπομίμησιν τῆς γῆς), which alters all things that fall into it. Consuming some things and increasing others, it made a dispersion of fine water and of aerial fire, the invisible and the visible, a secretion from the formed substance, in which all things are carried and come to light, each according to its allotted portion. And in this fire made three circuits, extending to each other inwards and outwards: one extending towards the cavities of the moist having the power of the moon; another extending towards the outer circumference, towards the solid enclosure having the power of the stars; the middle circuit extends both inwards and outwards [having the power of the sun].[54]

In this passage, identified by Jouanna as 'the first clear formulation in an entirely preserved Greek text of the micro/macrocosmic theory',[55] the author makes the case that fire forms the organs and other bodily structures in accordance and resemblance with the macrocosmic structures, especially in their shape or function (or both). The expression *apomimēsis* is often mistranslated as 'imitation', in the sense of making a copy of something that pre-exists as a paradigm (i.e. it presupposes an ontological priority of the model over its copy). This rendering works well for other authors, such as Plato, but it is inappropriate in the case of the Hippocratic text, since here *apomimēsis* (as well as *mimēsis* and the verb *mimeomai*) indicates a resemblance, likeness, or analogy, suggesting epistemological priority (i.e. the more obvious part of the analogy illustrates the less evident part, as a rule the macrocosmic process or

54 *Vict.* 1.10 (VI.484–86 L. = 134.5–16 Joly-Byl), trans. Jones (modified). The final words in brackets ('having the power of the sun,' ἡλίου δύναμιν ἔχουσιν) were added by Joly and Byl on the basis of a parallel passage in 4.89 (VI.644 L. = 220.22–23 Joly-Byl). See also Jouanna 1998.

55 Jouanna (1999) 463 n. 69.

structure illustrates some process or structure in the body), but not necessarily an ontological one.[56]

This is also evident in *On Sevens* (chapter 6), in which we read that all animals and plants on the earth 'have a nature similar to the world' (*natura similem habent mundo*) and are made of the same constituents.[57] Like the author of *On Regimen*, who successively mentions in his account water, sea, earth, aerial fire, moon, stars, and the solid enclosure (the sun can also be at least implied in the middle circuit), the author of *On Sevens* enumerates more or less the same items in chapter 6, and indicates for each its place in the macrocosm and specifies its analogue in the human body: (1) the earth (bones and flesh) and moist heat (marrow, brain, and semen); (2) water (the blood in the veins) and sea (the moisture in the intestines); (3) the outer air (breath); (4) the moon (the seat of reason); (5) the sun (the heat in the intestines and veins); (6) stars (the heat under the skin); and (7) the cold coat around the world (skin).[58]

As for the significance for medical practice of this knowledge of the macro-microcosmic analogies, the author of *On Sevens* suggests that it helps one to understand how fevers and acute diseases originate, and how they can be managed and also prevented,[59] although he does not provide any clarification of exactly what this help consists in. A possible clue, I suggest, can be found in the account of dreams that plays a significant role in both Hippocratic accounts. The author of *On Regimen* introduces the topic by saying that 'he who has learnt correctly about the signs that come in sleep will find that they have an important influence upon all things', and that 'whoever knows how to interpret these acts correctly knows a great part of wisdom.'[60] The author of *On Sevens* claims in chapter 40 that 'things seen in dreams' can be of use in diagnosis (mentioned alongside the complexion, the qualities of the tongue, eyes, urine, faeces, voice, and veins, and also the way in which one inhales, as well as other signs),[61] and in chapter 45, in which he gives more details about the diagnostic potential of dream visions, he sums up his position by stating that 'dreams show clearly which diseases are strong (*magna*) and which will come in the future.'[62]

56 Cf. Burkert (1972) 44–45, Bartoš (2014) and (2015) 132–38.

57 *Hebd.* 6 (VIII.637 L.). Cf. *Hebd.* 6 (IX.436 L.).

58 *Hebd.* 6 (VIII.637–38 L.), cf. *Hebd.* 6 (IX.436–37 L.).

59 *Hebd.* 12 (VIII.639 L.), cf. *Hebd.* 12 (IX.439 L.).

60 *Vict.* 4.86 (VI.640 L. = 218.12–13 Joly-Byl).

61 *Hebd.* 40 (VIII.660 L.), cf. *Hebd.* 40 (IX.458 L.).

62 *Hebd.* 45 (VIII.662 L.): *Somnia vero ostendunt morborum manifeste quidem que magna sunt et quae future sunt conturbat enim corpora.* Cf. IX.460 L. *Somnia vero ostendunt morbos manifeste quidem quae magna sunt et quae future sunt.*

Both authors provide almost identical explanations of how dreams can serve in diagnosis, based on the assumption that the soul is awake in sleep and sees everything that happens in the body. The dreaming soul, as the author of *On Regimen* puts it, 'has cognizance of all things – sees what is visible, hears what is audible, walks, touches, feels pain, ponders.'[63] The first key for understanding dreams has to do with whether one repeats in the dream one's daily practice, which indicates health, or whether the dream deviates from one's everyday waking experience, which is interpreted as a sign of pathology. The author of *On Regimen* puts it as follows:

> Such dreams as repeat in the night a man's actions or thoughts in the day-time, representing them as occurring naturally, just as they were done or planned during the day in a normal act – these are good for a man. They signify health, because the soul abides by the purposes of the day, and is overpowered neither by surfeit nor by depletion nor by any attack from without. But when dreams are contrary to the acts of the day, and there occurs about them some struggle or triumph, a disturbance in the body is indicated, a violent struggle meaning a violent mischief, a feeble struggle a less serious mischief. As to whether the act should be averted or not, I do not decide, but I do advise treatment of the body. For a disturbance of the soul has been caused by a secretion arising from some surfeit that has occurred.[64]

The analogy between the human body and the concentric tripartite structure of the universe (introduced in chapter 10) reappears in chapter 89 to provide an interpretive key to a specific sub-group of dream visions in which heavenly bodies appear. 'To see the sun, moon, heavens, and stars clear and bright, each in the proper order, is good,' claims the author, 'as it indicates physical health in all its signs, but this condition must be maintained by adhering to the regimen followed at the time.' But if there is any contrast between the dream and reality, it indicates 'a physical illness: a violent contrast a violent illness, a slighter contrast a lighter illness.' As the author reminds his readers, 'the outer circuit [in the body] belongs to the stars, the middle circuit to the sun, the circuit towards the cavities belongs to the moon',[65] and, therefore, the state of the heavenly bodies (as seen in dreams) also correlates with the condition

63 *Vict.* 4.86 (VI.640 L. = 218.9–11 Joly-Byl), trans. Jones.

64 *Vict.* 4.88 (VI.642–44 L. = 220.1–10 Joly-Byl), trans. Jones. Cf. *Hebd.* 45 (VIII.662 L.).

65 *Vict.* 4.89 (VI.644 L. = 220.18–23 Joly-Byl), trans. Jones (modified) ἄστρων μὲν οὖν ἡ ἔξω περίοδος, ἡλίου δὲ ἡ μέση, σελήνης δὲ ἡ πρὸς τὰ κοῖλα.

of the corresponding bodily parts. Thus heavenly bodies and other macrocosmic phenomena seen in dreams can serve as a clue for the diagnosis of the human body and, occasionally, even for locating pathological processes, on the assumption that we know what bodily part each of the macrocosmic objects and phenomena corresponds to. For instance, when a heavenly body seems to be dark and dull, and to move upwards, it indicates fluxes in the head; when it moves into the sea, it indicates diseases of the bowels; when into the earth, it shows that tumours are growing in the flesh.[66] Nor is it only heavenly bodies that can be interpreted according to this pattern: rivers, for instance, correlate with blood vessels, fruits with human semen, and springs and cisterns with the bladder (*Vict.* 4.90; cf. *Hebd.* 6). On the whole, all the correspondences between macrocosm and the human body are based on the assumption that all things in the body are made in analogy with the cosmos (ἀπομίμησις τοῦ ὅλου, *Vict.* 1.10, VI.484 L. = 134.5–6 Joly-Byl), and that the human body and its parts have a 'similar nature' (*natura similis*, *Hebd.* 6) to the cosmos and its parts. Both are made from the same constituents and, accordingly, they both suffer the same changes (*Hebd.* 12).[67]

In summary, as the accounts of human nature in the Hippocratic texts attest, the holistic method recommended by Socrates in the *Phaedrus* was employed by medical authors with remarkable flexibility. As I have attempted to illustrate here, three forms of holistic approach can be distinguished, along with three possible meanings of the term holistic. First, an account can be holistic in the sense that it treats each and every part together with the whole body ('therapeutic' holism). This approach is common to all proponents of dietetics and relates to the specifics of dietetic procedures that are, as a rule, applied to the whole body. Secondly, the dietetic account can be understood as holistic due to its consideration of the environmental influences on the human body ('environmental' holism). One must 'observe the risings and settings of stars' in order to forecast seasonal changes, which bring with them a potential pathogenic excess of hot, cold, wet, and dry. Being alert to these changes then allows one to proactively apply the opposing regimen, thus maintaining the bodily balance in a healthy state. On this view, the 'whole universe' stands primarily for weather conditions and regular seasonal changes.[68]

---

66 *Vict.* 4.89 (VI. 650 L. = 224.4–6 Joly-Byl). Cf. *Hebd.* 15 (VIII.641 L.; IX.440–41 L.).

67 *Hebd.* 12 (VIII.639 L.) *Cum sit ergo talis ejusmodi mundus ostendam et in egritudinis hec pati totum mundum et aliorrum omnium corpora.* Cf. IX.439 L. *Cum ergo ejusmodi sit mundus, ostendam et in ergitudine haec pati totius mundi et aliorum omnium corporum.*

68 Cf. *Hebd.* 23 (VIII.647 L.).

Finally, the accounts in *On Regimen* and *On Sevens* are holistic in the sense that they explain the structure of the human body as analogous to the structure of the whole cosmos ('cosmic' holism). From this point of view, a specific knowledge of cosmic structures is a necessary condition for (a) a proper understanding of the structure and development of the human body, and (b) a successful interpretation of the relevant dream images, which contributes substantially to the dietetic diagnosis. 'So with this knowledge about the heavenly bodies, precaution must be taken, with change of regimen …', as the author of *On Regimen* (*Vict.* 4.89) concludes. This kind of knowledge does not derive from the physician's knowledge of 'how to watch for change and excess in food, drink, wind, and the whole universe.' Rather, it draws on the soul's intimate knowledge of its own body and on the assumption that this knowledge is encoded in the visions seen in dreams. Accordingly, whoever learns about the structural and functional correspondences between macrocosmic phenomena and the individual parts of the human body can also decipher the particular signs of health and disease in dream visions and make use of them in dietetic therapy as well as prophylaxis.

Acknowledgments

I am grateful to the audience in London who heard an earlier version of this paper for an inspiring discussion of the topic; to Colin G. King, Chiara Thumiger and the anonymous reviewers for their helpful comments on previous drafts of this essay; and to the Czech Science Foundation (project 19-07091S) for its support of my research.

Bibliography

Bartoš, H. 'The Concept of Mimêsis in the Hippocratic De Victu.' *Classical Quarterly*, 64 (2014) 542–57.

Bartoš, H. *Philosophy and Dietetics in the Hippocratic On Regimen: A Delicate Balance of Health*. Leiden: Brill (2015).

Bartoš, H. 'Soul, Perception and Thought in the Hippocratic Corpus.' In *Philosophy of Mind in Antiquity: The History of the Philosophy of Mind, Volume 1*, ed. J. Sisko. London and New York: Routledge (2018) 64–83.

Bartoš, H. 'Aristotle's Biology and Early Medicine.' In *Cambridge Companion to Aristotle's Biology*, ed. S. Connell. Cambridge: Cambridge University Press (forthcoming).

Brisson, L. *Platon. Phèdre*. Paris: GF-Flammarion (1989).

Brisson, L. 'L'unité du Phèdre de Platon. Rhétorique et philosophie dans le Phèdre.' In *Understanding the Phaedrus. Proceedings of the Second Symposium Platonicum*, ed. L. Rosetti. Sankt Augustin: Academia Verlag (1992) 61–76.

Brown, E. 'Knowing the Whole: Comments on Gill, "Plato's Phaedrus and the Method of Hippocrates".' *The Modern Schoolman*, 80 (2003) 315–23.

Burkert, W. *Lore and Science in Early Pythagoreanism*. Cambridge MA and London: Harvard University Press (1972).

Cooksey, T. L. *Plato's 'Symposium': A Reader's Guide*. London and New York: Continuum (2010).

Ferrari, G. R. F. *Listening to the Cicadas: A Study of Plato's Phaedrus*. Cambridge: Cambridge University Press (1987).

Gill, M. L. 'Plato's Phaedrus and the Method of Hippocrates.' *The Modern Schoolman*, 80 (2003) 295–314.

Hackforth, R. *Plato's Phaedrus*. Cambridge: Cambridge University Press (1952).

Hutchinson, D. S. 'Doctrines of the Mean and the Debate Concerning Skills in Fourth-Century Medicine, Rhetoric and Ethics.' *Apeiron*, 21.2 (1988) 17–52.

Joly, R. 'La question hippocratique et le témoignage du *Phèdre*.' *Revue des Études Grecques*, 74 (1961) 69–92.

Jouanna, J. 'La Collection hippocratique et Platon (*Phèdre*, 269c–272a).' *Revue des Études Grecques*, 90 (1977) 15–28.

Jouanna, J. 'L'interprétation des rêves et la théorie micromacrocosmique dans le traité hippocratique *du Régime*: sémiotique et mimésis.' In *Text and Translation*, ed. K.-D. Fischer et al. Leiden: Brill (1998) 161–74.

Jouanna, J. *Hippocrates*. Trans. M. B. DeBevoise. Baltimore: Johns Hopkins University Press (1999).

Jouanna, J. (ed. and trans.) *Hippocrate: La nature de l'homme*. CMG 1.1.3. Berlin: Akademie-Verlag (2002).

Kucharski, P. 'La 'mèthode d'Hippocrate' dans le *Phèdre*.' *Revue des Études Grecques*, 52 (1939) 301–57.

Le Blay, F. 'Microcosm and Macrocosm: the Dual Direction of Analogy in Hippocratic Thought and the Meteorological Tradition.' In *Hippocrates in Context: Papers Read at the XIth International Hippocrates Colloquium, University of Newcastle Upon Tyne 27–31 August 2002*, ed. P. J. van der Eijk. Studies in Ancient Medicine 31. Leiden: Brill (2005) 251–69.

Lloyd, G. E. R. 'The Hippocratic Question.' *Classical Quarterly*, 25 (1975) 171–92.

Lommer, F. 'Hippokrates: Die Siebenzahl.' In *Die Werke des Hippokrates in neuer deutscher Übersetzung* Bd. 20, ed. R. Kapferer. Stuttgart: Hippokrates-Verlag Marquardt & Cie (1938) 83–125.

Mansfeld, J. *The Pseudo-Hippocratic Tract Peri Hebdomadon Chapters 1–11 and Greek Philosophy*, Assen: Van Gorcum & Prakke (1971).

Mansfeld, J. 'Plato and the Method of Hippocrates.' *Greek, Roman and Byzantine Studies*, 21 (1980) 341–62.

Roscher, W. *Die hippokratische Schrift von der Siebenzahl: in ihrer vierfachen Überlieferung*. Paderborn: F. Schöningh (1913).

Rowe, C. J. *Plato: Phaedrus. With translation and Commentary*. Warminster: Aris & Phillips (1986).

Smith, W. D. *The Hippocratic Tradition*. Ithaca NY: Cornell University Press (1979).

Smith, W. D. 'Regimen, κρῆσις, and the History of Dietetics.' In *Tratados Hipocráticos*, ed. J. A. López Férez. Madrid: Universidad Nacional de Educatión a Distancia (1992) 263–71.

Smith, W. D. 'The Genuine Hippocrates and his Theory of Therapy.' In *Aspetti della terapeia nel Corpus Hippocraticum*, ed. I. Garofalo et al. Florence: Olschki (1999) 107–18.

Thein, K. 'A Much Disputed "Whole" at *Phaedrus* 270.' *Croatian Journal of Philosophy*, 12.35 (2012) 139–52.

Thivel, A. 'Hippocrate vu par Platon.' *Diotima*, 19 (1991) 22–28.

van der Eijk, P. J. 'Divination, Prognosis and Prophylaxis: The Hippocratic Work "On Dreams" (De victu 4) and Its Near Eastern Background.' In *Magic and Rationality in Ancient Near Eastern and Graeco-Roman Medicine*, ed. H. F. J. Horstmanshoff et al. Leiden: Brill (2004) 187–218.

de Vries, G. J. *A Commentary on the Phaedrus of Plato*. Amsterdam: Hakkert (1969).

West, M. L. 'The Cosmology of Hippocrates' *De Hebdomadibus.' Classical Quarterly*, 21 (1971) 365–88.

Yunis, H. *Plato. Phaedrus*. Cambridge: Cambridge University Press (2011).

Primary Texts: Editions and Translations Used

Galen. *De elementis ex Hippocratis Sententia* (*Hipp.Elem.*). Ed. P. De Lacy. CMG V.1.2. Berlin: Akademie-Verlag (1996).

Galen. *In Hippocratis De Natura Hominis Commentaria* III. Ed. J. Mewaldt. CMG V.9.1. Leipzig and Berlin: Akademie-Verlag (1914).

Hippocratis De Victu Acutorum Commentaria IV, ed. G. Helmreich. CMG V.9.1. Leipzig and Berlin: Akademie-Verlag (1914).

Hermias Alexandrinus. *In Platonis Phaedrum Scholia*. Ed. P. Couvreur. Paris: E. Bouillon (1901).

Hippocrates. *Oeuvres complètes d'Hippocrate*. Ed. É. Littré. Paris: J. B. Baillière (1839–1861).

Hippocrates. *Airs, Waters, Places* (*Aër.*). Ed. and trans. W. H. S. Jones, in *Hippocrates*. Vol. 1. LCL 147. Cambridge MA: Harvard University Press (1923).

Hippocrates. *De Aere Locis Aquis* (*Aër.*). Ed. L. Heiberg. CMG I 1. Leipzig and Berlin: Akademie-Verlag (1927).

Hippocrate. *La nature de l'homme* (*Nat. Hom.*). Ed. and trans. J. Jouanna. CMG 1.1.3. Berlin: Akademie-Verlag (2002).

Hippocrates. *Nature of Man* (*Nat. Hom.*). Ed. and trans. W. H. S. Jones, in *Hippocrates*. Vol. 4. LCL 150. Cambridge MA: Harvard University Press (1931).

Hippocrate: Du Régime. (*Vict.*). Ed. and trans. R. Joly and S. Byl. CMG 1.2.4. 2nd edn. Berlin: Akademie-Verlag (2003).

Hippocrates. *Regimen.* (Vict.). Ed. and trans. W. H. S. Jones, in *Hippocrates*. Vol. 4. LCL 150. Cambridge MA: Harvard University Press (1931).

Plato. *Charmides*. Trans. R. K. Sprague, in *Plato: Complete Works*, ed. J. M. Cooper. Indianopolis and Cambridge: Hackett (1997).

Plato. *Phaedrus*. Trans. A. Nehamas and P. Woodruff, in *Plato: Complete Works*, ed. J. M. Cooper. Indianopolis and Cambridge: Hackett (1997).

CHAPTER 5

Holism and the Methodists

David Leith

Abstract

As far as the Methodist medical sect is concerned, the question of holism most conspicuously arises in connection with the topic of the affected part (ὁ πεπονθὼς τόπος, *locus affectus*) in disease, which was a variable that the Methodists ignored, or at least downplayed, in contrast to their rivals. Extant Methodist treatises are often found insisting that the whole body suffers in disease, and that it should accordingly be treated as a whole. In this sense, the Methodists can be said to have taken a kind of holistic approach to therapeutics. But their reasoning on the question of the affected part turns out to be nuanced, and their rivals' claims that they ignored the affected part altogether is something of a distortion. In this paper, I attempt to specify exactly what the Methodist position was on the question of the affected part in disease, what sort of holism this represented and how their approach may have developed out of more fundamental commitments. I argue that the application of their 'Method' led to a distinctive and noteworthy position on the issue of holism, one which deliberately encouraged the physician to minimise the significance of *differences* between diseases, including differences in the location of symptoms, and to focus rather on certain features which they share. Analysis of this position reveals some interesting characteristics of their approach to therapy in general, in particular their exploitation of the huge body of earlier therapeutic literature of the Classical and Hellenistic periods which they had inherited.

Ancient doctors who would have been identified as Rationalists or as Empiricists took into account a whole range of variables when deciding upon the correct course of therapy for their patients. Factors such as the time of year, the geographical location, the age, sex, constitution or habits of the patient, and so on, had a considerable impact on their choice of remedies to prescribe.[1] We are told, however, that the Methodist sect rejected all such variables as irrelevant: in their radical attempt to simplify therapeutics, they claimed that

1 See e.g. Gal., *SI* 3 (I.69–72 K.); cf. Cael. Aur., *Tard. Pass.* 3.8.108.

 | DOI:10.1163/9789004443143_007

treatment did not need to vary at all in response to these factors.[2] The question of holism, however, most conspicuously arises in connection with the topic of the affected part (ὁ πεπονθὼς τόπος, *locus affectus*) in disease. This was another variable that the Methodists ignored, or at least downplayed, in contrast to their rivals. In fact, their refusal to take into account the affected part is the first aspect of their doctrine Galen mentions in his critique of Methodism in chapter 6 of his *Sects for Beginners*:

> [1] The so-called Methodists, however, ... seem to me not only to disagree with the ancient sects as to the account of the art but, beyond that, also to change the practice of the art in many respects. They claim that neither the part affected has anything useful to offer towards an indication as to the appropriate treatment, nor the cause, nor the age, nor the season, nor the place, nor the consideration of the strength of the patient, nor his nature, nor his disposition.
>
> GALEN, *De sectis ad eos qui introducuntur* 6 (I.79 K.), trans. FREDE

In apparent confirmation of this, as we shall see below, extant Methodist treatises are often found insisting that the whole body suffers in disease, and that it should accordingly be treated as a whole. In this sense, the Methodists can be said to have taken a kind of holistic approach to therapeutics. But their reasoning on the question of the affected part turns out to be nuanced, and their rivals' claims that they ignored the affected part altogether is something of a distortion. In this paper, I shall attempt to specify exactly what the Methodist position was on the question of the affected part in disease, what sort of holism this represented and how their approach may have developed out of more fundamental commitments. As I shall argue, the application of their 'Method' led to a distinctive and noteworthy position on the issue of holism, one which deliberately encouraged the physician to minimise the significance of *differences* between diseases, including differences in the location of symptoms, and to focus rather on certain features which they share. Analysis of this position reveals some interesting characteristics of their approach to therapy in

2 The Methodists were particularly distinguished from their Rationalist and Empiricist adversaries in regard to their attitude to disease causation: not only did they reject as therapeutically irrelevant the hidden causes inferred by the Rationalists, but also the perceptible, antecedent causes (such as excessive food or drink consumption, overheating) taken into account by both Rationalists and Empiricists. Celsus, *praef.* 13–67, esp. 54–7, and Gal., *SI* 7 (I.84–87 K.) provide detailed and critical reports. For the Methodists' complex attitude to causation in disease, see esp. Lloyd (1983) 193–96, and van der Eijk (1999a)/(2005) 306–15.

general, in particular their exploitation of the huge body of earlier therapeutic literature of the Classical and Hellenistic periods which they had inherited.

The relevant evidence unfortunately comes mostly from a single source, Caelius Aurelianus. This Methodist physician produced, probably in the fifth century CE, a Latin version of two treatises, *On Acute Diseases* and *On Chronic Diseases*, which had been composed around 100 CE by his renowned Methodist predecessor Soranus of Ephesus.[3] Although there are general questions about the extent to which some fundamental features of Methodist doctrine may have changed over the centuries, I shall draw attention to corroborating evidence from other Methodist sources where appropriate and possible.[4] As far as I can see, there seems to be no particular reason to doubt that the Methodists' views on the affected part in disease, and their commitment to treating the body as a whole, remained fairly stable throughout the sect's history.

I begin with a brief review of the main principles of Methodism.[5] The sect was first developed by Themison of Laodicea in Rome in the early first century BCE, under the influence of his teacher, Asclepiades of Bithynia, the dominant medical authority in Rome at the time.[6] Asclepiades' theory conceived of the body as made up of invisible particles separated by void space, and hence as a porous, sponge-like substance whose density could be altered.[7] Against this background, the Methodists identified two common features (Greek κοινότητες) which they believed could be identified in any disease. One

3 On the relationship between Caelius and Soranus, and the difficult question of how closely Caelius' Latin represents Soranus' original Greek in *On Acute Diseases* and *On Chronic Diseases*, see the very helpful discussion in van der Eijk (1999b) 415–28, with further references. Urso (2003) and (2008) show that in the case of Caelius' translation of Soranus' *Gynaecia*, which can be compared with the original Greek, Caelius both abridges the source text, notably in doxographical passages, and expands upon it, but in the latter case consistently with a view to exegesis and clarification, making explicit aspects of Soranus' meaning that he sees as implied. For Soranus in general, see Hanson and Green (1994).

4 Tecusan (2004) 18–21 warns against taking unsympathetic ancient critiques of the Methodists as grounds for hypothesising significant developments within the sect, but also documents examples of, as she puts it, 'refinements on matters of detail' by successive generations of Methodists, representing 'permanent revisions but no drastic change' (p. 21). Pigeaud (1993) looks at the respective contributions of the pioneering Methodists Themison of Laodicea and Thessalus of Tralles, while van der Eijk (1999a)/(2005) focuses on Caelius Aurelianus and the question of how much his work reflects developments in Methodist ideas, particularly in regard to epistemological issues.

5 The fragments of the Methodists, besides Soranus, are collected in Tecusan (2004). For detailed discussions of Methodism, see also esp. Edelstein (1967); Frede (1987); Gourevitch (1991); Pigeaud (1991) and (1993); van der Eijk (1999a)/(2005).

6 For Asclepiades' influence, see most recently Flemming (2012).

7 I shall return to the possible significance of the Asclepiadean background below.

was a state of constriction, in which the body is too constricted or compacted to allow the proper movement of bodily fluids; another was a state of flux or looseness, in which fluids move too easily within the body and are excessively dissipated. Each and every disease, they believed, involves one or other of these common states, and in fact some diseases can involve both, with constriction affecting one part of the body, and flux another. Two features of these common features of disease were key. The first is the fact that they happen to be evident. It may have required some Methodist training to become fully practised in identifying constriction or flux correctly in every case, but nevertheless they were there for all to see, and not hidden states that needed to be inferred. The second is that they immediately and straightforwardly indicated to the doctor how they were to be treated, for excessive constriction was obviously to be counteracted by relaxing, and excessive flux by constriction. So the Methodists' focus on what is *common* to diseases, and the straightforward path it opened up to treatment, is basically what they referred to by their Method. With this background in mind, we can look more closely at what they had to say about the affected part in disease specifically.

1 The Methodist Approach to the Affected Part in Disease

Repeatedly in his writings *On Acute* and *On Chronic Diseases*, Caelius Aurelianus is found emphasising that in conditions such as phrenitis, lethargy, pleurisy, etc., it is the *whole* body that is affected, and not just one or more of its parts.[8] This is so important because of the implications for treatment: as Caelius notes, bodies which are *affected* as a whole need to be *treated* as a whole. I shall begin here with a sample of five passages from his works, covering distinct acute and chronic diseases, which focus on this issue of the level at which the body is affected:

> [2] (Phrenitis)
> Now we hold that the whole body suffers in common, for it is affected as a whole by fever. Fever is one of the signs that make up the indication of phrenitis, and for that reason we treat the whole body. But we say that the head suffers *more*, since the antecedent signs show it, such as its

8 For earlier discussions of the Methodists' approach to the affected part in disease, see Tecusan (2004) 10–11, esp. n. 13, and McDonald (2012) 70–74. Van der Eijk (1998) and (1999b) 442–45 draw attention to the ways in which Caelius' accounts of his predecessors' views on the affected part may depend on earlier doxographical sources.

heaviness, tension, pain, noises, ringing in the ears, dryness, impairment of the senses, etc.[9]

CAELIUS AURELIANUS, *Celeres Passiones* 1.8.55

[3] (Pleurisy)
Therefore when we see the disease pleurisy, we see that not just the pain in the side, but also the body as a whole suffers, as the acute fever indicates – for fevers belong to the whole body. We are right to say, however, that the pleural membrane suffers *more*, since the pains are localised there.

CAEL. AUR., *Cel. Pass.* 2.16.100

[4] (Cardiac disease)
Since we observe, in accordance with Soranus' judgement, that the whole body is relaxed into a state of looseness [*in solutionem laxari*], we maintain that it necessarily suffers as a whole. And we must not even argue about the part that suffers most, to avoid getting embroiled in an obscure inquiry [*in occulta quaestione*]. For neither the indication nor the treatment is altered by these, since we ought to apply remedies to all parts of the body.

CAEL. AUR., *Cel. Pass.* 2.34.183

[5] (Hydrophobia)
The part that suffers most [*praepatitur*] is the one which was injured by the bite. No one will deny that it is from here that the disease originates. And the whole body is affected, as we can show from what each of these authorities have said. For when different authorities claim that different parts suffer, they admit that all of them suffer. And this is corroborated by the symptoms which manifestly affect hydrophobic patients.

CAEL. AUR., *Cel. Pass.* 3.14.116

[6] (Dropsy)
As far as the types of dropsy are concerned, although we do not change the general treatment [*non generaliter mutemus curationem*], it is better to say that one type involves the whole body, as though penetrating among the rarefied gaps [*inter viarum raritatem*] in a sheet of papyrus or

9 Unless otherwise stated, translations are my own. For Caelius Aurelianus, I have benefited from the translation in Drabkin (1951).

> a sponge, named *leucophlegmatia* from the fluid ..., and that another type is located in the part of the body between the peritoneum and intestines.
>
> CAEL. AUR., *Tardae Passiones* 3.8.102

In each of these passages, specific reasons are given as to why these particular diseases are thought to affect the body as a whole. The most common reason adduced is the presence of fever, which is held to affect the body as a whole, presumably because the body exhibits an abnormal temperature throughout. Thus in passages [2] and [3] above, fever is cited as the indication that phrenitis and pleurisy affect the entire body. The cardiac disease, however, discussed in passage [4], is not always found with fever.[10] In the run-up to this passage, Caelius has reviewed an extensive debate among previous physicians as to whether the heart, the heart's membrane, the diaphragm, the oesophagus, the lungs, and so on, are the seat of the disease. For Caelius and Soranus, however, the fact that the entire body exhibits the common feature of flux or looseness is a clear sign that the whole body is affected. Hydrophobia, at passage [5], is a slightly different case again. Although the part which suffers most is acknowledged to be the part that was bitten by the hydrophobic animal in the first place, the wide range of symptoms that the disease subsequently presents, as well as the range of affected parts named by previous doctors, persuade Caelius that, again, the whole body comes to be affected.

The fact that we always find specific reasons of this sort implies that, although it is important to recognise when a condition affects the body as a whole, there is no expectation that this will always be the case. This implication appears to be confirmed in the analysis of dropsy in passage [6]: here Caelius identifies two principal forms of dropsy, one which affects the entire body, with the excessive fluids penetrating everywhere, and another type which is confined to the area between the peritoneum and intestines. As we shall see, the Methodists also recognise other genuinely localised conditions.

Yet it is important to note first that whenever Caelius identifies the whole body as the site of the disease, there is often also some comment on which part suffers most. The fact that the whole body is affected is rarely the end of the story. So with phrenitis, the head is believed to suffer more than the rest of the body (passage [2] above). Similarly, pleurisy affects the pleural membrane most, and, as we have seen, Caelius is clear that no one would want to deny that hydrophobia originates from the place in which the sufferer was bitten (passages [3] and [5]). At other times, the principal location of suffering cannot be determined with certainty. With the cardiac disease, for example, the

10 At least according to the Methodists: see Cael. Aur., *Cel. Pass.* 2.33.179.

extensive disagreement between earlier physicians is described as an obscure inquiry, one which will not in any case affect treatment (passage [4]). But for the most part, it *is* possible to identify the part that suffers most, and Caelius is scrupulous in naming it. His justifications for identifying this principally affected part are also listed, generally referring to a predominance of symptoms associated with a particular place. So in phrenitis the head suffers more, as witnessed by the heaviness, tension, pain and so on focused there, and in pleurisy the pleural membrane is believed to suffer more because of the pains experienced in that part. It is important to emphasise that these reasons are never connected with an account of the disease which appeals to its hidden *causes*, of the sort that a Rationalist doctor might give; the Methodists' reasons for prioritising an affected part are always based on directly observable phenomena (fevers, outward symptoms and so on).

As noted, for Caelius it is crucial that the body, when affected as a whole, must accordingly be treated as a whole. But the identification of the primarily affected parts does also have an impact on treatment. When we look at the detailed instructions for therapy in Caelius' treatises, we find that localised remedies, and specifically ones that are designed for the part primarily affected, are perfectly acceptable. Here are two examples, from sections on diseases we have already been considering:

> [7] (Treatment of phrenitis)
> If a state of looseness is combined with the state of stricture, so that loose bowels and sweating occur, treat the head in the manner described, using the previously mentioned fomentations, for the loss of reason is still due to the inflammation of the membranes of the brain. But treat the middle parts with cold, green olive oil.
>
> CAEL. AUR., *Cel. Pass.* 1.9.68

> [8] (Treatment of pleurisy)
> The parts which are in pain should be heated with warm cloths and, when the paroxysm has reached its peak, covered with clean wool wrung out in warm, sweet olive oil … The constant pain increases the discharge of fluids due to the sleeplessness and spoiled digestion … To the parts affected by pain apply cerates made with sweet olive oil or henna oil, mixed with fenugreek flour.
>
> CAEL. AUR., *Cel. Pass.* 2.18.103, 106, 112

So we see that, in phrenitis, the head is to be treated with fomentations because of the inflammation of the membranes of the brain, while in pleurisy the pain which showed that the pleural membrane suffers most in the disease is to be treated specifically with wool soaked in warm, sweet olive oil. Another clear example is dropsy, in which liquid collected in the abdominal cavity is sometimes drained directly through tapping.[11] Soranus' *Gynaecia* offers confirmation of Caelius' approach, recording a range of localised treatments for various uterine affections.[12] Identifying the part that suffers most can also play a role in diagnosis: for example, Caelius distinguishes melancholy from mania partly because in melancholy it is the oesophagus which suffers principally, while in mania it is the head.[13]

As we have also noted, the Methodists did not think that all conditions affect the whole body. There is plenty of room within Methodist pathology for genuinely localised conditions, in which the rest of the body is not thought to be affected. Obvious and extreme examples are conditions which are to be treated surgically. For surgery the Methodists proposed a distinct set of four common features, or *koinotētes*, which indicate treatment. These are firstly what is abnormal coming from outside the body, such as an arrow; then, within the body, what is abnormal in place, such as a broken bone; what is abnormal in size, such as an abscess; and finally what is abnormal through deficiency, such as a fistula.[14] These common features all immediately indicate the proper course of treatment, which obviously very much depends on which part of the body the abnormality is found. Another interesting example is expectoration of blood (ἀναγωγὴ τοῦ αἵματος, *sanguinis fluor*), which, although a condition stemming from an internal wound or abrasion, was standardly treated using dietetic remedies, as if a standard chronic disease, rather than with surgical techniques.[15] Caelius lists various possible locations for the origin of the blood in this condition, such as the top of the throat, the windpipe, the oesophagus, the lungs, and so on.[16] He then goes on to specify that the treatment must be applied either to this originating place itself, or to its neighbouring parts; we are then told that this is why it is important for the Methodist to ascertain the part from which the blood originates, 'and not, as some think, for the sake of altering the treatment, since generally we recommend that the same things

11 E.g. Cael. Aur., *Tard. Pass.* 3.8.122–35.

12 E.g. pessaries at Sor., *Gyn.* 3.23.2 (for uterine inflammation); 3.28.5 (for hysterical suffocation) (= 108.9, 111.16 Ilberg), etc.

13 Cael. Aur., *Tard. Pass.* 1.6.183 (additional reasons for distinguishing the two diseases are also given); cf. Urso (2018) 304–5. I am very grateful to the anonymous reader for drawing my attention to this diagnostic significance of the part which suffers most.

14 See ps.-Galen, *Introductio sive Medicus* 3.6 (XIV.681 K. = 7–8 Petit).

15 Cf. Cael. Aur., *Tard. Pass.* 2.12.145–46.

16 Cael. Aur., *Tard. Pass.* 2.11.127–36.

are applied to all (parts).’[17] Similarly certain remedies are to be applied to parts suffering from paralysis.[18] So the treatment itself (such as a warm cloth, or cold, green olive oil) is not to change according to the part affected, but merely where it is to be applied.

In general, then, the Methodists put considerable emphasis on determining whether a given condition affects the whole body, although specific reasons need to be pinpointed before such a conclusion can be reached. This emphasis is generally due to their conviction that bodies which are affected as a whole also need to be treated as a whole. At the same time, however, it often seems to be important to identify the part that is affected more than the rest of the body, and this *can* have an effect on treatment, even if only in determining where a remedy should be applied. Localised remedies are very much part of Methodist therapeutics. But we have also seen that there are a range of conditions which are themselves genuinely localised, and do not affect the body as a whole.

All this suggests that it would not be correct to say that the Methodists have a general, prior commitment to holism *per se*. Decisions to treat the body as a whole have to be reached through careful attendance to the particular condition and its symptoms. Nevertheless, there is a clear tendency to focus on the whole body at the expense of its parts. In this respect, Methodists often seem to find themselves critical of what they portray as their opponents’ misguided focus on the affected parts. They were criticised in turn by their opponents for what was presented, unfairly, as a simplistic approach to the question of the affected part in disease.

2 Affected Parts and the Methodist Common Features

So what exactly underlies this rather nuanced Methodist position on the question of the affected parts? In this next section, I shall attempt to relate their approach more clearly to the fundamentals of Methodist doctrine.

Not long before passage [7] above, which prescribed some localised remedies for phrenitis, Caelius discusses his predecessors’ approach to the treatment of this notorious disease. He observes that they were particularly

17 Cael. Aur., *Tard. Pass.* 2.11.128 *intelligimus locos ex quibus sangui<ni>s fluor vel lapsus fertur quod erit aptissimum ob adhibendam curationem iisdem vel eorum vicinis partibus, et non, ut quidam existimant, commutandae curationis causa, cum generaliter eadem cunctis adhibenda probamus.*

18 E.g. Cael. Aur., *Tard. Pass.* 2.1.49, *recorporativam curationem, quam Graeci metasyncriticam vocant, utilem approbamus partibus in passione constitutis.*

interested in identifying the affected part in phrenitis, so that they can apply appropriate localised remedies, and he reviews their attempts to define it based on physiological arguments on the location of the ruling part of the soul (the *hēgemonikon*).[19] For Caelius, however, such disputes are redundant from a therapeutic perspective. Here is what he has to say:

> [9] It has been asked what part suffers in cases of phrenitis, and especially by the leaders of other sects, so that they can prescribe remedies depending on the affected part and prepare localised remedies for the parts in question. We, however, do not change the general treatment [*generalem curationem*] on the basis of the [affected] parts or the adjacent places. For when it lies under the same genus [*sub eodem genere iacens*], a difference in the [affected] parts is not an essential one.
>
> CAEL. AUR., *Cel. Pass.* 1.8.53

The emphasis is here on revealing a method for identifying the aspects of a disease that are relevant for determining treatment. And given Caelius's Methodism, we would obviously expect the common features of constriction and flux to be the most relevant factors, overlooked by his rivals who mistakenly focus on the affected parts. This expectation seems to be confirmed by his use of the language of genus and differentiae of disease. For elsewhere, this is precisely how Soranus describes individual disease types and their relation to the common features. In a passage of his *Gynaecia*, Soranus refers to the different senses in which an unnatural *pathos*, or affection, can be meant:

> [10] In the case of [an affection, πάθος] against nature, sometimes it is meant in a general and generic sense [ὡς καθόλου καὶ γενικόν] – such as 'constriction' [οἷον τὸ στεγνόν] –, and sometimes in a particular and subordinate sense [μερικὸν καὶ ὑποβεβηκός] – such as the phrenitic or lethargic [affection].
>
> SORANUS, *Gynaecia* 3.1.2 (94 Ilberg)

So the common features, such as constriction, count as the genus or kind, whereas individual affections such as phrenitis or lethargy are subordinate to the common features, and represent *particular* affections or *species*.

Hence presumably what Caelius means about differences in the affected part is that variation in these does not affect the diagnosis of the generic common feature: a constricted body is a constricted body however you look at it.

19 Cael. Aur., *Cel. Pass.* 1.8.53, 56.

So once we have observed that a given disease is subsumed under the genus of one of the common features, then identification of distinct types within that genus would not affect the overall course of therapy. This is because what we need to know is that the common feature characterising this particular condition is of constriction, for example, which immediately indicates a relaxing course of treatment. It will make no difference to this basic insight to know whether the condition, say cardiac disease, is primarily located in the heart or the diaphragm – the relaxing course of treatment will still be called for (although one might wish to apply the relaxing treatment to different parts of the body). Caelius confirms that his Methodist predecessors took the same approach. According to him, certain followers of the prominent first century CE Methodist, Thessalus of Tralles, stated that 'a difference in the location must not alter the power of the common features.'[20]

But if the affected part is not supposed to affect the treatment that the common feature indicates, how do we make sense of the fact that in the detailed treatments which Caelius and other Methodists recommend, there are in fact localised remedies which *are* tailored to the needs of the parts that are primarily affected? The answer to this question is likely to have something to do with Caelius' careful specification that it is the *general* treatment that should remain uninfluenced by a consideration of the affected part. In his discussion of dropsy at passage [6] above, we saw that he refused to change the treatment '*generaliter*', 'generally', based on the different forms of the disease. Likewise, in passage [9], on phrenitis, it is the '*generalis curatio*', the 'general therapy', that is unaltered. Hence an implied distinction is drawn between the overall strategy used to treat a disease, and some of the specific details of treatment that go along with it. Often the distinction concerns the general type of remedy, which remains unchanged, and the specific locations to which it should be applied, which may be variable according to the part affected.[21]

Further light may be shed on Caelius' distinction between general and specific by looking at his recommendations for treating individual diseases. There are obviously many cases in which one's view on the affected part might suggest a particular type of remedy. Rationalist physicians especially tend to focus their treatments on the locations where they believe the cause of the disease resides: in passage [9] for example, Caelius emphasises this very point.

20 Cael. Aur., *Tard. Pass.* 1.12.145 *aliqui etiam Thessali sectatores recenti incisurae sive vulneri*[s] *passione<m> subici dixerunt: 'non enim oportet locorum differentia coenoteton mutare virtutem.'*

21 See *Cel. Pass.* 2.28.147–48 on peripneumonia, and the passages on expectoration of blood, discussed above in nn. 16 and 17, with text thereto (pp. 140–41).

Caelius' criticisms of Hippocrates elsewhere illustrate the point further, in his discussion of the treatment for ileus, or intestinal obstruction, recommended in the Hippocratic treatise *Diseases* 2. According to the Hippocratic author, the upper parts of the body should be cooled, and the whole body then warmed in a hot bath. As Caelius emphasises, this is due to the author's belief that ileus is caused by excessive heat in the upper parts, and chilling in the lower parts:

> [11] Among the ancient physicians, Hippocrates in Book 2 of his work *On Diseases* says that generally the upper parts should be cooled, and in particular emetic drugs prescribed and phlebotomy on the arm and head. He then recommends that the patient be placed in a tub filled with hot water ... He is influenced by his views concerning the causes [of the disease], for he believes or claims that it is caused by burning heat in the upper parts and chilling in the lower. Therefore he thinks that remedies with opposing effects should be prescribed, without seeing that the disease is brought about by inflammation [and therefore is a disease of stricture: cf. *Cel. Pass.* 3.17.146].
>
> CAEL. AUR., *Cel. Pass.* 3.17.153–55

The Methodist, by contrast, must always keep in mind the common feature which characterises the disease, and must reject any remedy that is counter-indicated by it. A particular localised treatment might well do some good in that particular place, or perhaps in the short term, but this is outweighed by the greater damage it would cause overall when the common feature is taken into account. And this is repeatedly the point of Caelius' criticisms of rival physicians. To take the same example from the Hippocratic treatment of ileus in *Diseases* 2, Caelius' objection is that ileus is characterised by constriction, since it involves the classically constricted symptom of inflammation. This would not respond well to the opposing therapies that the Hippocratic author recommends, especially the cooling treatment in the upper parts. The lesson is clear that remedies indicated by the affected part must always be over-ruled by remedies indicated by the common feature.

It follows, however, that if localised remedies happen to be *consistent* with the demands of the common feature, there should be no objection to employing them. And the localised remedies we looked at earlier would seem to confirm that this is in fact how the Methodists saw things. So in passages [7] and [8], the localised remedies for phrenitis and pleurisy which Caelius recommends are explicitly described as in line with the demands of the common feature. With phrenitis, in passage [7], since the membranes of the brain are inflamed and constricted, the head is to be treated using relaxing remedies, whereas the middle parts, which suffer from the common feature of flux, are to be treated with the constricting effects of cold, green olive oil. Similarly, in passage [8], the pain in the pleural membrane in pleurisy, since it causes sleeplessness and digestion, and thereby increases the constriction, must be treated locally by relaxing remedies. In all cases, Caelius stresses how these treatments are consistent with the overarching common feature. Decisions such as these would lead to an approach which produces a *general* therapy that is tied directly to the common features, but whose *specific* or *particular* remedies could in some cases be influenced by an awareness of the part affected most.

All sorts of different kinds of remedies might be suggested by the varied symptoms and features of an illness that a doctor takes note of – indeed, a huge range of different remedies *had* been suggested to various predecessors and rivals of the Methodists. Yet these remedies often turn out to have unforeseen consequences: they might appear to be helpful in some respects or in the short term, but then found out to exacerbate other symptoms of the disease and lead to later complications; they might conflict with one another and produce various unwanted effects on the body. The Methodist, however, has a method for discovering the most effective and safest remedies, by testing all suggested treatments against the demands of the predominant common feature. This leads to what might be called a sort of therapeutic calculus. Tensions between different indicated treatments can be negotiated by establishing a hierarchy of therapeutic criteria. The common feature is what must stand as the ultimate criterion, while other criteria should be viewed as subordinate. Within this hierarchy, the Methodist finds that the affected parts are typically among these subordinate criteria: localised remedies can certainly be applied to the part of the body that is affected most, but these must ultimately be checked for their effects in relation to the relevant common feature.

Indeed, Caelius' and Soranus' practice of systematically criticising the therapies prescribed by their predecessors can be read as a detailed exposition of the correct Methodist thought process when faced with a disease. Wesley Smith coined the term 'hamartography', or 'listing of errors', to label this practice in Soranus and Caelius.[22] Its purpose has generally been taken to be basically negative.[23] Caelius' criticisms are certainly copious and unrelenting, yet there is room for taking them as intended for a more positive purpose, and I would like to suggest that hamartography can be viewed as a key aspect

---

22 Smith (1979) 224.

23 See e.g. van der Eijk (1999b) 397–99, 433–39, esp. 437 '[t]he invariably negative reaction displayed by Caelius with regard to the views of the ancients suggests that the main, if not the only reason for discussing them, is to criticize and ridicule them.'

of the Method. More than just a self-indulgent harangue against the folly of one's predecessors, it could (also) represent a means of illustrating just how the Methodist must think through various possible therapies, by weighing up the pros and cons, with the common feature constantly in mind. A given treatment might look promising at first sight, but upon further reflection be revealed as harmful in light of the underlying common feature once identified, and this is what the Methodist must learn to be constantly on the lookout for. Everything, including the question of the affected part, must be subordinated to the demands of the common feature that represents the generic affection.

Even other Methodists sometimes fail to think properly Methodist thoughts. An example comes from the discussion on ileus again, where Thessalus is criticised for his reasoning in prescribing only a small amount of liquid to drink:

> [12] Thessalus, in the first book of his *On Regimen*, … says that we ought to prescribe <a small amount of> drink, since it may pass to the affected parts … But, arguing against Erasistratus in the second book, which he called 'Comparison', he says the following, clearly contradicting his words: 'For the amount of liquid should not change because of difference in the parts [affected], but based on the constriction or flux.' So it is inconsistent for him to believe that the quantity of drink should be diminished in sufferers from ileus because of the affected part. He should have clearly stated and shown how the quantity of drink should be diminished from a consideration of the acute disease.
>
> CAEL. AUR., *Cel. Pass.* 3.17.172–73

Thessalus' thought was apparently that the drink could descend to the affected parts, that is to the intestines, where it could cause problems if it were in too great a quantity. But Caelius points out that this is inconsistent with his own instructions, citing his statement elsewhere that it is the common features, i.e. 'constriction or flux', that should determine quantity of liquid, and not the affected part. It must be emphasised, however, that Caelius is happy that reducing the intake of drink is absolutely the right thing to do, and makes the same recommendation himself earlier on in his treatise.[24] Thessalus' treatment is quite correct; it is just the reasoning behind it that is questionable. This might look like mere nitpicking, and so it may be, but it perhaps begins to seem less so if read as an illustration for the trainee Methodist of the need to keep the

24 Cael. Aur., *Cel. Pass.* 3.17.148 'give him a little to drink in order to soothe him. For if he drinks a great deal, the inflammations are aggravated and the severity of the disease is increased.'

common features constantly in mind. The aim is always to ensure that the treatment be based on the correct criteria, and not on indications that have been shown in other cases to be unreliable.

Overall, then, the Methodists are concerned to relate all diseases treated by dietetics to the primary common features of constriction and flux, and hence to play down, though certainly not to eliminate, the significance of the affected part. The affected part can have an influence on treatment, but only when its significance is properly subordinated to the demands of the all-important common feature. The common feature will dictate the general therapeutic strategy, and hence specific types of treatment can be tested for their conformity with this. When rival physicians fail to appreciate this, and focus *unduly* on the affected part, they put themselves at serious risk of falling into error.

3 The Asclepiadean Body

It is hoped that these considerations may help to make further sense of the Methodists' direct pronouncements on the topic of the affected part in disease, and their quasi-holistic approach to treatment. But I also want to explore some deeper influences that may be operative in their conception of how diseases and remedies affect the body. In particular, I wish to evaluate the impact that Asclepiades of Bithynia's theory of matter may have had on the Methodists' emphasis on the porous and permeable nature of the body, and hence on their relative lack of interest in locating diseases in specific parts.

Having spent at least some time in Athens before coming to Rome, Asclepiades developed a systematic medical theory which drew extensively on Epicurean atomism.[25] According to his doctrine, the human body, as with everything in the universe, is made up of tiny, imperceptible particles called (*anarmoi*) *onkoi*. These are in perpetual motion, bouncing around forever in void space, without any providential intelligence at work in the universe to guide them. Health is maintained by the free and balanced motion of the *onkoi* through the void interstices (or *poroi*) within the body's structure, while disease is primarily the consequence of a blockage or impaction of *onkoi* in a particular part of the body, with different diseases resulting from blockages in different parts. Hence the specific localisation of pathological phenomena was absolutely fundamental to Asclepiades' approach to diagnosis and treatment.[26]

25 For Asclepiades' stay at Athens, see Cael. Aur., *Cel. Pass.* 2.22.129; for the influence of Epicureanism, see most recently Leith (2009) and (2012), responding esp. to Vallance (1990).

26 Vallance (1990) 93–122 offers a detailed reconstruction of Asclepiades' pathology.

A significant corollary of Asclepiades' particle physics, however, is that there are no absolutely impermeable structures within the body. All substances are made up of invisible particles separated by void gaps, and suitably sized particles, all in constant motion, will be able to pass through these gaps without constraint. Hence anatomical structures can never act as impassable boundaries for fluid substances, and will therefore be of secondary relevance for our understanding of human physiology. Galen offers a clear illustration of this point in his critique of Asclepiades' account of how urine makes its way into the bladder.[27] For Asclepiades, the liquid we drink, in the course of its passage through the body, becomes thinned and eventually turns into vapours (*atmoi*) which are fine enough to pass through the coat of the bladder. There, they condense again into liquid and become urine. In the first book of *On the Natural Faculties*, Galen the anatomist is of course outraged by Asclepiades' ignorance in believing the bladder to be like a sponge or piece of wool, rather than a completely impervious organ. But for Asclepiades, there are no completely impervious structures anywhere in the body, or indeed in the universe: any substance will have void gaps within it that can be infiltrated by particles of the right size. As Caelius Aurelianus reports, 'all things, [Asclepiades] says, which are situated in the interior parts of the body are in contact with each other by a hidden connection.'[28]

It is clear that Themison, who was Asclepiades' pupil, took on various aspects of his master's medical system, and among these seems to have been the basic conception of the body as a porous, sponge-like entity that is susceptible to constriction and rarefaction in its parts.[29] The Methodists of course denied that they were Rationalists of any sort, refusing to make use of hidden or obscure entities and causes in treatment.[30] They certainly distanced themselves

27 Gal., *De naturalibus facultatibus* 1.13 (II.30–35 K.).

28 Cael. Aur., *Cel. Pass.* 1.15.128. The Epicureans similarly emphasise that nothing is impermeable (except atoms): cf. e.g. Lucretius, *De rerum natura* 1.346–47 'however solid things may be thought to be, here is proof that you may discern them to be of less than solid consistency' (trans. by Rouse and Smith).

29 There is evidence that the Methodists deliberately kept some of the main features of Asclepiades' pathology, but shifted attention away from the elemental theory and focused instead on more vague talk of pores: cf. the modification made to Asclepiades' definition of cholera by certain Methodists reported at Cael. Aur., *Cel. Pass.* 3.19.189: 'certain members of our sect have given the same definition [as Asclepiades], taking away only 'impaction of *onkoi*' (*concursum corpusculorum*) and adding 'openness of pores' (*viarum raritatem*).'

30 See above n. 2.

from Asclepiades' fully developed physical theory.[31] Nevertheless, there are signs of their acceptance of the general principles of Asclepiades' conception of the body on some level. In fact, Galen would have us believe that Thessalus adopted the basic principles of Asclepiades' theory of matter in his treatise entitled the *Canon*.[32] Soranus similarly refers on occasion to the porosity of the body in Asclepiadean terms. He notes in his *Gynaecia* that the gaps which are perceptible only to reason will allow the dispersal of fumigations throughout the body, irrespective of what else may be going on physiologically, even citing in support Asclepiades' observation that a patient can perceive the flavour of rue when it is applied to the legs.[33] We also saw earlier, in passage [**6**], that Caelius distinguished a type of dropsy which permeates the entire body, through its gaps, as if it were a piece of papyrus or sponge. It will be remembered too that the Methodists refused to grant knowledge of anatomy any *therapeutic* value (whatever other kind of value it may have).[34]

I do not wish to get into the difficult and unresolved question of how the Methodists felt such views could be consistent with their anti-Rationalist

31 For Soranus' and especially Caelius Aurelianus' prominent criticism of Asclepiades, see von Staden (1999) and van der Eijk (1999b) 406–7, 425–26, 431–32. See Vallance (1990) 131–43 for an attempt to map the Methodists' common feature of constriction onto Asclepiades' theory of blockage (*enstasis*) as the cause of disease, and the common feature of laxity onto an alternative explanation Asclepiades reserved for certain conditions. However, most diseases in Asclepiades' pathology involve *both* blockage *and* a swift motion of particles towards the affected part, and I would interpret their Asclepiadean inheritance in more abstract terms.

32 Gal., *De methodo medendi* 4.4 (X.267–68 K.), '[b]ut as it is – for the term (sc. 'altering the compound', τὸ μετασυγκρίνειν) is a proper part of their madness, born of Asclepiades' hypothesis, like the rest of their views – they are surely bound to explain their own fantasies. But speaking of bodies being compounded and separated [συγκρίνεσθαι ... καὶ διακρίνεσθαι] is legitimate only for those who posit masses and interstices [ὄγκους καὶ πόρους] as primary elements, or atoms and void, or generally speaking impassive and unalterable bodies – and they do say such things, and continually use these terms. Indeed Thessalus establishes these starting-points in his *Canon*, but even there innovates in a certain way on the views of Themison and Asclepiades' (trans. Johnston and Horsley).

33 Sor., *Gyn.* 1.35 (24–25 Ilberg) (after observing Euenor's and Euryphon's prescription of fumigations to test whether a woman can conceive), '[a]ll this is wrong. For ... the substances made into suppositories and fumigations will be carried up through the gaps observable by reason (διὰ τῶν λόγῳ θεωρητῶν πόρων), even if a person is unable to conceive. Hence Asclepiades says that when a cerate made with rue is applied to a patient with ulcerated legs, they will have a perception of its quality because of its dispersal.'

34 See esp. Sor., *Gyn.* 1.5 (6 Ilberg); cf. e.g. Gal., *MM* 5.3 (X.319 K.). For further comment, see Lloyd (1983) 188–89, 192–93.

stance.[35] But it seems clear that, even if they did not commit themselves fully to the existence of imperceptible *onkoi* and void space, they did inherit from Asclepiades a general conception of the body as something fundamentally porous, and without impenetrable internal boundaries. Of course, the notion that substances will not be restricted to certain parts of the body, but can permeate it in its entirety, is particularly important for the present examination of the Methodists' holism, and their relative disinterest in localised pathologies. It also explains why they thought that remedies did not in general have to be applied locally in order to work.

4 Conclusion

I suggest, then, that from the outset Methodists were predisposed to think of the human body as something only very loosely partitioned, insofar as it is porous throughout and lacks solid internal boundaries. This prior conception of the body will have tended to favour a more holistic approach to pathology and therapeutics. Of course, this did not result in an extreme stance which banned all talk of affected parts. They were perfectly happy to recognise the obvious fact that some parts can suffer more than others when things go wrong in the body. But they were at pains to show how too much attention to the affected part could distract from the far more important *general* features of illness. The Methodists, and physicians of the Roman period in general, were heirs to a huge body of therapeutic recommendations for a range of well-defined pathological phenomena (phrenitis, lethargy, etc.). From this perspective, their task can be read as one of sifting the useful from the ineffective from among this morass, not (necessarily) of coming up with new treatments. Representing a simplified approach to medicine, their Method focused on the features that pathological phenomena had in common, and their framework of common features established a hierarchy of criteria by which to judge the efficacy of established therapies. Differences in the affected part in disease had suggested all sorts of remedies to their predecessors, but the Methodists found that such remedies often clashed with the indications provided by their all-important common features. Nevertheless, consideration of the affected part could suggest useful specific treatments, and helpful localised remedies, but what determined their usefulness ultimately was their conformity to the demands of the common feature involved. The affected part was to be used with great care: by

35 Cf. van der Eijk (1999a)/(2005) 308–10.

itself it could never be decisive for therapy, but there was certainly a place for it within the Method when properly handled.

Acknowledgments

I am very grateful to Chiara Thumiger as organiser of the conference and for her help in improving this paper, as well as to the original audience members for their questions and responses, especially Brooke Holmes. I am also indebted to the anonymous reader for extremely helpful comments and suggestions.

Bibliography

Edelstein, L. 'The Methodists.' In *Ancient Medicine: Selected Papers of Ludwig Edelstein*, ed. O. Temkin and C. L. Temkin. Baltimore: Johns Hopkins Press (1967) 173–91.

Flemming, R. 'Antiochus and Asclepiades: Medical and Philosophical Sectarianism at the End of the Hellenistic Era.' In *The Philosophy of Antiochus*, ed. D. Sedley. Cambridge: Cambridge University Press (2012) 55–79.

Frede, M. 'The Method of the So-called Methodical School of Medicine.' In M. Frede, *Essays in Ancient Philosophy*. Oxford: Oxford University Press (1987) 261–78.

Gourevitch, D. 'La pratique méthodique.' in *Les écoles médicales à Rome*, ed. P. Mudry and J. Pigeaud. Geneva: Librairie Droz (1991) 51–81.

Hanson, A. E., and M. Green. 'Soranus of Ephesus: Methodicorum princeps.' In *ANRW* II 37.2. Berlin: De Gruyter (1994) 968–1075.

Leith, D. 'The Qualitative Status of the *Onkoi* in Asclepiades' Theory of Matter.' *Oxford Studies in Ancient Philosophy*, 36 (2009) 283–320.

Leith, D. 'Pores and Void in Asclepiades' Physical Theory.' *Phronesis*, 57.2 (2012) 164–91.

Lloyd, G. E. R. *Science, Folklore and Ideology*. Cambridge: Cambridge University Press (1983).

McDonald, G. C. 'The "*Locus Affectus*" in Ancient Medical Theories of Disease.' In *Medicine and Space. Body, Surroundings and Borders in Antiquity and the Middle Ages*, ed. P. A. Baker, H. Nijdam and K. van't Land. Leiden and Boston: Brill (2012) 63–83.

Pigeaud, J. 'Les fondements du Méthodisme.' In *Les écoles médicales à Rome*, ed. P. Mudry and J. Pigeaud. Geneva: Droz (1991) 7–50.

Pigeaud, J. 'L'introduction du Méthodisme à Rome.' In *ANRW* II 37.1. Berlin: De Gruyter (1993) 565–99.

Smith, W. D. *The Hippocratic Tradition*. Ithaca: Cornell University Press (1979).

Tecusan, M. *The Fragments of the Methodists*. Volume One: Methodism outside Soranus, Studies in Ancient Medicine 24.1. Leiden and Boston: Brill (2004).

Urso, A. M. 'Riscritture di Sorano nel Mondo Latino Tardoantico. Il caso dei Gynaecia.' In *Galenismo e Medicina Tardoantica: fonti Greche, Latine e Arabe*, ed. I. Garofalo and A. Roselli, AION Quaderni 7. Naples (2003) 161–202.

Urso, A. M. 'Quando l'Esegesi Cambia il Testo: Traduzione e Riscrittura nei Gynaecia di Celio Aureliano.' In *Femmes en médecine. Actes de la Journée internationale d'étude organisée à l'Université René-Descartes-Paris V, le 17 mars 2006, en l'honneur de Danielle Gourevitch*, ed. V. Boudon-Millot, V. Dasen and B. Maire. Paris: De Boccard (2008) 205–22.

Urso, A. M. 'Mental Derangement in Methodist Nosography: What Caelius Aurelianus Had to Say.' In *Mental Illness in Ancient Medicine. From Celsus to Paul of Aegina*, ed. C. Thumiger and P. N. Singer. Studies in Ancient Medicine 50. Leiden and Boston: Brill (2018) 285–314.

Vallance, J. *The Lost Theory of Asclepiades of Bithynia*. Oxford: Oxford University Press (1990).

van der Eijk, P. J. 'Quelques remarques sur la méthode doxographique de Caelius Aurélien.' In *Maladie et maladies dans les textes latins antiques et médiévaux*, ed. C. Deroux. Brussels: Latomus (1998) 342–53.

van der Eijk, P. J. 'The Methodism of Caelius Aurelianus: Some Epistemological Issues.' In *Le traité des* Maladies Aiguës *et des* Maladies Chroniques *de Caelius Aurelianus: nouvelles approches*, ed. P. Mudry. Nantes: Institut Universitaire de France (1999a) 47–83. Repr. in P. J. van der Eijk, *Medicine and Philosophy in Classical Antiquity*. Cambridge: Cambridge University Press (2005) 299–327.

van der Eijk, P. J. 'Antiquarianism and Criticism: Forms and Functions of Medical Doxography in Methodism (Soranus, Caelius Aurelianus).' In *Ancient Histories of Medicine. Essays in Medical Doxography and Historiography in Classical Antiquity*, ed. P. J. van der Eijk. Studies in Ancient Medicine 31. Leiden, Boston and Köln: Brill (1999b) 397–452.

Von Staden, H. 'Caelius Aurelianus and the Hellenistic Epoch: Erasistratus, the Empiricists, and Herophilus.' In *Le traité des* Maladies Aiguës *et des* Maladies Chroniques *de Caelius Aurelianus: nouvelles approches*, ed. P. Mudry. Nantes: Institut Universitaire de France (1999) 85–119.

Primary Texts: Editions and Translations Used

Caelii Aureliani Celerum Passionum libri III, Tardarum Passionum Libri V. 2 vols. Ed. G. Bendz, *Corpus Medicorum Latinorum* VI, 1. Berlin: Akademie Verlag (1990–1993).

Claudii Galeni Opera Omnia. 22 vols. Ed. C. G. Kühn. Leipzig: Cnobloch (1821–1833).

Galien. *Le médecin. Introduction*. Ed. C. Petit. Paris: Les Belles Lettres (2009).
Sorani Gynaeciorum libri IV, De Signis Fracturarum, De Fasciis, Vita Hippocratis Secundum Soranum. Ed. J. Ilberg, *Corpus Medicorum Graecorum* IV. Leipzig and Berlin (1927).

Caelius Aurelianus. *On Acute Diseases and on Chronic Diseases*. Ed. and trans. I. E. Drabkin. Chicago University Press (1951).
Galen. *Three Treatises on the Nature of Science*. Trans. R. Walzer and M. Frede. Indianapolis: Hackett Publishing Company (1985).
Galen. *Method of Medicine*. Trans. I. Johnston and G. H. R. Horsley. Cambridge MA and London: Harvard University Press (2011).
Lucretius. *On the Nature of Things*. Trans. W. H. D. Rouse. Revised by M. F. Smith. Cambridge MA and London: Harvard University Press (1924).

CHAPTER 6

Is Graeco-Roman Medicine Holistic? Galen and Ancient Medical-Philosophical Debates

P. N. Singer

Abstract

The chapter attempts to analyse what can sensibly be understood by the term 'holism', which is very frequently used in relation to ancient medicine. It identifies three fundamental senses of the term – (1) unity of mind and body, (2) a unitary conception of the body itself, (3) unity of the body with its larger environment or cosmos – and considers ways in which both ancient medical theory and ancient diagnostic and clinical practice do or do not correspond with those conceptions. The paper focuses on Galen, but also contextualizes his approach within the Graeco-Roman medical and philosophical tradition, and compares it with others available in the ancient world, including those of Celsus and the Methodists. It is argued that a complex and nuanced picture emerges, within which, however, attention to overall states of the body tends to predominate over localization, and there are intricate accounts of the mutual dependence of 'soul' and 'body.'

1 Introduction

Graeco-Roman medical thought, in common with other 'alternative' or non-western medical traditions, is very often stated to offer a holistic approach to health, and is (almost equally often) celebrated for that. But the terms 'holism' and 'holistic' tend to be used vaguely, or at least without any accompanying definition. (Further on these problems, and in particular on those arising from modern projections of 'holism' onto Hippocrates, see Helen King's chapter in this volume.) In this paper I want to be more precise about the way, or rather the ways, in which the term may be applied to ancient medical thought, and to consider the practical significance of the holisms, or arguments in relation to holism, thus identified – both how they affected clinical practice and how they were used to express rivalries or disputes over competence. My focus here will not be on the second point, that of the value judgement in relation to the various holisms we may encounter, although some remarks relevant to that may be offered in passing. My aims rather are:

(1) to pin down what we mean by holism, and in particular its different possible senses as relevant to the Graeco-Roman material;
(2) to consider which (if any) of these Galen's therapeutic approach conforms to, and in what ways this is important for his approach to health;
(3) to consider also the limitations to holism in Galen, that is, important senses in which his approach seems to go in a very different direction from some of the senses of holism identified;
(4) to put this Galenic approach in relation to other ancient medical approaches.

To begin with, then, I suggest three main senses of 'holism' of particular relevance to Graeco-Roman medicine:

(a) mind–body holism: mind (or soul) and body are, in an important clinical sense, a unity;
(b) whole-body holism: the whole body must be considered in any pathological state; this sense includes, or may be divided into, two further senses:
    (b1) the whole body must be considered in medical diagnosis;
    (b2) the body as a whole, rather than individual parts, are the focus of medical treatment;
(c) one-with-the-cosmos holism: we as human beings are part of a larger whole, conceived in terms of our environment or of the cosmos in an even larger sense, in a way which is importantly relevant to health.

The paper will proceed, then, by considering Graeco-Roman thought on health, disease, diagnosis and clinical treatment in relation to each of the above senses of holism. In each case we shall examine Galen first, and in most detail, but will also consider the relationship of the Galenic model to other models and debates within ancient medicine and philosophy, considering both the classical (Hippocratic and Platonic) background and practitioners closer to Galen's own time, in the first and second centuries CE.

2 Mind–Body Holism

2.1 *Galenic Complexity*

The Galenic picture here is a somewhat complex one. There are two important senses in which Galen presents the pathology and treatment of the soul, or mind,[1] as a separate domain from that of (the rest of) the body, and thus moves in a fundamentally different direction from (a)-type holism.[2] First, there is a clear Galenic category of medically-defined illnesses which are (in our terms) mental or neurological: the 'medical psychic impairments'[3] – such items as *mania, lēthargos, paraphrosynē, epilēpsia,* or *melancholia.* These are understood essentially as impairments of brain function. The diagnostic distinctions between them consist in the differences in cognitive, behavioural or neurological disorders which they present; to this extent their pathology is conceptually distinct from that of the rest of the body. Their aetiology, meanwhile, depends (largely[4]) on the same system, that of the hot, cold, wet and dry and their imbalances, which underpins Galen's system in general.

For example, *paraphrosynē* or 'derangement' is understood as an impairment of the soul's 'leading-faculty' (*hēgemonikon*), located in the brain. This admits of further diagnostic distinctions, depending on precisely which function of the brain is impaired. Here as with other 'mental' disturbances, the aetiology depends closely on the opposition of excessive heat, leading to over-excited states (e.g. *mania*) and excessive cold, leading to depressed ones (e.g. *lēthargos, melancholia*).[5]

In both these respects, then – the diagnostic use of differential mental impairment and the focus on physical aetiologies – Galen's account of medical psychic impairment begins to look not very dissimilar from a standard contemporary one. It is only 'holistic' in the minimal sense that bodily factors have an effect on the soul or mind.

---

1 These two terms cannot, of course, be taken as co-extensive. (For the problem of locating an ancient category of 'mental', or of mapping the ancient discourse on to modern terminology, see now e.g. Thumiger and Singer (2018) 18–24.) But, at the risk of simplification, we may say that there is, *at least in pathological contexts*, a rough equivalence between the domains covered by Galen's *psychē* (and cognates) and those covered by our terms 'mental' and 'psychological' – though the provisos must be made, both of the overlap with our category of 'neurological' and of the distinct nature of the *ethical* discourse on the soul, on which see further below.

2 For a fuller account of Galen's variety of approaches to and therapy for soul pathology, see Singer (2018); and cf. Devinant (2018).

3 I adopt this terminology (cf. Singer 2018) to separate this distinctly medical category from the *pathē psychēs* considered as emotions or affections, and also to do justice to the imprecise equivalence between the Greek term and our 'psychological' or 'mental.'

4 As we shall see further below, there is also acknowledgement of the possibility of psychogenic causes of some of these items.

5 See in particular Galen, *Distinctions in Symptoms* (*Symp. Diff.*) 3 (VII.55–62 K. = 216–26 Gundert) and *Affected Places* (*Loc. Aff.*) 3.6–12 (VIII.160–204 K.), in conjunction with Singer (2018) 386–93; also Devinant (2018); Julião (2018).

The second – and again, clinically crucial – sense in which Galen seems to be markedly non-holistic is in his *ethical*, as opposed to medical, account of 'psychotherapy.' Here, he presents the diagnosis and treatment of the passions or affections of the soul (*pathē psychēs*),[6] as a separate discipline, different in kind from the rest of medicine. In *Affections and Errors of the Soul* and *Avoiding Distress*, he offers the reader, or potential patient, a range of quasi-medical interventions for the cure of the soul, which are quite distinct from the typical medical interventions 'for the body' (diet, exercise, drugs, blood-letting). Here the clinical techniques are rather: interaction with a personal supervisor to provide impartial criticism of one's irrational behaviour; self-examination; visualization of the relative attractiveness of virtuous and vicious behaviour; self-training to anticipate negative outcomes; certain kinds of daily reading or recitation. These kinds of intervention or discipline, sometimes called the therapy of the word, are evidenced also in other authors, for example Plutarch, Seneca, Marcus Aurelius, Epictetus.[7]

In the interests of concision, the following extract from *Affections* will suffice to exemplify this separate domain of the *pathē psychēs* – quasi-medical, but involving philosophical rather than expert medical intervention:

> The affections of the soul (πάθη ψυχῆς) are … rage, anger, fear, distress, envy, vehement desire (θυμὸς καὶ ὀργὴ καὶ φόβος καὶ λύπη καὶ φθόνος καὶ ἐπιθυμία σφοδρά) … How should one excise these affections? … If you find such a person [*sc.* who will speak the truth to you] … ask him to make evident to you directly which … affections he sees in you, emphasizing the gratitude you will feel towards him: he will be your saviour, even more so than the man who saves you when you have a bodily sickness (νοσοῦντα τὸ σῶμα).
>
> GALEN, *Affections and Errors of the Soul* (*Aff. Pecc. Dig.*) 1.3 (V.9 K. = 7–8 de Boer)[8]

6 The choice of English translation for *pathos* is problematic. While 'affection' (the option chosen here) is less than idiomatic, 'passion' is misleadingly dramatic and 'emotion', conversely, too neutral: for Galen a *pathos psychēs* is always a negative event, though they vary in severity. For Galen on the *pathē* see Manuli (1988); Hankinson (1993); Gill (2010); Kaufman (2014); Singer (2013); Singer (2019); Singer (forthcoming b).

7 The Galenic works appear in English translation with substantial notes and introductions discussing the therapeutic techniques in question, and their philosophical background, in Singer (2013). For discussion of them see especially Gill (2010), further Singer (2018), esp. 394–99; Singer (2019).

8 Translations are my own unless otherwise stated. However, published translations of the texts quoted are in any case mentioned in the bibliography at the end of the chapter, for the reader's ease of reference.

But there are other Galenic texts which might be considered to offer something more like (a)-type holism, texts which *either* suggest that the soul actually is identical with the body, or bodily in its fundamental nature, *or* present a more reciprocal, or closely 'intertwined', causal relationship between body and soul than that suggested at the end of the first paragraph of this section, above.

Famously, Galen posits a form of soul–body identity thesis (albeit in a work whose overall thesis, and title, correspond rather to a more straightforward soul–body *dependence* thesis):

> … it is preferable to say, not that it is slave to the body, but that this is actually what the mortal part of the soul is: the mixture of the body (τὴν κρᾶσιν τοῦ σώματος).
>
> GALEN, *The Soul's Dependence on the Body* (*QAM*) 4 (IV.782 K. = 26 Bazou)

This is followed a few lines later (IV.783 K. = 27 Bazou) by the argument, albeit in a dialectical context, that the substance or essence (*ousia*) of the soul should be equated with a bodily mixture (*krasis*). There has been much discussion of this apparent statement of an identity thesis, and of its relationship with Galen's overall views.[9] It will suffice here to observe that Galen is at the very least strongly drawn towards a fundamentally physical understanding of the soul, in a way evidenced not just by philosophical pronouncements such as that above, but also by remarks offered in the context of clinical discussions – and also of physiological discussions, where he highlights the fundamental role of a form of breath or *pneuma* in accounts of the soul's activities.[10]

Of particular interest for our present discussion are the *practical* claims made, for example that diet and physical activity, via the mixture they produce in the body, actually provide a basis for ethical improvement:

> The capacities of the soul depend on the mixtures of the body (ταῖς τοῦ σώματος κράσεσιν ἕπεσθαι τὰς δυνάμεις τῆς ψυχῆς) … we derive good-mixture from our food and drink and other daily activities, and on

9 Amid much recent literature, see especially: Lloyd (1988); Hankinson (1991a), (1991b), (2006); Vegetti (1999); Von Staden (2000), (2011); Tieleman (2003); Donini (2008); Gill (2010); Singer (2013) 18–33 and 335–69; Havrda (2017).

10 E.g. at *Causes of Symptoms* (*Caus. Symp.*) 2.5 (VII.191 K.), where he asserts that the soul either uses *pneuma*, blood and heat as its primary instruments or actually *is* those physical things. So, Galen toys with a thesis of soul–*pneuma* identity too, but seems ultimately to reject it, and indeed *consistently* refrains from committing himself on 'the substance of the soul': see Frede (2003); Donini (2008); Singer (2013) 340 nn. 19 and 21; Singer (forthcoming a); and further on *pneuma* in Galen see Julius Rocca's chapter in this volume.

> the basis of this mixture are then able to improve the virtue of the soul (εἰς ἀρετὴν τῇ ψυχῇ συντελέσομεν).
>
> GALEN, *QAM* 1 (IV.767–68 K. = 7 Bazou)

A further analysis comes near the end of the same work:

> This part [*sc.* negative outside influences] accounts for bad habits … and false opinions (ἐθισμοί τε … μοχθηροὶ … καὶ δόξαι ψευδεῖς) … while if we are educated by good, upright individuals we acquire correct opinions and good habits. But it is on mixtures that depend cleverness and foolishness (ἀγχίνοιά τε καὶ μωρία) … and the mixtures themselves are consequent on genetic factors and a daily regime involving good humoral fluid (εὐχύμοις διαίταις). And these mutually reinforce each other (συναυξάνειν ἄλληλα) … People become quick-tempered because of a hot mixture, but then through their quickness of temper inflame their innate heat (ἔμφυτον θερμασίαν); conversely, those who are well-balanced (σύμμετροι) in their mixture have well-balanced motions (κινήσεις) of the soul and are assisted towards good humoral mixture (εὐχυμίαν).
>
> GALEN, *QAM* 11 (IV.820–21 K. = 87–88 Bazou)

We have here a complex interaction of factors – nature, training and outside influence, habit, established soul characteristics – contributing to the ethical and cognitive health of the human being; moreover, a close *reciprocal* relationship is envisaged between the physical factors from which soul characteristics are ultimately derived and those developed characteristics themselves. We may well interpret this reciprocal, or closely 'intertwined', causal relationship between body and soul, as broadly in line with (a)-type holism.

There seems, then, to be a tension in Galenic thought, between, on the one hand, two therapeutic approaches – that found in his account of medically-defined psychic impairments, and that found in his ethical 'psychotherapeutics' – which *both* in different ways see the *psychē* as something to be diagnosed and cured as an entity separate from the rest of the body, and another approach which tends to regard the health of body and health of soul as fundamentally inextricable.

We shall proceed now to consider some further texts which elaborate this 'inextricability' view, in the context of the maintenance of human health. Before doing so, we should address the problem of what may seem like a second tension, *within* those texts which advance such an inextricability view. For on the one hand we have the apparent identity statements, or theoretical statements of a fundamentally physical nature of the soul, considered above; and on the other we have a number of passages, still emphasizing the close interconnectedness of soul and body, but doing so while talking in an untheorized way of soul and body – and their health – as separate items.

This second tension is, I suggest, fairly readily resolvable, in practical if not in detailed theoretical terms. Here it may be helpful to introduce the concept of 'pragmatic dualism.' That is: you may believe, theoretically or ultimately, that mind and body are parts or aspects of a single entity. But you may still find it useful, in everyday and indeed in clinical contexts, to speak of mind and body and their interaction. This, I would suggest, is common linguistic practice also in contemporary medicine. The mind, and the mental – and the distinction between them and the body or the physical – are concepts regularly employed in everyday communication, including in interactions between doctors and patients. And they continue to be employed even by individuals whose theoretical view may be that mind is reducible to body, that they are ultimately one. So, using dualist language in this sense may not be in conflict with (a)-type holism. One may be using 'pragmatic dualism' in ordinary language to specify particular subsets of event or experience ('of the soul', 'of the body'), even while regarding the two as aspects or inextricably linked parts of what is, in the most important clinical sense, a unity.

Particularly interesting in this context is Galen's large work on everyday healthy living, *Matters of Health*. Here, there is an undeniably physical basis to most of what Galen is saying about the soul. However, in the context of an account of two sets of experiences and interventions which can be seen, in a practical everyday sense, as different in kind, we will end up talking quite a lot about the soul and the body as different things, and indeed about their interaction. But a strong statement of such interaction, even if it uses the pragmatically dualistic language, may still count as some kind of mind – body, or (a)-type, holism.

For example, Galen has a strong and detailed view about the way in which a range of mental or emotional experiences – rage, worry, distress, weeping, resultant insomnia – may negatively affect physical health.

> ... baths; rages (θυμοί); worries (φροντίδες); distress (λῦπαι); and all such things which pretty nearly transform the mixture through their every shift ...
>
> GALEN, *Matters of Health* (*San. Tu.*) 1.5 (VI.28 K. = 14 Koch)

> For, indeed, rage, weeping, anger, distress, worry which is more than it should be, as well as significant sleeplessness (ἀγρυπνία) arising from them, provoke fevers, and become the starting-points of major diseases,

> just as, conversely, an idle intellect (ἀργὴ διάνοια), mindlessness (ἄνοια) and a soul which is completely lacking in spirit (ἄθυμος) often bring about poor colour (ἀχροίας) and ill-nourishment (ἀτροφίας) through feebleness of the innate heat.
>
> GALEN, *San. Tu.* 1.8 (VI.40–41 K. = 19–20 Koch)

On the one hand, there is here a clearly-defined separate category, that of the *pathē psychēs*, which are different in kind from diet, exercise and baths; on the other, they are listed indiscriminately alongside those latter kinds of factor. And, crucially, the mechanism by which they affect physical health is the same: these mental disturbances disrupt the balance by causing excessive heat, cold, or dryness, just as the wrong diet or baths will.

Indeed, Galen further elaborates this understanding of emotional disturbance, of the *pathē psychēs*, as functioning within a physical model of explanation:

> Now, rage (θυμός) is not simply an increase, but as it were a kind of boiling of the hot in the heart ... The internal heat increases in those suffering shame (τοῖς αἰδεσθεῖσιν) too, as all of the hot first of all courses together to the inside ... For in shame the breath (πνεῦμα) ... is stirred about all over the place both inside and about itself, along with all the blood, just as it is in people suffering anxiety (τῶν ἀγωνιώντων).
>
> GALEN, *San. Tu.* 2.9 (VI.138–39 K. = 61 Koch)

> It is possible to observe its [*sc.* the internal heat's] motions manifestly in many other affections, but especially those of the soul (ἐν ἄλλοις τε πολλοῖς καὶ μάλιστα τοῖς ψυχικοῖς παθέσιν).
>
> GALEN, *Caus. Symp.* 2.5 (VII.191 K.)

There is an inextricable relationship between the *pathē* of the soul – or at least an important set of them – and the physiological complex of innate heat, blood and *pneuma*, a relationship explored by Galen in considerable detail.[11] This enables one to observe bodily changes which are specific to particular emotional states, and thus even to diagnose such states on that basis.

On the other hand, it can be crucial for diagnosis and treatment to know whether a particular state has its origin in the soul or in the body. An example is the lovesick woman in *Prognosis*. The case, and Galen's quasi-theatrical

11 For further discussion and a fuller range of the most relevant Galenic texts, see Singer (2017).

success in his self-presentation of it, are well known. Here, I simply draw attention to one feature of the case in Galen's account of it, namely the either – or nature of his differential diagnosis. After his first consultation, Galen says,

> I decided she was suffering from *one of two things*: from a depression caused by black bile (μελαγχολικῶς δυσθυμεῖν) or from some distress (λυπουμένην) she was unwilling to confess.
>
> GALEN, *Prognosis* (*Praen.*) 6 Nutton (XIV.631 K. = 100–102; trans. NUTTON, slightly adapted)

The answer turns out to be the latter: the woman is eaten up by passion for a dancer of the name of Pylades – as Galen dramatically demonstrates by taking her pulse at the moment that this name is mentioned. But the point is that in a case where symptoms may look very similar, it is of clinical importance to establish which the underlying cause was: a physical one or a psychogenic one. Relevant material could be added here from the *Commentary on Hippocrates' Epidemics VI*, where Galen describes a number of cases of psychogenic illness, involving in particular forms of anxiety, grief, obsession or delusion, several of them with fatal outcomes.[12] In one sense, such cases again emphasize the separateness of the psychic as a diagnostic category; but at the same time they serve to show again the inextricable nature of the soul–body organism.

One could, given more space, add further Galenic passages which elaborate on this intertwined or reciprocal interaction between soul and body. Galen asserts the value of a good daily regime for the character as well as the body; but at the same time claims to have cured people suffering from a variety of physical conditions by attending to 'unbalanced motions' arising in the soul.[13] In the latter context, he also gives detailed prescriptions for various imperfect conditions of the soul, ranging from musical activities and poetry composition to sporting activities including fighting and hunting. He summarizes the point:

> … the person who is capable of employing these arts [*sc.* those related to music and physical exercise] will best educate both body and soul.
>
> GALEN, *San. Tu.* 1.7 (VI.37 K. = 18 Koch)

The notion that emerges of a mind–body complex, with an intricate causal intertwining of health of 'soul' and health of 'body', seems to give us one strong sense of holism to which Galen does subscribe, and perhaps also – to return

12 See especially Hipp. *Epid. VI* ch. 8 (485–87 Pfaff).

13 *San. Tu.* 1.6 (VI.32–33 K. = 16 Koch); 1.8 (VI.39–42 K. = 19–20 Koch).

briefly to the evaluative question – one where contemporary readers may find the approach fruitful or at least suggestive.

2.2 *Hippocratic and Platonic Background*

The legacy of Hippocratic and Platonic models seems especially important here. The former is relevant in the following way. The Hippocratic Corpus in general terms lacks a clearly defined notion of the mental or (with few exceptions) the soul, and therefore does not tend to regard mental disorders as different in category or fundamental character from any other disorders.[14] More specifically, a range of Hippocratic texts dealing with diagnosis, disease causation, or the maintenance of health presents lists of physical and (in our terms) psychological factors and/or symptoms alongside each other, in a way very similar to that which we observed above in Galen's *Matters of Health*. Indeed, Galen's approach in this area – both the identification of relevant factors affecting health, and the prescriptions, both crucially centring on diet, exercise and physical environment – is clearly fundamentally moulded by that Hippocratic discourse.[15] (And we might wish to say that his approach in this area represents the most 'intertwined' or holistic part of his work.)

The parallelism that we have observed in some Galenic texts between health of body and health of soul, meanwhile, has a clear Platonic heritage. Such a parallel is a recurrent feature of many Platonic dialogues, as is the additional specification – also observed above in Galen – that the former is regarded as the domain of the doctor and the latter that of the philosopher. A crucial text for the elaboration of the parallel is Plato's *Gorgias*, which uses the example of medicine, both to assert the status and value of true arts or sciences in contradistinction to false ones, and to indicate the existence of an equivalent or higher expertise concerned with the goods of the soul – the domain of justice, in which the expert will be the philosopher. Galen engages closely with that text, quoting from it and following its argument in detail, in his other important work on the definition of and proper approach to health, *Thrasybulus*.[16] He finds support here for his claims for the elevated status and scientific nature of the art of medicine. Yet, at the same time, this is a text which tends to point to a clear distinction between the domains of health of soul and health of body.

---

14 See Singer (1992); Gundert (2000); Thumiger (2013) and (2017).

15 One may point to the presence of 'psychological' and 'physical' symptoms alongside each other, for example in lists of symptoms in the *Epidemics* (see further the literature cited in the previous note). And see n. 24 below on the (unacknowledged) importance to Galen of the Hippocratic text *Regimen*.

16 See esp. *Thras.* 34–36 (V.872–76 K. = 81–83 Helmreich).

In this context it is worth considering Plato's own direct contributions to the discussion of holism. Two texts are of particular relevance: *Charmides* (on which see further chapter 8 below) and *Phaedrus*. The argument of *Charmides* (156b–57a) proceeds by a progressive expansion of the 'whole' that is relevant to the clinical context. First, it is suggested that the doctor curing an eye complaint must not just know about the eyes, but also about the whole head; then, that he must in fact know about the whole body; finally, it is proposed that understanding of the whole body will be incomplete or inadequate without attention to the soul too, such attention being, in fact the starting-point for successful medicine. Here, then, the soul – body unity is the relevant 'whole' (τοῦ ὅλου, 156e) which medicine must address. In *Phaedrus*, meanwhile, Socrates praises 'Hippocrates' for, precisely, a kind of holism, that is to say an insistence on investigation into the nature of *the whole*. Unfortunately, it is not clear, and certainly not agreed by modern scholarship, precisely which 'whole' is in question here. The argument at this point has developed (again) from a parallelism between the domains of soul and body (270b); it is then asserted that 'it is impossible to understand the nature of the soul without the nature of the whole' (270c). Is it knowledge of the soul in its entirety that is meant, or knowledge of the entire soul–body unity, or indeed knowledge of the whole cosmos? What is clear, however, is that Plato is asserting – and attributing to Hippocrates – the view that proper scientific knowledge must proceed from an understanding of (followed by appropriate subdivision of) the relevant 'whole' in question.

Galen responds directly to this passage from *Phaedrus*, though in the context of scientific method rather than that of the soul–body relationship: he takes it to support his own views on correct procedure in the study of nature.[17] His response to Plato's statement of holism understood specifically in relation to the soul–body complex is perhaps less clear, or at least less explicit. We might wish to say that the holism of *Charmides* is tendentially reversed by that of Galen's *The Soul's Dependence on the Body*. In the former, medical expertise seems ultimately to be subsumed under that of the philosopher; in the latter, it is the doctor who turns out to have the understanding which is most relevant, also in ethical contexts.[18]

---

17 E.g. in his *Commentary on Hippocrates' Nature of the Human Being* (*HNH*) 1 (XV.4–5 K. = 4–5 Mewaldt). Interestingly in relation to the *Charmides* argument, Galen explicitly attacks (for example in *Parts of Medicine*) doctors with a specialism confined to one particular part of the body. That attack is doubtless to be understood partially in socio-medical terms – Galen the educated, encyclopaedic intellectual asserting his superiority over mere artisan practitioners.

18 It is a complicating factor in Galen's case that he wishes at times to present himself also as a philosopher. So, the demarcation of a distinct medical and philosophical expertise

Yet, as already suggested, neither of those is the whole story, since both Plato and Galen operate in many of their discussions with a clear division and parallelism between the two areas of expertise.

2.3 *Areas of Competence: Doctor versus Philosopher?*

These complexities in the relationship between the Platonic–Galenic medical–philosophical discourse lead us on to another point. The doctor, Galen says, is interested in the health of the soul, and should therefore have a wide range of musical and cultural knowledge:

> The character of the soul (τὸ τῆς ψυχῆς ἦθος) is destroyed (διαφθείρεται) by bad habits (μοχθηρῶν ἐθισμῶν) in food, drink, physical exercise, things watched and heard, and music as a whole. Indeed, the person who undertakes the art of health should be experienced in all these, and should *not think that it is only the business of the philosopher to shape the character of the soul* (πλάττειν ἦθος ψυχῆς); *but rather his because of something greater*, that is the health of the soul itself (τὴν τῆς ψυχῆς αὐτῆς ὑγείαν), and the doctor's for the sake of the body's not being dragged with it into sickness.
>
> GALEN, *San. Tu.* 1.8 (VI.40 K. = 19 Koch)

In the doctor's case, then, such knowledge has an ultimately *bodily* aim. You might have thought that such things as music, entertainment and performance arts would be beyond the doctor's ken. This is not the case. Nor is it the case, however, that such knowledge belongs, properly speaking, in the doctor's domain. The doctor's expertise in 'soul' matters is here an instrumental one: he must interest himself in them because of their impact on the health of the body. It is the philosopher who would be expected to have an interest in the soul 'for the sake of something' higher – that is to say, presumably, for the sake of the soul in its own right, for its moral or ethical health.

But this Platonic parallelism has very particular consequences in the later philosophical–medical tradition: the idea that doctors can and should interest themselves in philosophical matters turns out to be a highly controversial one, reflecting an ongoing dispute over competence in the Graeco-Roman intellectual and healthcare world. It seems probable, as Sean Coughlin suggests, that Athenaeus of Attalia was a pivotal figure in this history, drawing on both the medical tradition and Platonic discourse, prefiguring, possibly indeed

would not deprive Galen of his competence: he may have two distinct areas of competence, in two different personas.

influencing, Galen's synthetic, Platonist-cum-medical approach.[19] There were both doctors who believed that doctors should not delve into philosophy (apparently Soranus was also one of these[20]) and philosophers who rejected physical health as an appropriate topic for their debates. A near-contemporary of Galen's, Plutarch, gives evidence of this debate.

> ZEUXIPPUS … in medicine that man [Glaucus] is, as Homer has it, 'one who is worth many others', yet he is hostile towards philosophy … He was just attacking us, proclaiming that … we were responsible for a great … confusion, daring to discourse on the healthy daily regime (διαίτης ὑγιείνης). For he stated that the border between philosophers and doctors should be as distinct as that between Mysians and Phrygians.
> MOSCHION. And yet I would gladly have heard this and the other discussions.
> ZEUXIPPUS. Well, you are a philosopher by nature, Moschion, and do not object to a philosopher who is interested in medicine; indeed, you get angry with one who thinks it more appropriate to be seen laying claim to the knowledge of geometry, dialectic and music than wanting to learn 'that which has been here established as good or as bad', for the body.
> PLUTARCH, *Precepts on Health*, *Moralia* 122b–e

Plutarch here presents us (a) with the figure of such an anti-philosophical doctor, Glaucus, who believes in a strong separation between medicine and philosophy, (b) with the notion that certain philosophers confine their interests to geometry and dialectic rather than bodily health, but also (c) with the actual characters of the dialogue, Zeuxippus and Moschion, respectively a philosopher who *does* take a strong interest in matters of health and a doctor who is 'a philosopher' by nature – and, of course, with the notion of a fruitful conversation between them.

Both within medicine and within philosophy, then, one could have an argument, not just on that conventional bone of contention, the relationship of soul and body, but also as to how *holistic one's own discipline actually is or should be*. Should the philosopher interest himself to know about dietary interventions, because they may have an influence on the soul – or, if you like, the person as a whole? Is it appropriate, or arrogant and carpet-bagging, of

19 See Coughlin (2018).

20 Soranus, *Gynaecology* 2.57.2–3 (93 Ilberg), cited by Coughlin (2018) 112. Competence conflicts between medicine and philosophy are explored further, especially in the context of Stoic authors and Caelius Aurelianus, by Ahonen (2018); cf. Polito (2016).

the doctor to say things about the soul or mind, the traditional domain of the philosopher?

2.4 *Mental Illness: Causal and Therapeutic Complexity*

Within Galen, we have been considering the question of mind–body holism mainly in relation to the question of the *pathē psychēs* and how these (and the philosophical discourse around them) interact with the body (and with medical approaches to it). We also briefly considered Galen's approach to the medical psychic impairments.

We should consider, then, how Galen's approach in this latter context here may contrast with that of his contemporaries or near-contemporaries. For while Galen's clinical approach to the medical psychic impairments is largely based on physical interventions – diet, sleep, exercise, and so on in milder cases; drugs and blood-letting in more severe ones – there are also somewhat different clinical tendencies within the medical culture of the period – tendencies which seem to take account of or interact with the patient in a broader sense than simply in terms of aberrations in bodily mixture, and might in that sense be considered holistic in ways which Galen's clinical practice is not.

The encyclopaedist and medical author Celsus, for example, having made a distinction between different varieties of *insania*, suggests a number of interventions which involve attention to the individualities of patient experience, and to the patient's environment. Advice is given as to the extent to which a deranged patient is to be agreed with or indulged, as opposed to corrected; techniques are suggested to engage the patient's interest; suggestions are made for varieties of music as story-telling, as well as for the creation of an appropriate environment, especially in terms of light and darkness.[21]

And similar therapeutic approaches can be found in Aretaeus, Caelius Aurelianus and Rufus. Aretaeus advises peace and quiet, and a simple physical environment, to counteract the over-excited mental state of *phrenitis*, and gives a reverse kind of prescription for the depressed state of *lēthargos*. Caelius offers detailed prescriptions, in terms of the appropriate kinds of language and intellectual interaction (including reading aloud to the patient with deliberate errors; theatrical entertainments; vocal exercises) for different levels or phases of *furor* (equivalent to Greek *mania*).[22]

---

21 Celsus 3.18 (123–26 Marx), discussed by Thumiger and Singer (2018) 11–14.

22 See Aretaeus 5.1 (91–92 Hude) and 5.2 (esp. 98 Hude); Caelius, *Acute Diseases* 1.11.98–99 (76 Bendz); 1.11.80–82 (66–68 Bendz); *Chronic Diseases* 1.5.156–57 (522–24 Bendz) and 1.5.162–67 (562–68 Bendz); and cf. 1.5.175–79 (534–36 Bendz).

It is probably important not to exaggerate the differences here, or the prominence of this cognitive or interactive model: passages such as those just considered remain, within the texts of Celsus, Caelius and Aretaeus, the exception rather than the norm. Yet is fair to say that, at points at least, a therapeutic approach is suggested which is interestingly different from that based entirely on dietary or pharmaceutical interventions.

2.5 *Summary*

In summary we may say that (a)-type holism exists at least in the sense that, in certain important diagnostic and clinical contexts, soul and body are inextricably interconnected; but that there is a potential conflict between this 'interconnectedness' and various statements of mind–body parallelism or dualism – even if this may in some contexts be understood, as I have suggested said, as a merely 'pragmatic dualism.' There is, also, a perceived tension or conflict as to how holistic – or, alternatively, dualistically divided, the disciplines of medicine and philosophy are, or should be. Finally, the extent to which soul and body attract different types of clinical treatment is different in different medical authors of the imperial period.

3 Whole-Body Holism

3.1 *Galenic Medicine: Whole Body or Affected Part?*

I turn then to my second main category, 'whole-body holism.' The following passage gives a brief encapsulation[23] of the way in which human health is understood in terms of a state of the body as a whole, in turn understood ultimately as a balance of the fundamental qualities, hot, wet, cold and dry which compose it.

> ... while the health of the uniform (ὁμοιομερῶν) parts, as they are called, consists in some kind of good balance (συμμετρία) of cold, hot, dry and wet, that of the organic (ὀργανικῶν) parts is brought about from the composition, amount, magnitude and shaping (συνθέσεώς τε καὶ ποσότητος καὶ πηλικότητος καὶ διαπλάσεως) of the uniform ones. So, too, the person who is capable of preserving these will be the good preserver of health.
>
> GALEN, *San. Tu.* 1.1 (VI.1 K. = 3 Koch)

23 Further texts of particular relevance here are *Causes of Diseases* and *Distinctions in Diseases*, which – with some elaboration and some variations – offer a fundamentally similar account of the levels of analysis within the body.

Though the specifics of the model (the division into the levels of organic and uniform parts, the underlying conception of mixture) are Galenic, the notion that health and disease consist in some kind of balance or imbalance of the fundamental constituents of the body again has clear Hippocratic ancestry; indeed, the notion is, in different forms, pervasive in ancient medical thought.[24] To give just two central examples of Galenic texts which seem to foreground this (b)-type holism, both *Matters of Health* and *Mixtures* prominently feature the notion of *overall states* of the body as explanations for individual patient characteristics and pathologies. So too, a wide range of Hippocratic texts (prominently e.g. *The Nature of the Human Being*, *The Sacred Disease*, *Affections*, *Regimen*) present some combination as fluids as the fundamental constituents of the human body and/or as responsible for health and disease.[25]

But how do such apparently holistic notions fit with the importance of determining the *locus affectus* – the precise organ or place in a body which is affected, or which is the underlying cause of a condition?[26] The latter notion is also one which Galen insists on and elaborates at considerable length, not least (unsurprisingly) in his work entitled *Affected Places*: here, it is crucial to diagnosis and treatment to identify, not just a general, overall state of the body, but the location or origin of the ailment.

> One must always start with the organ of the damaged activity (βεβλαμμένης ἐνεργείας), and then find out which type of damage it is … and, if it is one that has already become established, whether the effective cause of the impairment (τῆς ποιούσης τὸ πάθος αἰτίας) is contained within the part or is passing through it …

24 The Anonymus Londinensis offers a more precise doxographical distinction, between texts that rely on a theory of elements and those that rely on a theory of residues. For the prevalence of theories of balance in ancient theories of health – and also for the specific similarity of Galen's views in this area to those of the Hippocratic *Regimen*, even though he does not explicitly acknowledge it – see Grimaudo (2008).

25 So, for example, in *Mixtures* (*Temp.*) 2.6, the progress from childhood to old age is understood as a gradual process of cooling and drying, therefore the old are prone to 'cold diseases'; different overall disease-types, understood in terms of the model hot–cold–wet–dry, derive from environmental conditions that have those qualities (cf. *Commentary on Aphorisms* (*Hipp. Aph.*) 6.67 (XVIIIA.78–79 K.), for a patient with a yearly onset of melancholy); and an overall process of drying-plus-heating is a predisposing cause of fever. For this last phenomenon, in addition to the passages cited from *Matters of Health*, cf. *Causes of Diseases* (*Caus. Morb.*) 2 (VII.4 K.), and the passages gathered in the Appendix of Singer (2017).

26 On the significance, and disputed nature, of this concept in ancient medical thought, see also McDonald (2011).

> A further distinction we should make is between impairments (πάθη) which arise through sympathy with another part and those which arise by 'idiopathy' …
>
> GALEN, *Loc. Aff.* 1.2 (VIII.22 K. = 252 Gärtner); 1.3 (VIII.30 K. = 260 Gärtner)

As seen from these quotations, Galen does more than just emphasize the importance of bodily location. He makes precise distinctions in terms of original or primary location and the secondarily or sympathetically affected part – distinctions which will have crucial consequences for treatment.

There are, moreover, important diagnostic distinctions to be made *within* particular bodily locations, between the solid structures and the fluids or residues that arise within them. This can be seen from the following two passages, the first designed to correct a common misconception to do with old age, the second arising in the context of a fascinating Galenic attempt to make precise aetiological distinctions within the pathology of the brain and of mental disorder.

> … some well-reputed doctors … maintain that old age is wet … deceived by the quantity of the *residues* (περιττωμάτων). For their eyes water, their noses fill with mucus, and a large amount of saliva gathers … their lungs, too, are full of this kind of fluid (χυμοῦ) … None of these things, however, contradicts the proposition that the *bodies* of the old are dry.
>
> GALEN, *Temp.* 2.2 (I.580 K. = 45 Helmreich, trans. Singer and van der Eijk, p. 110)

> … each disposition (διαθέσεως), too, will have two versions, one arising from the wet or dry fluids (χυμοῖς), the other from the bodies themselves, in the case where the solid bodies reach the same state of bad-mixture (δυσκρασίας) as the fluids (ὑγροῖς).
>
> GALEN, *Loc. Aff.* 3.6 (VIII.163 K.)

3.2 *Galen versus the Others*

It is not only that Galen insists on this kind of analysis; such an analysis also provides a bone of contention between him and rival ancient physicians, in particular the Methodists but also others who insist, rather, on talking of states of the whole body and *not* of the part affected. In the following passages we may observe such arguments advanced by Methodists both *in propria persona* and through the lens of Galen's criticism. (A much fuller and more nuanced account of the Methodists' views in this area is given by David Leith, in chapter 5 above.)

> Soranus ... states that the *whole body* is troubled by the ailment (*passione*) [*sc. peripneumonia*], but the lung more violently ... [Such an enquiry] is useless from the point of view of cure, since this is in no way compromised by a lack of precise knowledge of locations, for it is the whole body which we feel to suffer. Nor should the nature of the remedies be altered in relation to the place affected; this should remain the same as long as the disease itself remains.
>
> CAELIUS AURELIANUS, *Acute Diseases* 2.28.147–48 (232 Bendz)

> [In *insania*] the entire nervous apparatus (*nervositas*) suffers (*patitur*) ... but the head suffers more (*magis*) ...
>
> CAELIUS AURELIANUS, *Chronic Diseases* 1.5.152 (520 Bendz)

> [A Methodist:] Why should one consider the parts of the body? Are these not valueless for the indication of treatment? ... Since the nature of the part does not in any way alter the mode of treatment ... consideration of the part will, obviously, be pointless.
>
> GALEN, *Sects for Beginners* (*SI*) 7 (I.86–87 K. = 18 Helmreich)

The Methodists are well known to have reduced all illnesses to certain commonalities (*koinotētes*), understood in terms of constriction or looseness. Evidence such as the above suggests that they went further and insisted on these commonalities as states of the whole body rather than of specific locations. Soranus (first century BCE/CE), or Caelius Aurelianus (fifth century CE), is prepared to admit of a part which suffers *more*, or more violently. But at the same time there is a resistance to the notion of the *locus affectus* as such, and an insistence that even the notion of a part which *patitur magis* is irrelevant to treatment. This insistence may seem odds with another well-known feature of Methodist medicine, namely the presentation of diseases, in the texts, in a 'head-to-toe' order. The Methodist view appears to be that local manifestations of an illness are relevant features, of value for diagnosis, but that all diseases are nevertheless diseases of the whole body, and must be treated accordingly.

Another view of interest in this connection is that of Celsus. By contrast with the Methodists, Celsus does not insist on the non-local nature of diseases in general. He does, however, define a specific category of diseases as being, precisely, diseases of the body as a whole, rather than arising in particular parts.[27]

---

27 For further discussion of Celsus' diagnostic divisions, see now Thumiger and Singer (2018) 7–15.

> I shall divide all [*sc.* diseases] into those which appear to subsist in the body as a whole (*in totis corporibus consistere videntur*) and those which arise in particular parts (*oriuntur in partibus*).
>
> CELSUS 3.1 (101 Marx)

For Celsus, then, not all diseases, but an important subset of them, are without specific location. This subset includes both fevers – that most prominent, indeed almost omnipresent, entity in ancient medicine – and mental aberrations, ailments of the soul.

An interesting consideration here is that the notion that either mental aberrations of a certain kind or fevers might be defined as diseases of the whole body is one that Galen could in principle largely have agreed with. In the case of the medical psychic impairments, especially those involving paralysis or lethargy, the condition as Galen describes it certainly has a powerful effect on the whole body.[28] And with fevers too we seem to have a condition which involves the whole body: he tells us, indeed, that the cause of fever is that a pathological level of heat has become extended through the body as a whole.[29] It is striking, then, that he nevertheless does not *explicitly* conceptualize, as Celsus does (and as Caelius and the Methodists do in a much more sweeping way) the notion of diseases, or of certain diseases, being 'of the whole body.'

In any case, we have seen clear limitations to Galenic (b)-type holism: in certain contexts, at least, it is important to insist on precise location *against* opposing notions of diseases as belonging to the body as a whole. And – to touch again briefly on the evaluative point – we may very well find this limitation a positive thing: it would surely be difficult to deny that, in at least some medical contexts, precise knowledge of the location and physiology involved in a disease is, to put it at its mildest, something worth having. On the other hand, to what extent does Galen really operate such a precise, local analysis? It is, perhaps, enlightening to consider the polemical or competitive context. To what end does Galen spend so long in *Affected Places* and elsewhere insisting on detailed knowledge of internal parts, of physiology, of the *locus affectus* – and how much difference does it make in practice?

Let us consider one particular case upon which Galen expends a lot of energy, both in *Affected Places* and elsewhere, namely the importance of understanding that the brain is the location of mental or psychological

28 See e.g. *Symp. Diff.* (VII.58–59 K. = 221–22 Gundert), with the discussion of Singer (2018) 388–40.

29 *Caus. Morb.* 2 (VII.4 K.).

aberrations – those, precisely, of the *hēgemonikon* or leading-faculty of the soul. Galen recurs to this theme often and at considerable length.

> The fact that all ailments of the leading activities (τὰ τῶν ἡγεμονικῶν ἐνεργειῶν πάθη) arise in the brain is agreed by all doctors, as long as they do not think one thing in their soul but say another, as the result of the argumentative compulsion of a sect ... such argumentativeness ... is unforgiveable amongst those with long experience in medical matters. For they bathe the head in all cases of infirmity arising from sleeplessness, as also in all cases of delirium, *phrenitis* and *lēthargos*. Archigenes applies medicaments to the head in cases of damage to the memory, too ...
>
> GALEN, *Loc. Aff.* 3.7 (VIII.166–67 K.)

How crazy and incoherent, cries Galen, are his rival physicians, those who claim in theory to believe that the seat of the soul is the heart, but then when an ailment of the soul comes along apply their remedies to the head! Archigenes is a particular butt of this polemic. Why on earth do he and others apply remedies – embrocations, in particular – to the head if the head is not the seat of the illness in question? And of course we may very well feel that Galen – even if he does undoubtedly over-egg his pudding – is on pretty solid ground here. Yet it is at least arguable, as Orly Lewis has suggested, that it is Galen who is distorting the picture: that he is representing a whole repertory of traditional remedies as 'directed towards the brain', which are in fact better understood as, precisely, part of a (b)-type holistic approach which sought to heat or cool the whole body.[30] It seems, moreover, highly probable that he is borrowing strongly from precisely those physicians with whom he claims to have a strong theoretical opposition. That is to say, he may very well be strongly indebted to Archigenes for the actual range and choice of remedies used. That, of course, does not in itself affect the validity or invalidity of his claim; but one should at least consider the counter-argument that the fact that some (though by no means all) remedies were applied to the head in such cases need not entail any particular view on the location of the *hēgemonikon* – either on Galen's part or on that of his rivals. The underlying principle might be, precisely, one which views psychological aberration and its treatment as implicating the body *as a whole*.

But let us consider the Galenic approach more broadly. We have seen evidence of his insistence on the identification of the *locus affectus*, and on a distinction between solid structures and fluids or residues. Yet, again, when

30 See Lewis (2018).

we come to practice, most of Galen's actual interventions – diet, drugs, venesection – seem to be addressed towards an alteration of the state of the body as a whole. One must of course make certain exceptions, e.g. for the treatment of wounds; and one must consider seriously some of the specifications made in *Affected Places* already observed. Still, one is left with a suspicion that some of Galen's most precise specifications of the part of the body affected, and the aetiology by which this affects other parts or structures, are not followed up in very great detail or may not have very profound consequences for actual therapy. The suspicion may, indeed, arise that such specifications are motivated at least partly by polemical rather than practical considerations – that is to say, by Galen's desire to distinguish himself ideologically from the Methodists and, more generally, to assert the superior level of his own detailed knowledge of the internal structures and functioning of the human body.

Certainly, Galen insists that one must tailor interventions specifically to the *individual* nature, with particular attention to a person's natural endowments, previous habits, age, etc.; and all these factors receive a great deal of attention in *Matters of Health*. But considerations arising from distinctions between different parts or functions within the body receive much less. The following passage on old age summarizes Galen's approach through much of this work, and indeed elsewhere.

> One should, in all cases, attempt correction through the opposing imbalance. Age, itself, is cold and dry ... Its correction takes place through those things which moisten and heat, such as hot baths ... the drinking of wine ...
>
> GALEN, *San. Tu.* 5.3 (VI.319 K. = 141 Koch)

It seems to me that this approach – essentially consistent with our (b)-type holism – is fairly representative of much of Galen's practice.

3.3 *Further Aspects of Galenic Holism: Diagnosis, Fever, Pulse*

A little should be said concerning the further sub-distinction, suggested at the outset, between (b1)- and (b2)-type holism. In particular, one might want to argue for (b1)-type holism – the strong diagnostic relevance of features observed throughout the whole body – while holding to a much less holistic view with regard to the location and treatment of a disease. Two things seem particularly relevant, here, in relation to Galen. One is that he certainly would wish to claim – again in a way strongly indebted to the Hippocratic tradition – that a whole range of factors, observable in different parts of the body, and by different senses, are potentially relevant to diagnosis. The extended account of the *facies Hippocratica* and other fatal signs in the *Commentary on Hippocrates' Prognostic*, combining the Hippocratic tradition with Galen's own claims to both precise and wide-ranging observation, provides a particularly pertinent, and rich, example.[31] The other is to consider the centrality of the pulse, as a diagnostic and prognostic tool, on the one hand, and on the other of fever as a disease category, within Galen's medical thought and practice.

The pulse is a diagnostic indicator that both belongs to the whole body – it can in principle be taken anywhere in the body, as Galen himself emphasizes – and reveals information about the state of the body as a whole. Now, it is of course true that certain specific types of pulse, taken in conjunction with other diagnostic indicators, will help identify particular, localized ailments. But it is also true that fever (as the object of diagnosis) is almost as prominent in Galen as pulse (as the tool of diagnosis): the two may in a sense be seen as counterparts. So, for example, in that work which functions as both advertisement and summary by Galen of his own clinical practice, *Prognosis*, it is above all – leaving aside considerations 'external' to the art[32] – the pulse which Galen presents as the focus of his diagnostic skill. And, in terms of diseases described, it is – leaving aside certain psychogenic pathological states – fever that appears as the central diagnostic category. This twin dominance of pulse and fever is then further reinforced by the particular works of his own to which Galen points us in this work: the series of works on the pulse, and the treatises *Crises*, *Critical Days* and *Distinct Types of Fever*.[33] Between them these explicate the diagnostic or semiotic 'science' of which he has, in *Prognosis*, given practical exemplification.

And indeed, the above groups of works occupy a central place in Galen's diagnostic and clinical output. Given that the pulse is a diagnostic indicator

---

31 *Hipp. Prog.* 1.5–42 (XVIIIB.22–109 K. = 209–58 Heeg). Especially relevant here are the fact that the specific bodily features observed in the face enable one to infer facts about the state of the body as a whole; and the fact that other signs, arising in different parts of the body (e.g. sleeplessness, loose bowels, hunger, XVIIIB.32 K. = 214 Heeg; the pulse, XVIIIB.38 K. = 217 Heeg; delirious hallucinations, XVIIIB.71–75 K. = 236–38 Heeg; respiration, XVIIIB.76–77 K. = 238–39 Heeg) are brought in to confirm or clarify the diagnosis arising from observation of the face. Indeed, Galen *explicitly* emphasizes the connection between signs from the face and those from the rest of the body at XVIIIB.55–56 K. = 227 Heeg.

32 Galen's own term (ἔξωθεν) at *Prognosis by the Pulse* (*Praes. Puls.*) 1.1 (IX.216 K.).

33 These latter works are mentioned as crucial at *Praen.* 9–10 (XIV.651–52 K. = 120 Nutton and XIV.657 K. = 126 Nutton) and ch. 12 (XIV.664 K. = 132 Nutton); the pulse works at 14 (XIV.671 K. = 138–40 Nutton).

of the whole-body state, and that fevers are, as we have suggested, whole-body illnesses, this emphasis in Galen's writing again supports a strong sense of both (2a)- and (2b)-type holism.

3.4 *Summary*

Here again, it would be difficult to deny that a somewhat complex picture has emerged. Undoubtedly, certain other doctors or medical schools emphasize the whole-body approach to health and disease more strongly and more explicitly than does Galen; and in some contexts that represents an explicit point on which he attacks them. It is also true that – again in certain contexts – the *locus affectus* is of central importance to Galen's argument. But it also seems to be true that we lose much if we ignore the polemical aspect of that argument; and that, in terms of actual interventions and dietary recommendations, what Galen offers tends toward a model in which he to quite a large extent conceptualizes health, as well as disease, diagnosis and treatment, in relation to the body as a whole.

4 One-with-the-Cosmos Holism

We as human beings are part of, and composed of the same fundamental elements as, the world around us. In a sense, of course, this is obvious. But Galenic (like most varieties of Hippocratic) medicine arguably makes the connection closer and more palpable. It does this in two ways especially. First, it emphasizes the essential qualitative identity of our bodies with simpler organisms and other objects in the outside world: both within our bodies and outside them, the hot, cold, wet and dry are not only the ultimate, but also very frequently the clinically most relevant, constituents. The transition from talk of the heat or dryness of our bodies to talk of those same qualities in plants, meats, drugs, etc., is – as we have already observed in *Mixtures* and *Matters of Health*, to which could be added *The Properties of Foodstuffs* – a seamless one. Secondly, it emphasizes the fundamental importance to health and ill-health of the immediate environment, in the sense of the seasons and the ambient air.

So much seems clear; and this embeddedness of human natures within their biological and meteorological environment undoubtedly provides one of the stronger senses in which the term 'holistic' may reasonably be applied to the ancient medical discourse.

Grander, or more elevated, accounts of the sense in which we are 'one with the cosmos' are offered by the philosophical and ethical, rather than strictly medical, tradition. For example, the notion of our fundamental oneness with nature, our connectedness with the cosmos, is a key feature of Stoic thought. This can be understood both in terms of our physical or environmental nature (we function within and should take account of the larger ecological entity) and our nature as rational beings (our rational nature provides a connection with the universe as a whole, which is to be understood as a rationally ordered entity).[34]

Such considerations may at first sight seem less relevant to our enquiry. But in at least one context Galen does want to insist strongly on our connectedness with the universe, conceived in terms of a higher or transcendent rationality:

> What part of the cosmos could be of less worth than the earthly one? And yet even here, some intelligence arrives from the heavenly bodies – bodies whose contemplation leads one at once to wonder at the beauty of their substance, of the sun … of the moon … of the stars.… just as the substance (οὐσία) of their bodies is purer (καθερωτέρα), there exists an intelligence which is to precisely that same degree better and more complete. When we see that in slime, in mud, in marshes, or in rotting plants and fruits, there nonetheless arise animals which provide a wonderful indication of the intelligence that constructs them (τοῦ κατασκεύσαντος αὐτὰ νοῦ), what must one think is the case of the heavenly bodies? … it seems to me that a considerable intelligence is extended (οὐκ ὀλίγος τις ἐκτετάσθαι δοκεῖ νοῦς) even through the actual air that surrounds us; it would not otherwise be able by nature to partake of the sun's ray nor of its power.
>
> GALEN, *On the Function of the Parts of the Body* (*UP*) 17.1 (IV.358–60 K. = ii.446–47 Helmreich)

Galen is here talking in terms which have strong Platonist echoes, although there is, certainly, a distinct lack of precision in the theory as expounded here.[35]

34 Recent scholarship on Stoicism has emphasized these features both as central elements of Stoicism and as ones which can be attractively interpreted within a twenty-first century worldview. See e.g. Gill (2014), as well as https://modernstoicism.com/#_ednref25.

35 Fundamental to the study of this text is Frede (2003), who, while admitting the 'tantalizingly vague' (111) nature of Galen's remarks, also explores in depth their connections with other late antique philosophical and scientific views, and shows how Galen is here asserting the all-pervasive explanatory power of the sun in the physical universe, as well as its causal relationship with the Demiurgic intellect, on the one hand, and the composition of bodies and their fundamental elements, on the other. (Some aspects of Galen's relationship with Platonists of his time are also discussed by Singer (2014).) A broader point of relevance to our argument, though it cannot be considered further here, is the sense in which Neoplatonist thought may itself be understood as holistic (rather than, as

But it seems to me that there is a profound sense in which what is in play here is another form of holism – one again belonging within our type (c), and one to which Galen, even if he is unclear about the metaphysical detail, profoundly subscribes. That is, the sense in which our intelligence, or indeed the intelligence of any being on the earth – to the extent that it has intelligence – connects us with the stars, with the divine intelligence. That may not be something that Galen, or any medical author, is prepared to elaborate in detail; but some such account is, in fact, central simultaneously to Galen's teleological and to his physical world view.

Moreover, it is possible to bring things down to earth a little. There is, as we have already seen, (c)-type holism in the sense of the fundamental continuity between our own, human natures and that of the rest of the natural world. But there is a further point, too. Galen understands human beings as belonging, in both physical and epistemological terms, at the centre of the universe. It is not just that we represent a sort of optimal or central case of the mixture which also accounts for the composition of all things in the natural world. It is simultaneously the case that this central position of human beings within the cosmos has consequences for the role of our rationality within the universe. Human beings are ideally constructed and positioned to observe and evaluate everything else in the natural world.[36]

So, in fact, a proper understanding of our cosmic nature – of the way in which both our rationality and our physicality are connected with those of the universe as a whole – is central, not just to Galen's theological views but also to his scientific project. It is some such account – a cosmically holistic account, if you like – which explains how it is that we are able to discuss these matters rationally in the first place; to engage successfully in the project of observation, analysis and diagnosis; to conceptualize and take care of our health.

Acknowledgments

I am grateful to Chiara Thumiger for the invitation to participate in the conference 'Ancient Holisms' in London in 2017, as well as to the participants at that event for helpful and congenial interaction. I also express my gratitude to the

it typically is, dualistic), because of the fundamental understanding of Intellect and Soul as explanatory principles that pervade the entire cosmos, including the biological and human world.

36 For Galen's assertion of both points, see esp. *Temp.* 1.9 (I.563–65 K. = 34–35 Helmreich), with the notes of Singer and van der Eijk (2018) ad loc.

Wellcome Trust, by which I was funded for the research project within which the present paper took shape.

Bibliography

Adamson, P., Hansberger, R. and Wilberding, J. (eds.) *Philosophical Themes in Galen. Bulletin of the Institute of Classical Studies* Supplement 114. London: Institute of Classical Studies (2014).

Ahonen, M. 'Making the Distinction: the Stoic View of Mental Illness.' In *Mental Illness in Ancient Medicine: from Celsus to Paul of Aegina, Studies in Ancient Medicine* 50, ed. C. Thumiger and P. N. Singer. Leiden: Brill (2018) 343–62.

Barnes, J., J. Jouanna and V. Barras (eds.) *Galien et la philosophie: huit exposés suivis de discussions. Entretiens sur l'antiquité classique* 49. Vandoeuvres: Fondation Hardt (2003).

Coughlin, S. 'Athenaeus of Attalia on the Psychological Causes of Bodily Health.' In *Mental Illness in Ancient Medicine: from Celsus to Paul of Aegina*. Studies in Ancient Medicine 50, ed. C. Thumiger and P. N. Singer. Leiden: Brill (2018) 109–42.

Devinant, J. 'Mental Disorders and Psychological Suffering in Galen's Cases.' In *Mental Illness in Ancient Medicine: from Celsus to Paul of Aegina*, Studies in Ancient Medicine 50, ed. C. Thumiger and P. N. Singer. Leiden: Brill (2018) 198–221.

Donini, P.-L. 'Psychology.' In *The Cambridge Companion to Galen*, ed. R. J. Hankinson. Cambridge: Cambridge University Press (2008) 184–209.

Frede, M. 'Galen's Theology.' In *Galien et la philosophie: huit exposés suivis de discussions. Entretiens sur l'antiquité classique* 49, ed. J. Barnes, J. Jouanna and V. Barras. Vandoeuvres: Fondation Hardt (2003) 73–129.

Gill, C. *Naturalistic Psychology in Galen and Stoicism*. Oxford: Oxford University Press (2010).

Gill, C. 'Introduction.' In *Epictetus: The Discourses*. Trans. R. Hard. Oxford: Oxford University Press (2014).

Grimaudo, S. *Difendere la Salute: Igiene e Disciplina del Soggetto nel De Sanitate Tuenda di Galeno*. Elenchos: A Collection of Texts and Studies on Ancient Philosophy 49. Palermo: Bibliopolis (2008).

Gundert, B. 'Soma and Pysche in Hippocratic Medicine.' In *Psyche and Soma: Physicians and Metaphysicians on the Mind–Body Problem from Antiquity to Enlightenment*, ed. J. P. Wright and P. Potter. Oxford: Oxford University Press (2000) 13–35.

Hankinson, R. J. 'Galen's Anatomy of the Soul.' *Phronesis*, 36 (1991a) 197–233.

Hankinson, R. J. 'Greek Medical Models of Mind.' In *Psychology, Companions to Ancient Thought* 2, ed. S. Everson. Cambridge: Cambridge University Press (1991b) 194–217.

Hankinson, R. J. 'Actions and Passions: Affection, Emotion and Moral Self-Management in Galen's Philosophical Psychology.' In *Passions and Perceptions: Studies in Hellenistic Philosophy of Mind*, ed. J. Brunschwig and M. Nussbaum. Cambridge: Cambridge University Press (1993) 184–222.

Hankinson, R. J. 'Body and Soul in Galen.' In *Common to Body and Soul: Philosophical Approaches to Explaining Living Behaviour in Greco-Roman Antiquity*, ed. R. A. H. King. Berlin: De Gruyter (2006) 232–58.

Hankinson, R. J. (ed.) *The Cambridge Companion to Galen*. Cambridge: Cambridge University Press (2008).

Havrda, M. 'Body and Cosmos in Galen's Account of the Soul.' *Phronesis*, 62 (2017) 69–89.

Johnston, I. (trans. with introduction) *Galen on Diseases and Symptoms*. Cambridge: Cambridge University Press (2006).

Julião, R. 'Galen on Memory, Forgetting and Memory Loss.' In *Mental Illness in Ancient Medicine: from Celsus to Paul of Aegina*, Studies in Ancient Medicine 50, ed. C. Thumiger and P. N. Singer. Leiden: Brill (2018) 222–44.

Kaufman, D. H. 'Galen on the Therapy of Distress and the Limits of Emotional Therapy.' *Oxford Studies in Ancient Philosophy*, 47 (2014) 275–96.

Lewis, O. 'Archigenes of Apamea's Treatment of Mental Diseases.' In *Mental Illness in Ancient Medicine: from Celsus to Paul of Aegina*. Studies in Ancient Medicine 50, ed. C. Thumiger and P. N. Singer. Leiden: Brill (2018) 143–75.

Lloyd, G. E. R. 'Scholarship, Authority and Argument in Galen's Quod animi mores.' In *Le Opere Psicologiche di Galeno: Atti del Terzo Colloquio Galenico Internazionale, Pavia, 10–12 settembre 1986*, ed. P. Manuli and M. Vegetti. Naples: Bibliopolis (1988) 11–42.

Manuli, P. 'La passione nel De placitis Hippocratis et Platonis.' In *Le Opere Psicologiche di Galeno: Atti del Terzo Colloquio Galenico Internazionale, Pavia, 10–12 settembre 1986*, ed. P. Manuli and M. Vegetti, M. Naples: Bibliopolis (1988) 185–214.

Manuli, P. and Vegetti, M. (eds.) *Le Opere Psicologiche di Galeno: Atti del Terzo Colloquio Galenico Internazionale, Pavia, 10–12 settembre 1986*. Naples: Bibliopolis (1988).

McDonald, G. C. 'The "locus affectus" in Ancient Medical Theories of Disease.' In *Medicine and Space: Body, Surroundings and Borders in Antiquity and the Middle Ages*. Visualising the Middle Ages 4, ed. P. A. Baker, H. Nijdam and K. van 't Land. Leiden: Brill (2011) 63–83.

Petit, C. (ed.) *Galen's Treatise* Περὶ ἀλυπίας *(De indolentia) in Context: A Tale of Resilience. Studies in Ancient Medicine* 52. Leiden: Brill (2019).

Petridou, G. and Thumiger, C. (eds.) *Homo Patiens: Approaches to the Patient in the Ancient World*. Studies in Ancient Medicine 45. Leiden: Brill (2015).

Polito, R. 'Competence Conflicts between Philosophy and Medicine: Caelius Aurelianus and the Stoics on Mental Diseases.' *Classical Quarterly*, NS 66 (2016) 358–69.

Singer, P. N. 'Some Hippocratic Mind–Body Problems.' In *Tratados Ipocraticos: Estudios acerca de su Contenido, Forma E Influencia: Actas del VIIe Colloque International Hippocratique*, ed. J. A. López Férez. Madrid: Universidad Nacional de Educación a Distancia (1992) 131–43.

Singer, P. N. (ed.) *Galen: Psychological Writings. Avoiding Distress; Character Traits; The Affection and Errors Peculiar to Each Person's Soul; The Capacities of the Soul Depend on the Mixtures of the Body*, translated with introductions and notes by V. Nutton, D. Davies and P. N. Singer, with the collaboration of P. Tassinari. Cambridge: Cambridge University Press (2013).

Singer, P. N. 'Galen and the Philosophers: Philosophical Engagement, Shadowy Contemporaries, Aristotelian Transformations.' In *Philosophical Themes in Galen. Bulletin of the Institute of Classical Studies* Supplement 114, ed. P. Adamson, R. Hansberger and J. Wilberding. London: Institute of Classical Studies (2014) 7–38.

Singer, P. N. 'The Essence of Rage: Galen on Emotional Disturbances and their Physical Correlates.' In *Selfhood and the Soul: Essays on Ancient Thought and Literature in Honour of Christopher Gill*, ed. R. Seaford, J. Wilkins and M. Wright. Oxford: Oxford University Press (2017) 161–96.

Singer, P. N. 'Galen's Pathological Soul: Diagnosis and Therapy in Ethical and Medical Texts and Contexts.' In *Mental Illness in Ancient Medicine: from Celsus to Paul of Aegina*. Studies in Ancient Medicine 50, ed. C. Thumiger and P. N. Singer. Leiden: Brill (2018) 381–420.

Singer, P. N. 'A New Distress: Galen's Ethics in Peri Alupias and Beyond.' In *Galen's Treatise* Περὶ ἀλυπίας *(De indolentia) in Context: A Tale of Resilience*. Studies in Ancient Medicine 52, ed. C. Petit. Leiden: Brill (2019) 180–98.

Singer, P. N. 'Galen on Pneuma: Between Metaphysical Speculation and Anatomical Theory.' In *Pneuma After Aristotle*, ed. S. Coughlin, D. Leith and O. Lewis. Berlin: Edition Topoi (forthcoming a).

Singer, P. N. 'What is a Pathos? Where Medicine meets Philosophy.' In *Medical Understandings of Emotions*, Ancient Emotions 2, ed. G. Kazantzidis and D. Spatharas. Berlin: De Gruyter (forthcoming b).

Singer, P. N., and P. J. van der Eijk. *Galen: Works on Human Nature, vol. I: Mixtures (De Temperamentis), Translated with Introduction and Notes*. Cambridge: Cambridge University Press (2018).

Thumiger, C. 'The Early Greek Medical Vocabulary of Insanity.' In *Mental Disorders in the Classical World*. Columbia Studies in the Classical Tradition 38, ed. W. V. Harris. Leiden: Brill (2013).

Thumiger, C. *A History of the Mind and Mental Health in Classical Greek Medical Thought*. Cambridge: Cambridge University Press (2017).

Thumiger, C., and P. N. Singer (eds.) *Mental Illness in Ancient Medicine: from Celsus to Paul of Aegina*. Studies in Ancient Medicine 50. Leiden: Brill (2018).

Tieleman, T. 'Galen's Psychology.' In *Galien et la philosophie: huit exposés suivis de discussions*. Entretiens sur l'antiquité classique 49, ed. J. Barnes, J. Jouanna and V. Barras. Vandoeuvres: Fondation Hardt (2003) 131–69.

Vegetti, M. 'Tradition and Truth: Forms of Philosophical–Scientific Historiography in Galen's De placitis.' In *Ancient Histories of Medicine: Essays in Medical Doxography and Historiography in Classical Antiquity*, ed. P. J. van der Eijk. Leiden: Brill (1999) 333–57.

Von Staden, H. 'Body, Soul, and Nerves: Epicurus, Herophilus, Erasistratus, the Stoics, and Galen.' In *Psyche and Soma: Physicians and Metaphysicians on the Mind–Body Problem from Antiquity to Enlightenment*, ed. J. P. Wright and P. Potter. Oxford: Oxford University Press (2000) 79–116.

Von Staden, H. 'The Physiology and Therapy of Anger: Galen on Medicine, the Soul, and Nature.' In *Islamic Philosophy, Science, Culture, and Religion: Studies in Honor of Dimitri Gutas*, ed. F. Opwis and D. Reisman. Leiden: Brill (2011) 63–87.

Wilkins, J. M. 'Treatment of the Man: Galen's Preventive Medicine in the De sanitate tuenda.' In *Homo Patiens: Approaches to the Patient in the Ancient World*, Studies in Ancient Medicine 45, ed. G. Petridou and C. Thumiger. Leiden: Brill (2015) 411–31.

Wright, J. P., and P. Potter (eds.) *Psyche and Soma: Physicians and Metaphysicians on the Mind – Body Problem from Antiquity to Enlightenment*. Oxford: Oxford University Press (2000).

Websites

https://modernstoicism.com (accessed 7 October 2020)

http://humanities.exeter.ac.uk/history/research/centres/medicalhistory/projects/healthcareandwellbeing/ (accessed 7 October 2020)

Primary Texts: Editions and Translations Used

Aretaeus. Ed. C. Hude, CMG II (1923/1958)

Caelius Aurelianus. *Acute Diseases* and *Chronic Diseases*. Ed. G. Bendz (with German translation by I. Pape). CML VI 1, 2 vols. (1990/1993). Ed. and trans. I. E. Drabkin, *Caelius Aurelianus On Acute Diseases and On Chronic Diseases*. Chicago: Chicago University Press (1950).

Celsus. *De Medicina*. Ed. F. Marx, CML I (1915). Ed. and trans. W. G. Spencer, 3 vols. Loeb Classical Library. Cambridge MA: Harvard University Press (1935/1938).

Galen. *Affected Places* (= *Loc. Aff.*). In K. VIII. Books 1 and 2 ed. F. Gärtner, CMG V 6,1,1 (2015).

Galen. *Affections and Errors of the Soul* (= *Aff. Pecc. Dig.* 1 and 2). In K. V. Ed. W. de Boer, CMG V 4,1,1 (1937). Trans. in Singer (2013).

Galen. *Avoiding Distress* (= *Ind.*) Ed. V. Boudon-Millot and J. Jouanna, with A. Pietrobelli, *Ne pas se chagriner*, Paris: Les Belles Lettres (2010). Trans. V. Nutton in Singer (2013).
Galen. *Causes of Diseases* (= *Caus. Morb.*). In K. VII. Trans. in Johnston (2006).
Galen. *Causes of Symptoms* (= *Caus. Symp.*). In K. VII. Trans. in Johnston (2006).
Galen. *Commentary on Hippocrates' Aphorisms* (= *Hipp. Aph.*). In K. XVIIIA. Book 6 ed. C. Savino, CMG V 12,6 (2020).
Galen. *Commentary on Hippocrates' Epidemics VI*. In K. XVIIA–B (partial). Ed. including German translation of surviving Arabic portion E. Wenkebach and F. Pfaff, CMG V 10,2,2 (1956).
Galen. *Commentary on Hippocrates' Prognostic* (= *Hipp. Prog.*). In K. XVIIIB. Ed. J. Heeg CMG, V 9,2 (1915).
Galen. *Commentary on Hippocrates' Nature of the Human Being* (= *HNH*). In K. XV. Ed. J. Mewaldt, CMG V 9,1 (1914).
Galen. *Distinctions in Diseases* (= *Morb. Diff.*). In K. VII. Trans. in Johnston (2006).
Galen. *Distinctions in Symptoms* (= *Symp. Diff.*). In K. VII. Ed. B. Gundert, CMG V 5,1 (2009). Trans. in Johnston (2006).
Galen. *On the Function of the Parts of the Body* (= *UP*). In K. III–IV. Ed. G. Helmreich, *Galeni De usu partium*, 2 vols., Leipzig: Teubner (1907/1909). Trans. M. T. May, *Galen On the Usefulness of the Parts of the Body*, 2 vols. Ithaca: Cornell University Press (1968).
Galen. *Matters of Health* (= *San. Tu.*). In K. VI. Ed. K. Koch, CMG V 4,2 (1923). Trans. I. Johnston, *Galen: Hygiene*, 2 vols. Loeb Classical Library. Cambridge MA: Harvard University Press (2017/2018).
Galen. *Mixtures* (= *Temp.*). In K. I. Ed. G. Helmreich, *Galeni De temperamentis libri III*. Leipzig: Teubner (1904). Trans. in Singer and van der Eijk (2018).
Galen. *Prognosis* (= *Praen.*). In K. XIV. Ed. with English translation V. Nutton, CMG V 8,1 (1979).
Galen. *Prognosis by the Pulse* (= *Praes. Puls*). In K. IX.
Galen. *Sects for Beginners* (= *SI*). In K. I. Ed. G. Helmreich, *Claudii Galeni Pergameni Scripta minora*, vol. III. Leipzig: Teubner (1893). Trans. in M. Frede and R. Walzer, *Galen: Three Treatises on the Nature of Science*. Indianapolis: Hackett (1985).
Galen. *The Soul's Dependence on the Body* (= *QAM*). In K. IV. Ed. A. Bazou, Γαληνοῦ Ὅτι ταῖς τοῦ σώματος κράσεσιν αἱ τῆς ψυχῆς δυνάμεις ἕπονται. Athens: Academy of Athens (2011). Trans. in Singer (2013).
Galen. *Thrasybulus* (= *Thras.*). In K. V. Ed. G. Helmreich, *Claudii Galeni Pergameni Scripta Minora*, vol. III. Leipzig: Teubner (1893).
Plutarch. *Precepts for Health*. Ed. and trans. F. C. Babbitt, *Plutarch: Moralia*, vol. II. Loeb Classical Library. Cambridge MA: Harvard University Press (1928).
Soranus. *Gynaecology*. Ed. J. Ilberg, *Sorani Gynaeciorum libri IV*, CMG IV (1927).

CHAPTER 7

Holism of Body and Mind in Hippocratic Medicine and Greek Tragedy

Elizabeth Craik

Abstract

It is contended that ancient Greek medicine is fundamentally 'holistic' in the literal sense that it views the human organism as a complete mental and somatic unity; and it is further argued that these ideas are not purely medical but are rooted in early Greek language and thought: a systemic and synoptic view of the body in health and disease and of the mind in order and disorder can be traced in many texts of creative as well as medical writers. It is seen that the most vital physical organs (concrete) identified by different Hippocratic authors coincide and correspond with the very same bodily parts that are associated by the Attic tragedians with significant (abstract) mental and emotional activity. Through a close analysis of terminology in plays including Aeschylus' *Prometheus Bound* and Euripides' *Hippolytos* a new understanding of usage is reached. Terms discussed include *kardia*, *thymos*, *phrenes*, *hepar*, *myelos* and *psyche*.

1 Preamble: Views of Holism; Stance Adopted in this Study

The popular modern, often somewhat vague, use of the term 'holistic' to delineate a range of medical ideas and procedures perceived to take an unconventional approach to the whole body need not concern us here. The designation, in common with the terms 'alternative' or 'complementary' with which it is often loosely associated, tends to have a pejorative tone in the discourse of professional medical practitioners, who find all these 'alternative' methods 'unscientific', that is to say without a scientific basis in observation and testing; though conversely such terms may be strongly commendatory in the parlance of the minority who pursue them. Modern advocates of methods such as those followed in homeopathy – homeopathy in particular with its avowedly Greek roots – frequently lay claim to ancient authority for their views. It might be contended that all of modern medicine, including its more 'scientific' branches, has roots in the *techne* ('art', 'craft') of the ancients; but this debate is too wide to be pursued here. In more standard modern medical usage, a 'holistic' view

 | DOI:10.1163/9789004443143_009

of the patient – based on a wide interpretation of *holos* ('whole') – is commonly understood to take cognizance of external factors, including social and economic considerations, as well as of disease and physical conditions. In the analysis of ancient evidence presented in this chapter, 'holistic' is interpreted in a more restricted literal sense, without reference to peripheral or extraneous concerns arising from the general circumstances of the patient.

At the same time, the internal personal condition of the individual is here considered in its entirety: not only all physical elements but also, in conjunction with these, total psychological makeup – including emotional charge – is regarded as relevant. It is contended that ancient Greek medicine is fundamentally 'holistic' in this particular literal sense, in that it views the human organism as a complete mental and somatic unity. It is argued in this chapter that these ideas are not purely medical, but are rooted in Greek language and thought. Seen already in Homeric epic, they come to penetrate and permeate general intellectual discourse, with the result that, in common with Hippocratic medicine, Attic tragedy of the fifth century views the human organism in holistic terms: all bodily parts are thought to be inter-related and, further, body and mind are seen as inseparable for both practical and theoretical purposes. Thus, throughout both medical and non-medical writing, a systemic and synoptic view of bodily disease and mental disorder is to be found. In the ensuing sections of the chapter, such a wide-ranging presentation of human existence, constitution and function, both physical and psychological, is identified and analysed in certain texts of medical and tragic writers.

2 Introduction: Interaction of Medicine and Tragedy; Ideas of Body and Mind

First, it is appropriate to contextualise, at least briefly, the arguments advanced here. Selective brevity is essential, as the bibliography of previous work on tragedy and medicine, a topic of long-standing scholarly interest, is vast;[1] and the bibliography of the relatively new subject of mind and body in medical and other texts is considerable and fast growing also.[2] The view, based on modern scholarly consensus, that mental or emotional disturbance may trigger a physical disorder and so present visible symptoms is implicit throughout this

1 See, for example, Guardasole (2000), Craik (2001) and Kosak (2004).

2 See the contributions of Gundert (2002), Cairns (2017) and Thumiger (2017); also Thumiger and Singer (2018). On the particular case of phrenitis, see McDonald (2009). On emotions, see Cairns and Nelis (2017); also Kazantzidis (forthcoming).

chapter. This study innovates in seeking to examine the presence and location of such symptoms (symptoms that render mental or emotional problems visible) in particular parts of the body, and to explore the significance of these parts through a close analysis of terminology. It innovates also in seeking to juxtapose and correlate the views expressed in medical and literary authors on the subject, with particular reference to tragedy. It is found that there is a remarkable coincidence between the key vital organs listed in several Hippocratic works (of manifestly different authorship) and the main bodily parts associated with mental activity or emotional function in different creative literary texts: significant coincident terms are *kardia*, *thymos*, *phrenes*, *hepar*, *myelos* and *psyche*. It is discovered that, in some cases, medical usage casts light on the underlying sense of poetic terminology and illumines nuance.

That there were close contacts and considerable interaction in many elements of the cultural and intellectual environment of classical Greece is indubitable. In small city-states, of which Athens was only one, writers and thinkers shared platforms, patronage and audiences. In addition, all Greek thought in life, literature and ideals drew, directly or indirectly, on Homeric epic, the much admired and habitually cited *fons et origo* of Greek education. Homer's formidable grasp of human anatomy has long been recognised; and, in particular, the knowledge displayed of which bodily parts were vital and which places, if sustaining wounds, would prove beyond cure, has been much remarked. This anatomical awareness was conjoined with ideas about the location of mental function in the physical body.[3] From this, it is readily apparent that fundamentally holistic views already prevailed even in the heroic age. These views are the common foundation of the various views explored in this chapter. In considering matters of life and death – fundamental to the mind-body conjunction – a pressing quest is identification and isolation of the physical location of consciousness. For this, we find a complex nexus of terms, in which *psyche* ('breath of life', 'soul'; but see further below) is dominant. The terms *kardia* ('heart') and *thymos* ('spirit'; but see further below) – anatomically of course distinct but alike located in the region of the *phrenes* ('midriff') – are in oral formulaic diction used almost interchangeably with reference to mental function. These terms of 'psychic organs', along with the term *psyche* itself, are a 'family rather than independent variables.'[4]

Before confining the discussion to medical and tragic texts, it is worth glancing at pre-Socratic ideas, a significant stepping-stone from Homeric to classical

3 See already Onians (1951).

4 For this terminology, see Cairns (2014), a valuable analysis of usage with full bibliography; see also Jahn (1987).

thought in medicine as well as in philosophy and in literature. Passages relevant to our concerns appear in debate attributed to Democritus on the location of perception and the senses in the *psyche* or the *nous* ('mind') or elsewhere (DK 68 A 33 = Diogenes 9. 45–49). Questions regarding the nature and the operation of connections between sense perception and intellectual cognition, fundamental to an understanding of the epistemology and biology of human understanding, constituted an ongoing medical debate.[5] Theories of the *psyche* are central to Plato's thought also: famously, the tripartite *psyche* delineated in *Republic* Book 4 contained the rational element with which we learn, the appetitive element concerned with desire, and – allied with but differentiated from the desirous or appetitive – the passionate element concerned with such emotions as anger. A rich vein of speculation is seen in *Timaeus*, where a wide-ranging debate on the formation and nature of the body extends to the nature, place and function of the mind within the body. Plato differentiated between illnesses involving the body and illnesses centred on the *psyche* (*Ti.* 86b 1–7); but at the same time viewed both as the proper concern of doctors, who nevertheless tended to ignore the *psyche* (156d).

That there was two-way influence between tragic and medical writers is readily demonstrable. The debt of tragedy to medicine is more commonly remarked than the converse: much has been written on the tragedians' familiarity with 'technical' terminology and the vocabulary of disease, little on the debt of medical writers to dramatic texts. However, as a corrective to this commonly held view that the direction of influence is principally from medical prose to tragic verse, we may note evident tragic elements in medical writing: in form, there is metrical patterning, including runs of quite complex lyric metres; in expression, there is use of poetic vocabulary and descriptive terms for aberrant states such as 'madness'; in content and tenor there is a common parallelism in presentation between case histories and tragic plots, seen in the pattern of medical *crisis* (turning point in disease leading to recovery or to deterioration) equivalent to tragic *peripeteia* (critical pivot in plot leading to a good or a bad outcome), also in the use of the term *hamartia* ('error') for both medical lapse and tragic flaw and the term *pathos* ('suffering') allied with death in both genres.[6]

Two particular examples may be given to illustrate the close character of mutual influence and interaction, the first of tragic content probably derived from medicine and the second of medical content apparently based on tragedy. Firstly, in Euripides' *Hippolytos*, produced in 428 BCE, the ideas expressed

5 See Lo Presti (2007).
6 See Craik (2015) 75 and 190.

by Phaedra's Nurse (declaring a contrast between the doctor, who has to take physical and mental pains to benefit the patient, and the patient, who is subject to physical pain only) are similar to those expressed at the beginning of the Hippocratic treatise *On Winds* (noting a contrast between the pains endured by the doctor and the benefits accruing to the patient); in addition, an indicative if not conclusive consideration, the language is markedly similar (E. *Hipp.* 186–89; [Hp.] *Flat.* 1 = VI.90 L). There may be a gnomic element in this parallel: the preamble of *On Winds* was much quoted in late antiquity by Christian as well as pagan writers.[7] Secondly, the author of the Hippocratic work *On Diseases* 4 describes the restricted geographical flourishing of the medical plant silphium in terms strongly reminiscent of Sophocles' description in *Oedipus Coloneus*, posthumously produced in 401 BCE, of the spontaneous generation of the olive on the acropolis of Athens ([Hp.] *Morb.* 4. 34 = VII.546 L.; S. *OC* 694–98).[8]

3 Medical Texts: Evidence of Holism

General holistic views can readily be identified in multifarious medical texts of different authorship and date, as well as in many Hippocratic works. It is evident that the conventional orthodoxy of disease aetiology and therapy is based on an essentially holistic view of the body: disease in its different manifestations is believed to have a common origin in flux from the belly to the head, with ensuing flux from the head to some affected bodily part. Treatment is considered to depend on the identification and elimination of matter regarded as excessive (typically too hot, too cold, too wet, or too dry) or as peccant (typically bilious or phlegmatic) in character, and on the restoration of overall bodily balance. To achieve this, the part affected, or alternatively the body as a whole, is treated by immediate expedients such as purging, in conjunction with longer-term measures such as digestive manipulation, to reduce or thin down the body.[9] Thus, attention to the particular *locus affectus*, the bodily part involved, is commonly combined with, or even subordinate to, general delocalised attention to the whole body. The fundamental idea of bodily intercommunication is given palmary, perhaps proverbial, expression in two very different texts, the practical medical vademecum *On Places in Man* and the theoretical anatomical treatise *On Bones* as follows: 'There is no beginning

7 See Anastassiou and Irmer (2006), pp. 251–52 and 255–57.

8 See Lonie (1981) *ad loc.*

9 The technical term for this procedure (*ischnainein*) occurs in Aristophanic comedy and general literary usage; see Craik (1998) 150.

in the body; but everything is alike beginning and end. For when a circle has been drawn its beginning is not to be found' (*Loc. Hom.* 1 = VI.276 L.; *Oss.* 11 = IX.182 L.). In a wide range of works – *Epidemics; On Places in Man; On Diseases in Women; On Regimen; On the Nature of Man* – we find both substantival and adjectival corroboration that a holistic view of bodily connections was widespread: there are *koinoniai* ('associations') in parts of the body; the body is a *homoethnie* ('organic unity') in which pain may be referred from one part to another, a concomitant telling concept; the adjectives *homotropos* ('of like character') and *homophylos* ('of like nature') are applied to bodily components (*Epid.* 2.1.6 = V.76 L.; *Loc. Hom.* 1 = VI.276 L., *Mul.* 2.174 = VIII.354 L.; *Vict.* 1.6 = VI.478 L.; *Nat. Hom.* 3 = VI.38 L.). We may glance at the word *physis*, an overarching term used of the bodily organism or constitution as a structural entirety. The term can be concrete as well as abstract, 'human form', fundamentally a 'human being' (*Morb.* 4.32 = VII.542 L.).[10] The importance of the body's own 'original constitution' is continuously asserted in the surgical procedures of *Fractures* and *Articulations*;[11] and consideration of this complete state is enjoined also in *Epidemics* (2.1.8 = V.80 L.).

For more specific views, we turn to the visionary treatise *Airs, Waters and Places*, one of the best known and most commonly cited in the entire Hippocratic corpus. This treatise is not purely medical in subject matter but can be viewed rather as a unique innovatory study of climatology in relation to medicine. It is an aspect of the carefully consistent structuralist arguments employed in this work that the entire makeup, physical and mental, of all peoples is presented as subject to conditioning by their different environmental circumstances. Different peoples have different inherent characteristics, all alike dependent on their different geographical and meteorological settings: all peoples are made up of homogeneous stereotypes, subject to an ineluctable overall blueprint that underlies and shapes mind and body alike. Holistic views of the innate character to be traced in different peoples are integrally interlaced in the author's world-view. (See especially *Aer.* 16 = II.62–66 L.) We may note here a further crossing-point between tragedy and medical writing: the stereotypical peoples of 'Asia' envisaged by the author of *Airs, Waters and Places* are analogous to the stereotypical eastern barbarians and slaves commonly presented in tragic scenario. Such ethnic stereotyping is marked in the contrast between Greek moderation and oriental extravagance to be seen in Aeschylus' *Persians*, while interest in distant places and peoples is evident in accounts of the mythical wanderings of Io in Aeschylus' *Suppliants* and

10 φύσις ἀνθρωποειδής.
11 ἀρχαίη φύσις.

Prometheus Bound.[12] Further, in late Euripidean plays, such as *Orestes*, exotic localities are envisaged in staging and there is exaggerated characterisation of foreigners, especially as slaves.

In *Epidemics*, a series of practitioners' notes based on case histories, we find a corollary to the theoretical holism of *Airs, Waters and Places*. Here there is evidence for holistic views with a more pragmatic basis. Medical judgment relies time and again on assessment and interpretation of mental and physical states in conjunction. If in tragedy it is from bodies and what they do that we read the mind,[13] so in medicine it may be from perceived or postulated mental states that we read the body. A physician of *Epidemics* 1 and 3, identified by some with the historical Hippocrates,[14] makes references to and allowances for mental and emotional states, such as grief and depression, as causative factors in illness. Problematic features are listed as 'not eating, feeling dispirited, not sleeping, irritation and being out of sorts' (*Epid.* 3, case 2 = III.112 L.).[15] The doctors of *Epidemics* 2, 4 and 6 make references to physiognomy as a determinant of character and health; they trace various bodily interconnections; and they write of 'signs', both emotional and physical (*Epid.* 2.1.8; 2.1.10; 2.3.15 = V.80, 82, 136 L.; VI.2.17 = V.286 L.).[16]

4 Medical Texts: Identification and Terminology of Vital Parts

There are recurrent, though not totally consistent, elements in the identification of vital parts advanced by physicians. Commonly included are *enkephalos* ('brain'), *hepar* ('liver') and *kardia* ('heart'); also significant are *myelos* (CSF, that is 'cerebro-spinal fluid') and *phrenes* ('mind' or 'mental diaphragm', an area of the diaphragm or midriff). It is notable that the very same vital parts and key features – especially *kardia, phrenes* and *hepar* – that act as dynamic elements in the overall physical function of the body are simultaneously centres of mental or emotional activity, that is of thought or feeling. In these instances, physical function is allied with cognitive and emotional function; concrete merges with abstract. In medical texts, there is the same implicit blurring of terminology and ideas as that which is apparent in philosophical and literary texts.

12 See in general Hall (1989), and more particularly Collard (2008), especially at xcii.
13 See Cairns (2017) 261.
14 On questions of Hippocratic authorship, see Jouanna (2013).
15 ἀπόσιτος, ἄθυμος, ἄγρυπνος, ὀργαί, δυσφορίαι.
16 See Craik (2015) 86.

The most clear key lists of vital parts are presented in these three works: *On Diseases* 1, *Koan Prognoses* and *On Diseases of Girls* (*Morb.* 1.3 = VI.144 L.; *Coac.* 499 = V.698 L.; *Virg.* = VIII.468 L.). Although these works differ considerably in genre and are unlikely to be of similar provenance or date, they evince broad agreement over vital bodily parts. In the nosological treatise *On Diseases* 1, death is said to ensue 'if a person is wounded in brain or spinal fluid or liver or mental diaphragm or bladder, or vessel of flowing blood (sc. artery), or heart.'[17] In the aphoristic collection *Koan Prognoses*, wounds are mortal 'if one is injured in brain or spinal fluid or liver or diaphragm, or heart or bladder or one of the large blood vessels' (also wounds to trachea and lung if breathing is impeded; also to intestines if large and transverse rather than minor and straight).[18] In the gynaecological piece *On Diseases of Girls*, a contrast is made between pins and needles in the lower limbs, harmless as the blood returns speedily there, and that part of the body is not crucial; 'whereas from heart and diaphragm it flows back slowly; for the vessels are slanting and the place is crucial, prone to derangement and mania.'[19]

We may note that in medical writers' perception, vital fluids described as 'forms of the moist' or (in some texts) as 'humours' are variously defined and located. Two key formulations are expressed, one in *On Diseases* 4 and one in *On the Nature of Man*: blood, phlegm, water, bile (*Morb.* 4.33 = VII.542–44 L.) or blood, phlegm, yellow bile, black bile (*Nat. Hom.* 4 = VI.38–40 L.). In *On Diseases* 4 and frequently, but not invariably, elsewhere, blood is associated with the heart, phlegm is associated with the head, water is associated with the spleen, and bile is associated with the liver. However, the fundamental emotion *orge* or *cholos* ('anger') usually associated with bile and the liver is occasionally associated rather with blood and the heart. The main bodily fluids are not fully distinct but potentially linked in pathology. These fundamental bodily fluids are associated to some degree, though not with complete consistency, with character and experience. Thus, it appears that the long humoral tradition of western thought and imagination is foreshadowed in the holistic ideas of ancient medicine: particular organs or parts are especially associated with humours and character. In the same way, an association between bodily vital parts and mental attributes is commonly present, expressed by metaphor and metonymy.

17 ἤν τις ἐγκέφαλον τρωθῇ ἢ ῥαχίτην μυελόν, ἢ ἧπαρ ἢ φρένας ἢ κύστιν ἢ φλέβα αἱμόρροον, ἢ καρδίην.

18 ἤν τις ἐγκέφαλον τρωθῇ ἢ ῥαχίτην μυελὸν ἢ ἧπαρ ἢ φρένας ἢ καρδίην ἢ κύστιν ἢ φλέβα τῶν παχειῶν …

19 ἐκ δὲ τῆς καρδίης καὶ τῶν φρενῶν βραδέως παλιρροεῖ· ἐπικάρσιαι γὰρ αἱ φλέβες καὶ ὁ τόπος ἐπίκαιρος ἔς τε παραφροσύνην καὶ μανίην ἕτοιμος.

This question is implicit: are these important terms in origin physical, concrete and anatomical/medical, adopted and adapted to have an abstract mental/emotional sense in literary contexts, perhaps also in spoken usage? Or alternatively does the burgeoning *techne* of medicine give a more specific sense to terms already current? In other words, to what extent do we find borrowings and coinages drawn from medicine; or alternatively to what extent are apparent borrowings/coinages initiated by medicine? A third possibility is here advocated: that, rather, there is an ongoing significant linguistic synergy reflecting the reality, both popular and intellectual, that mental and somatic functions are allied, rather than distinguished. Indeed, as seen above, this reality is apparent already in Homeric epic. We need not suppose that literary texts are derivative, drawing on medical sources; we need not give undue weight to the effect of medical neologism; rather there is ongoing mutual interaction in the use of a common language, subject to considerable conservatism as well as constant change.

In the following part of this chapter, two tragedies selected for particular attention are discussed: Aeschylus' *Prometheus Bound* and Euripides' *Hippolytos*. Many other plays of Aeschylus, Sophocles and Euripides are of comparable interest with regard to the terminology of mind and body; but the chosen works display an unusually wide-ranging and particularly effective poetic imagination in the use and adaptation of a range of terms. With regard to Aeschylus' *Prometheus Bound*, the term *kardia* (for which *kear* is a tragic variant) is discussed in conjunction with the term *thymos* (for which a new interpretation is advocated). Then, with regard to Euripides' *Hippolytos*, the term *psyche* (contrasted with the strongly physical term *demas* and allied with the emotionally suggestive term *myelos*) is discussed. The association of the liver, *hepar*, with anger, *cholos*, is discussed in relation to both texts.

5 Tragic Texts: 1, Aeschylus' *Prometheus Bound*

Aeschylus' *Prometheus Bound* has as its subject the vengeance of Zeus on the defiant Titan Prometheus. It is a multi-layered play of loose yet complex plot: at the beginning Prometheus is fettered to a cliff in the Caucasus, where the chorus and a succession of characters then pass by and address him. The characterisation is inventive and diverse: Hephaestus appears initially, to effect the fettering of Prometheus; Hermes arrives finally to make predictions; in the body of the play Prometheus is counselled and comforted by a chorus of sea-nymphs (Oceanids), by their father the demigod Oceanus, and by the wretched young girl Io, forced to wander helplessly in the guise of a heifer through Hera's jealous hostility. The staging is remarkable in the improbable setting of a distant and deserted Scythian region, in the striking aerial entry of the chorus and, above all, in the enforced static inaction throughout of the monumental protagonist. The unity of the play, centred on the Titanic hero, is reinforced by strong thematic elements. One theme is that of 'suffering' (variously expressed in near-synonymous terms as *ponos*, *athlon*, *nosos*, *mochthos*, *pemone*): the underlying universal suffering of mortals; the extreme physical torment of Prometheus; the extraordinary distress of Io. All are in desperate need of a 'cure' or 'release' (*pharmakon*).

Another theme, explored in more detail here, is that of 'anger.' The protagonist Prometheus and his adversary Zeus are alike obdurate in their rage. This theme is expressed in constant terminology of 'anger' (*cholos* 29, 199, 370, 376; *orge* 80, 315, 378, 678; also *thymos* as at 380). The terminology is redolent of the physical body as well as expressive of psychological sentiment. The term *cholos* is connected with the liver, sharing with the cognate *chole* the sense 'gall' or 'bile.' The term *orge* suggests swelling, in particular the emotional swelling engendered by anger but also – in certain passages – the physical swelling presenting in the diseased body.[20] The more complex term *thymos*, further discussed below, suggests the heat of anger, in its etymological derivation, cognate with *zesis* ('boiling') and sharing a root with *fumus* ('smoke').

One passage of *Prometheus Bound* quoted below (A. *PV* 376–80), an exchange between Prometheus and Oceanus, may be singled out as having a peculiarly dense collocation of medical language, in conjunction with metaphorical expression and extended imagery; it well demonstrates the inextricable connection and close interaction of mind and body.[21] In this passage, bodily parts are not just connected with, but are quite conjoined with, emotional processes. It is supposed that the physical *kear* – and with it the *thymos* – can receive therapy to bring about mental and emotional amelioration and change. It is visualised that the heart and spirit may be treated to remove excessive or undesirable elements (here anger, peculiarly connected with the spirit), in precisely the way that the body may be treated to remove excessive or peccant matter. The requisite therapeutic procedures are described as softening and reducing these parts and all is expressed in language (notably the verb *ischnainein*) identical with that found in medical texts. As is noted above, such treatment of the body, typically as a whole, is standard in Greek medical practice.

20 The synonymous verbs ὀργᾶν, σφριγᾶν ('to swell') can be good but are more often bad in nuance. See Craik (1998) 15.

21 Thomson (1932) 154–55, commentary on the lines, in his numbering 393–96, remains unsurpassed in understanding and explication of this passage.

Prometheus: 'I shall suffer until Zeus is sated with anger' (*cholos*).
Oceanus: 'Do you not realise, Prometheus, that words are healers of troubled rage?' (*orge*)
Prometheus: 'Yes, if one softens the heart' (*kear*) 'at the right time and does not forcibly reduce the swollen spirit' (*thymos*).[22]

The precise sense of *thymos* used in close conjunction with *kear* is debatable and translation is hazardous, but it is evident that the terms are almost synonymous in hendiadys, with reference to heart and spirit. At the same time, as noted above, the popular sense of *thymos* 'anger' is implicit: metonymy is key to the overall effect of this richly imagistic formulation. The anatomical location of the heart is well known. The anatomical location of the *thymos* has, it seems, been completely disregarded in modern scholarship on this text (as on others). But, like the heart, the *thymos* is a particular part of the body and has a precise place in the thorax: it is a gland lying near the throat, close to the heart certainly familiar to Greek doctors.[23] The novel suggestion is here offered that the common form and abstract sense of *thymos*/θυμός ('spirit') is intrinsically connected with the rarer anatomical form and sense of *thymos* ('thymus gland'). Indeed it may be suggested that, in a society familiar with the double usage, the inherent physical sense of *thymos* was always felt to underlie the mental sense. That the sense 'thymus gland' has been overlooked is doubtless because in general usage the connotation 'spirit' or 'anger' dominates. (In Plato's influential formulation, *thymos* is the passionate aspect of the tripartite *psyche* concerned with such emotions as anger.) In addition, general unfamiliarity with terminology viewed as technical and peculiar to medicine may play a part. A further reason must lie in the conventions of accentuation: the noun θυμός ('spirit', 'anger') has been regarded as quite different from the noun θύμος ('thymus gland'). While the difference in accent has surely contributed to general disregard of the interpretation put forward here, a parallel exists. The patent pun in Sophocles' *Philoctetes* on the differently accented forms of *bios* βίος ('life') and βιός ('bow') demonstrates that such words were not, or not always, clearly differentiated in punctuation (S. *Ph.* 931).[24]

Though primarily anatomical, the term *thymos* is better known in ancient culinary contexts. The thymus glands, two white fatty glands situated below the throat, are a type of offal (similar to kidneys or liver) regarded as a delicacy, especially when sourced from young animals such as calves and lambs. The

22 ἐάν τις ἐν καιρῷ γε μαλθάσσῃ κέαρ / καὶ μὴ σφριγῶντα θυμὸν ἰσχαίνῃ βίᾳ.

23 On the extensive ancient knowledge of glands, see Craik (2009).

24 ἀπεστέρηκας τὸν βίον τὰ τόξ' ἑλών.

modern culinary term is 'sweetbreads.' The thymus glands in humans too are relatively large in youth: lobes at the base of the neck extending into the thorax near the heart. If there is a reference here to the physical *thymos* (gland) along with the clear reference to the physical *kear* or *kardia* (heart) to which it lies close the impact of the dense medical metaphor is much enhanced. This suggestion may be thought less bold when it is noted that Eustathius identified the same sense of *thymos* in Homer: Eustathius comments on *Il.* 20. 402–6 that the *thymos* is a gland in the region of the collarbones.[25] The action of the *thymos* is implicit in many Hippocratic passages, especially though not only in *Epidemics*. The negated term ἀθυμίαι denotes suicidal thoughts or lack of spirit and courage by contrast with being *thymoeides*, 'having spirit.' The clearest statement that the *thymos* is envisaged as a physical entity in relation with other bodily parts (heart, lung and head) but also as intimately connected with sentiment and emotion (anger, equanimity) is found in a passage of *Epidemics* 6 (*Epid.* 6. 5. 5 [5. 316 L.]): 'Matters related to the *thymos* are as follows: sharp temper draws the heart and the lung in on themselves and draws hot and moist to the head; good temper relaxes the heart.'[26]

The pervasive play on the notion that body and mind are bound together appears also in narrative of the predicament of Io, who is simultaneously physically and mentally changed, being turned into a heifer and rendered mad (A. *PV* 673–74):

> Io: 'At once body' (*morphē*, lit. 'shape') 'and mind' (*phrenes* lit. 'diaphragm') 'were distorted.'

And the punning expression (A. *PV* 692) 'chill the *psyche*' in the chorus' reaction of pity for the sufferings and outrages of Io demonstrates the application of somatic sensation to mental or emotional feelings: concrete bodily chill and abstract mental chill are conflated.[27]

Towards the end of the play, Hermes predicts that an eagle will feast on Prometheus' dark liver (A. *PV* 1025).[28] The fate of Prometheus' liver is important in the after-history of the myth, as an eagle keeps returning to gnaw the Titan's regenerated liver (Cic. *Tusc. Disp.* 2.23–25).

---

25 I am indebted to Douglas Cairns for drawing my attention to this precedent.

26 ὁκόσα δὲ ἐκ θυμοῦ, ταῦτα· ὀξυθυμίη ἀνασπᾷ καρδίην καὶ πλεύμονα ἐς ἑωυτὰ καὶ ἐς κεφαλὴν τὰ θερμὰ καὶ τὸ ὑγρόν· ἡ δ' εὐθυμίη ἀφίει καρδίην. See the similar approach of Arist. *Probl.* 889a 15–25.

27 In ψυχεῖν ψυχάν the text and metre are insecure but the play on *psyche* is clear.

28 κελαινόβρωτον δ' ἧπαρ ἐκθοινήσεται. The translation 'dark' is disputed but this is here unimportant.

In view of Prometheus' unremitting rage, there is a clear symbolism to be seen in that it is the liver, with its general association with bile and anger, which is affected. The association of bile with liver is fundamental in anatomy and in popular usage; as noted above, the senses bile and anger coexist. In passing, we may remark that the liver can be regenerated: it is an organ uniquely able to renew itself. It is likely that Aeschylus and his contemporaries were aware of this extraordinary physical fact.

6 Tragic Texts: 2, Euripides *Hippolytos*

Euripides' play *Hippolytos*, produced in 428 BCE, centres on the ineluctable passion felt by Phaedra, wife of King Theseus, for her stepson Hippolytus; the reactions to this of characters and chorus are delineated and the fatal results described. This play is very different in its human sentiments from *Prometheus Bound* with its monumental heroic protagonist. But here too there is a wealth of figurative language and the terminology of physical and mental function is fundamentally the same: in general remarkable aspects of expression, physical coalesces with mental and emotional. First it may be emphasised that the term *psyche* is important in the language of the play. Different ancient writers in different contexts use the term *psyche* ('breath', 'soul') in different ways, with different nuances. It is, however, always central to the individual's being. In the medical treatise *On Regimen* the word is peculiarly difficult to pin down, as it embraces both 'vital stuff' (concrete) and 'animation' (abstract).[29] This range is similar to the duality of the other terms, *kardia* and *thymos*, traced above in Aeschylus' *Prometheus Bound*. But in the welter of usage, an underlying significance of *psyche* is always constant. Although seen as fundamentally separate from *soma* ('body'), *psyche* is at the same time fundamentally linked with life in the body. However, it has etymological links also – as seen above with regard to a passage in *Prometheus Bound* (A. *PV* 692) – with the sensation of coldness. The two senses 'breath' and 'soul' suggest an inherent connection with the transition from the warmth of life to the coldness of death.

With reference to Phaedra in the parodos (121–69) and elsewhere, a clear and telling distinction is made between usage of *psyche* and *demas*: both designations are applied to Phaedra as a living person, but the former has an emotional charge, while the latter is purely physical in application. The chorus introduce Phaedra with the description that 'her *psyche* is bound in

29 See Craik (2015) 272–73; cf. van der Eijk (2005) 127–28.

bed' (160).[30] By contrast, in the context of Phaedra's emaciated state brought about by fasting, the word *demas* is used (131, 138); similarly, as the parodos ends with the anapaestic approach of the Nurse, the word *demas* describes Phaedra's extreme pallor (175). Then in a lyric exchange Phaedra enjoins her Nurse to raise her *demas* and the Nurse uses the same word with reference to that action (198, 204). Yet alongside this usage, the Nurse's deep emotional involvement is evident in that her *psyche* longs for information (173); this is still further seen in her declaration to Phaedra that it is safer if affections do not penetrate to the 'inmost *myelos* of the *psyche*' (255).[31]

Implicit in this usage of *psyche* is the little-observed but significant Greek view of the *psyche* as the locus of erotic emotion. The function of the lungs and heart in respiration was not fully understood, but it was clearly recognised that lungs were important in breathing and so to life. Erotic emotions were related not to the *kardia* but to the *psyche* and the lungs. This is corroborated by Sophoclean usage: from *Phaidra*, the *psyche* of men, women and also of gods is affected by omnipotent power of Eros; from an unidentified play, Love is absorbed in the lungs of all with *psyche*.[32] The rich imagery of the expression 'inmost *myelos* of the *psyche*' (255) must be understood with reference to this view. There are strong associative elements at play. It was noted above that *myelos* is one of the vital parts identified in medical texts. It is cerebro-spinal fluid originating in the brain and coursing down the back of the body, not – despite a common misconception and mistranslation – invariably to be identified with bone marrow, as well observed by the author of the Hippocratic treatise *On Flesh* (*Carn.* 4 = VIII.588 L.). There is an association in medical texts between *myelos* and reproductive fluids. In *Hippolytos*, physical and emotional connotations are intricately mingled.[33] A similar concentration of associative power may be seen in the celebrated passage about two types of *aidos* (385–7) here too, through an obvious linguistic association, the sexual organs and sexual feeling are strikingly aligned.[34]

Also, as in *Prometheus Bound*, the liver is regarded as the seat of anger. In regarding himself as struck 'right to the liver' (1070) by his father, Hippolytus implies that anger on his part against Theseus has been induced, or is warranted: in locating the injury at the liver Hippolytos refers not to the liver as

30 εὐναία δέδεται ψυχά Barrett magisterially comments 'to object that a ψυχά cannot be in bed would be pettifogging; ψυχά becomes almost synonymous with Ph. herself.'

31 μαθεῖν ἔραται ψυχή 173; πρὸς ἄκρον μυελὸν ψυχῆς 255.

32 fr. 684 ἔρως … ψυχὰς ταράσσει … and fr. 941 ἐντήκεται γὰρ πλευμόνων ὅσοις ἔνι ψυχή.

33 See Craik (2008).

34 See Craik (1993).

a tender spot, painful if struck; but to the liver as seat of the anger he feels aroused in him.[35]

7 Conclusion

It has been argued in this chapter that a systemic and synoptic view of bodily disease and mental disorder – as similarly of healthy function in mind and body – is pervasively present in both medical and non-medical writing; that distinctions are constantly blurred between the physical and the mental or emotional, body and mind being linked in terminology as in thought. In this we see not the interaction of separable concepts but rather a consistent silent synergy in which metaphor shades into metonymy: key terms for bodily parts serve as key terms also for the location of mental functions and emotional feelings. A holistic view of mind and body is omnipresent in that the key physical organs identified by Hippocratic writers correspond with the significant bodily parts associated in the Attic tragedians with mental and emotional activity. The key organ *hepar* is the seat of the primal emotion anger. The *psyche* crucial to, or identified with, life is allied with the *kardia* and *thymos* situated with the lungs in the *phrenes*. The *myelos* crucial to reproductive life is allied allusively with the *psyche*.

Acknowledgments

I am grateful to Douglas Cairns for valuable comments on this paper, and to Chiara Thumiger for assiduous editorial activity. All translations from Greek are my own.

Bibliography

Anastassiou, A. and Irmer, D. *Testimonien zum Corpus Hippocraticum*, Teil I. Göttingen: Vandenhoeck & Ruprecht (2006).

Cairns, D. 'ψυχή, θυμός, and Metaphor in Homer and Plato.' *Études platoniciennes*, 11 (2014). Open access, available at http://etudesplatoniciennes.revues.org/566.

35 But contrast Cairns (2017) 252 'simply the idea that the pain … is like being struck in the liver by a weapon', not 'the liver as metonymous seat of emotions.'

Cairns, D. 'Mind, Metaphor, and Emotion in Euripides (*Hippolytus*) and Seneca (*Phaedra*).' *Maia*, 69.2 (2017) 247–67.

Cairns, D. and Nelis, D. (eds.) *Emotions in the Classical World: Methods, Approaches, and Directions.* Stuttgart: Steiner (2017).

Craik, E. M. 'αἰδώς in Euripides' *Hippolytos*: Review and Reinterpretation.' *JHS*, 113 (1993) 45–59.

Craik, E. M. *Hippocrates.* Places in Man, *Edited and Translated with Introduction and Commentary*. Oxford: Oxford University Press (1998).

Craik, E. M. 'Medical Reference in Euripides.' *BICS*, 45 (2001) 81–95.

Craik, E. M. 'Myelos: Matters of Life and Death.' *Acta Classica Supplement* II. Pretoria: V&R Printing Works (2008) 64–73.

Craik, E. M. *The Hippocratic Treatise* On Glands. Studies in Ancient Medicine 36. Leiden and Boston: Brill (2009).

Craik, E. M. *The 'Hippocratic' Corpus. Content and Context.* London: Routledge (2015).

Guardasole, A. *Tragedia e Medicina nell'Atene del V Secolo A.C.* Naples: Auria Editore (2000).

Gundert, B. 'Soma and Psyche in Hippocratic Medicine.' In *Psyche and Soma. Physicians and Metaphysicians on the Mind-Body Problem from Antiquity to Enlightenment*, ed. J. P. Wright and P. Potter. Oxford: Oxford University Press (2002) 13–36.

Hall, E. *Inventing the Barbarian*. Oxford: Oxford University Press (1989).

Jahn, T. *Zum Wortfeld 'Seele-Geist' in der Sprache Homers. Zetemata* Heft 3. Munich: Beck (1987).

Kazantzidis, G. *Medical Understandings of the Emotions in Classical Antiquity*. Berlin: De Gruyter (forthcoming).

Kosak, J. C. *Heroic Measures: Hippocratic Medicine in the Making of Euripidean Tragedy*. Studies in Ancient Medicine 30. Leiden and Boston: Brill (2004).

Lo Presti, R. 'The Ambiguous Role of Perception.' *Acta Classica*, 50 (2017) 129–46.

Lonie, I. M. *The Hippocratic Treatises 'On Generation,' 'On the Nature of the Child,' 'Diseases* IV.' Berlin: De Gruyter (1981).

McDonald, G. C. *Concepts and Treatments of Phrenitis in Ancient Medicine*. Dissertation University of Newcastle (2009).

Onians, R. B. *The Origins of European Thought about the Body, the Soul, the World, Time, and Fate*. Cambridge: Cambridge University Press (1951).

Thumiger, C. *A History of the Mind and Mental Health in Classical Greek Medical Thought*. Cambridge: Cambridge University Press (2017).

Thumiger, C. and Singer, P. N. (eds.) *Mental Illness in Ancient Medicine from Celsus to Paul of Aegina*. Studies in Ancient Medicine 50 Leiden and Boston: Brill (2018).

van der Eijk, P. J. *Medicine and Philosophy in Classical Antiquity*. Cambridge: Cambridge University Press (2005).

Primary Texts: Editions and Translations Used

Aeschylus. *Aeschylus. Persians and Other Plays*. Trans. C. Collard. Oxford: Oxford University Press (2008).

Aeschylus. *The Prometheus Bound, Edited with Introduction, Commentary and Translation*. Ed. G. Thomson. Cambridge: Cambridge University Press (1932).

Euripides. *Euripides. Hippolytos*. Ed. W. S. Barrett. Oxford: Oxford University Press (1964).

Hippocrates. *Oeuvres complètes d'Hippocrate*. Ed. É. Littré. Paris: J. B. Baillière (1839–61).

Hippocrates. *Pronostic*. Ed. J. Jouanna. Paris: Les Belles Lettres (2013).

Plato. *A Commentary on Plato's Timaeus*. Ed. A. E. Taylor. Oxford: Oxford University Press (1928).

CHAPTER 8

Plato's *Charmides* on Philosophy as Holistic Medical Practice

Giouli Korobili and Konstantinos Stefou

Abstract

In a well-known passage from the *Charmides* (155a8–58e5), Socrates is seen to extend the holistic principle that underlies good Greek medical practice in order to cover an as yet neglected factor, the soul. Specifically, he assumes the role of representing Zalmoxian medical art, and challenges the holistic conception on which contemporary doctors base their practice, mainly the idea that the well-being of a bodily part depends on the simultaneous treatment of both that part and the whole (the body as a whole). In introducing the factor 'soul', Socrates appears to promote a novel holistic concept of human nature and to modify the idea described above as follows: the well-being of a body depends on the simultaneous treatment of both that part (the body) and the whole (the soul). Yet this modified version has spawned much controversy: how are we to understand the body as a part of the soul? In this paper, we offer a fresh interpretation of the passage, holding that the soul is both part and whole, depending on the viewing angle. That is to say, the soul, when viewed in relation to man altogether, namely the soul-body compound, appears as one part of the whole but still the ruling element which, under normal circumstances, presides over the good of the whole. When viewed, however, under conditions where the harmonious coexistence between soul and body has been disturbed, making it illegitimate to speak of a harmonious whole, the soul takes on the role of the whole in order to restore the disassembled whole to its previous state of equilibrium.

1 Introduction

Plato's *Charmides*, largely due to its apparent inconclusiveness, renders itself vulnerable to accusations of lack of philosophical weight or doctrinal content. Like all other so-called 'Socratic', aporetic dialogues, it embarks upon a quest for a definition of a particular virtue, in this case σωφροσύνη,[1] but ends in what

1 Perhaps best translated 'temperance.'

 | DOI:10.1163/9789004443143_010

seems to be failure. When we look closer, however, many of the factors that seem initially perplexing form parts of a literary design constructed to promote a positive conclusion, which the reader is meant to extract from the dialogue itself. In the light of this interpretative approach, this paper offers a fresh and comprehensive look at the *Charmides*, centred on its ideas about 'wholeness.' It focuses especially on enigmatic passages which not only introduce, explicitly or implicitly, the notion of a whole consisting of parts, but also, through the holistic conceptions they encompass, while approving or opposing them, constitute the very core of Socrates' argumentative strategy in this Platonic dialogue.[2] Among these conceptions, what will be shown to be Socrates' novel holistic concept of human nature takes up the lion's share of the discussion.

But the nature of this concept has not yet been fully clarified. The basic problem is created by a well-known passage from the *Charmides* (155a8–58e5) in which Socrates draws on the holistic principle that underlies good Greek medical practice in order to differentiate it from the theory and practice of Zalmoxian medicine. According to the former, if a bodily part is going to be well, both that part and the whole (the body as a whole) must be treated at the same time. Yet the extended holistic version presented by Zalmoxian medical art introduces a new vital factor, soul, which appears on a first reading to modify the principle described above as follows: if a body is going to be well, both that part (the body) and the whole (the soul) must be cured at the same time. This modified version has greatly troubled scholars: how are we to understand the body as a part of the soul, at a literal level? Or should we try to decipher the figurative language of these lines?

This major interpretative difficulty has spawned considerable controversy, which can be briefly summarized as follows: some scholars deny that there can be any sort of whole-part relationship between soul and body, and they thus concentrate their attention on the causal priority of the former over the latter. Others take pains to retain the significance of the whole-part relationship by arguing that the relevant whole is not the soul, but the soul-body composite. Others seek to give due weight to both causal priority and the whole-part relationship, claiming that the relevant whole is the soul, and that the focus of attention in our passage moves from the whole (soul) towards the part, and, most notably, towards each bodily part individually.[3] In view of this scholarly

2 For discussion focusing on such passages as integral parts of the dialogue as a whole, see Hyland (1981) 35; Van der Ben (1985) 14.

3 Scholarly opinions can generally be divided into two groups: (a) those that de-emphasise the importance attached to the whole-part relationship in favour of the notion of causal priority that runs throughout the text; and (b) those that seek to preserve the importance of the

controversy over the conception of the whole that the *Charmides* presents,[4] a close interpretative reading of this much-debated passage, along with its immediate textual surroundings, is a *desideratum* which the present paper aims to address in order to establish a clearer picture of Socrates' holistic views of human nature. Our ultimate aim is to show that, when we elucidate the *twofold* nature of the concept of 'whole' presented in the *Charmides*, the overall significance of the dialogue is clarified as a model of holistic enquiry for the human search for *eudaimonia*.

2 Some Important Preliminary Remarks

2.1 *Accompanying the Body: towards a Holistic Conception of the Human Person*

The dramatic action of the *Charmides* is set in the gymnasium of Taureas in Athens, to which Socrates has just returned from the battle of Potidaea around the year 429 BCE. While his interlocutors, Chaerephon and Critias in particular, show a tremendous desire to hear news of the war, Socrates himself hastens to shift the subject of the conversation by introducing the key concept 'philosophy', yet without making perfectly clear, at least at the outset, its relation to the immediate context:

> **T1**: 'I in my turn began to question them [...] about the present state of philosophy and about the young men, whether there were any who had become distinguished for wisdom (σοφίᾳ) or beauty (κάλλει) or both (ἀμφοτέροις)' (153d2–5).
>
> trans. SPRAGUE[5]

whole-part relationship, eventually at the expense of the idea of the soul's priority over the body, on which see Tuozzo (2011) 119–20. Tuozzo goes on to propose a third approach which, he maintains, gives equal weight to both notions. Drawing on a passage from the *Theaetetus* (203–205), Tuozzo claims that our passage employs a fundamental distinction between πᾶν and ὅλον: while the latter refers to something other than a mere sum of parts, the former is a 'generalized way of referring to all the different parts of the human being' (121). Although the interpretation offered in this paper starts from the same principle, the need to attribute equal importance to both the whole-part relationship and causal priority, it nonetheless rests on radically different premises, as will be seen shortly. Discussions of the controversial passage include Anagnastopoulos (1972) 219–20; Hogan (1976); Steiner (1992) 34; Robinson (1995) 7–8; Hazebroucq (1997) 131; Rowe (1998) 88; McPherran (2004); Levine (2016) 66–68.

4 A good survey of the controversy is offered by Tuozzo (2011) 118–21.

5 Unless otherwise noted, quotations in English from the *Chrm.* are taken from the Sprague (1997) translation.

Note that Socrates' initial question simultaneously puts three issues on the table: pre-eminence in (a) wisdom, (b) beauty or (c) both. But it is the addition of (c) that opens up the possibility that the other two terms, wisdom and beauty, which in their first (co-)occurrence appear unrelated, might be interconnected or even form a set of parts making up a whole. Critias' subsequent response, however, limits the focus to (b) external or physical beauty, as can be seen from the fact that he draws attention to the impact of Charmides' (bodily) excellence on the crowd of admirers.[6]

In cautious opposition to this uniform praise of Charmides' surpassing physical beauty, Socrates advances a conception of the 'irresistible' person (ἄμαχον, 154d7) as someone whose perfect body is *accompanied by a well-formed soul* (τὴν ψυχὴν […] εὖ πεφυκώς, 154e1).[7] This holistic approach to irresistibility, in which an excellent soul is attached to an excellent body, raises two main questions: (a) what exactly is the place of the soul in such a whole? And, accordingly, (b) how should we understand the sense of the expression 'to have a well-formed soul' (τὴν ψυχὴν εὖ πεφυκώς), and what is Socrates' intention in using this expression? The latter question in particular generates a plethora of sub-issues. For example, might the expression τὴν ψυχὴν εὖ πεφυκώς be employed to convey the idea of a naturally, intrinsically, well-shaped soul? Or should we take it as denoting a soul that is capable of adjusting itself either to serve some particular function or to ensure the smooth operation of the

6 ἐρασταὶ […] τοῦ δοκοῦντος καλλίστου εἶναι, 154a5–6 ('admirers […] of the one who is thought to be the handsomest young man'); cf. 154c3. This restrictive admission, however, produces a careful critique of the very criterion for excellence that so far has taken pride of place. More specifically, expressions such as ὥσπερ ἄγαλμα ('as if he were a statue') or τὸ εἶδος πάγκαλος ('entirely beautiful in form') (154c8, 154d5), as employed by Critias, seem properly construed as introducing the notion of gradations in beauty and should make us wonder whether they are meant to serve as allusive pointers to other sorts of perfection which, based on the distinction of 153d4–5 (T1), have everything to do with wisdom or with both beauty and wisdom. Socrates, on the other hand, sees no problem in making use of the terms καλός and φαῦλος with reference to physical beauty and its opposite state, respectively. But he hastens to concede his inability to assess excellence on the basis of the criterion specified so far, since beauty, to his eyes, appears as a feature shared by almost everyone who has reached young adulthood (σχεδὸν γάρ τί μοι πάντες οἱ ἐν τῇ ἡλικίᾳ καλοὶ φαίνονται, 154b9–10). It is as though Socrates wants to diminish its noteworthiness within the spectrum of human admiration, dislodge it from its central position as the true object of praise, and eventually turn the spotlight in a different direction as yet only alluded to.

7 Here, in succession to ἀμφοτέροις (T1) and πάγκαλος (on which, see the preceding note) that we met earlier, the words ἔτι (154d7) and προσόν (154d8) seem to be used to point again to a very particular addition, psychic well-orderedness, which, although ironically presented as something trivial (σμικρόν τι, 154d8), is of the utmost importance for the attainment of manly indomitability.

whole? Or perhaps neither of the above is the case, and this formulation is simply intended to signal the aristocratic lineage of a noble man's soul. The latter option seems to be supported by Socrates' subsequent remark, which attempts to forge a link between Charmides' well-formed soul and Critias' household (154e3), implying that the presence of the former is entailed by the presence of the latter – a suggestion, however, that should not be taken at face value.[8]

Lest his remarks create a different impression at this point, Critias hastens to affirm Charmides' pre-eminence in respect to psychic well-orderedness.[9] This affirmation has the following important implications: (a) psychic well-orderedness is presented as self-evidently granted by noble birth alone; and (b) the state of being 'a fine and good person' (καλὸς καὶ ἀγαθός, hereafter *kalokagathia*), though often used to denote a combination of physical and ethical excellence,[10] seems to be assigned a two-fold sense, according to which we are entitled to speak of a fine and good person sometimes with respect to the body and sometimes with respect to the soul. But is it possible to speak of *kalokagathia* in respect to both entities? Let us linger a bit more on this second point. Based solely on Critias' emphasis on the two-fold character of *kalokagathia*, in conjunction with the earlier suggestion that physical beauty comes in degrees,[11] the reader might come away with the impression that *kalokagathia* in the body can be independent of that of the soul, or vice versa. Yet in view of Socrates' insistence on a rather inclusive, whole-oriented phraseology, one can hardly fail to recognise the direction in which his efforts have pointed so far, towards *a different conception of kalokagathia*, one that is the result of the *state of the whole* but which has implications both *for that whole and for its parts*.

Through his introduction of an additional factor, therefore, along with what was until then deemed the main one in the discussion of Charmides' excellence, Socrates manages to deflect the focus away from physical beauty and towards recognising the need to strip the youth's soul and look at it before contemplating his body.[12] If nothing else, this shift in focus establishes a kind of priority of the soul over the body, but it does not by itself offer further details about the nature of that priority. So why does Socrates stress the need for an inspection of the soul before that of the body? We can infer that behind

8 As is shown by the use of particles such as που (154e2) or γε (154e2), which are meant not only to qualify the expression, but to impart a fine ironic complexion to it.

9 Cf. 154e4.

10 Cf. Lampert (2010) 161.

11 Cf. 154d5.

12 οὐκ ἀπεδύσαμεν [...] ἐθεασάμεθα πρότερον τοῦ εἴδους, 154e5–6.

this shift lies his belief in the causal superiority of the soul over the body.[13] More will be said about this in *3.1*. Another crucial question concerns the way in which such a stripping-test is to be carried out. The answer offered in these lines is clear: through engagement in dialectical discussion, for which good will is counted among the essential qualities.[14] Yet irrespective of the degree of Charmides' readiness to participate in a discussion centred on the status of his soul,[15] this introductory part of the dialogue must be viewed as a serious effort to establish a very interesting claim upon which both interlocutors seem ready to agree: *that φιλοσοφία, philosophy or love of wisdom, consists in being willing to engage in dialectical inquiry, that is, being ready to strip one's soul in order to be inspected with respect to its well-orderedness.*

2.2 *De-localising a Disease Affecting a Bodily Part*

The soul's priority over the body, as well as the peculiarities of its treatment, are in fact gradually teased out through the discussion occasioned by Charmides' entrance into the circle of discussants. Charmides has recently been troubled by a physical ailment, a headache, for which Socrates must now pretend to know the remedy. Yet Socrates' acquiescence in the rules of this 'pretending' game is certainly at odds with his subsequent dialectical performance, in which, as will be seen, not only does he not pretend to be a medical practitioner, but he introduces a type of holistic medicine that aims to correct current practice.[16] This apparent inconsistency makes readers who have an overall view of the discussion sense the presence of a delicate irony; but anyone familiar with the episode might ask themselves about the proper criteria for distinguishing between a genuine and a false doctor, as well as about what the object of true medical treatment should be. Skepticism regarding Socrates' assumed role is further accentuated by his brief description of the effects of Charmides' enormous physical attractiveness upon his judgment.[17]

This humorous interlude seems intended to serve a twofold purpose. It stresses the devastating impact of 'being outside oneself'[18] and thus misguided

13 Cf. Pl. *Grg.* 463e–64a, 477b–c, 496e, 501c, 513e.

14 Cf. *Grg.* 487a3.

15 About which Critias speaks with much more confidence (ἐπεί τοι καὶ ἔστιν φιλόσοφός τε […], 154e8; 'since he is surely a philosopher, and […]', trans. Sprague, modified) than Socrates does (πάντως γάρ που […], 154e6; 'for anyhow, I suppose, […]', our trans.).

16 Cf. 158e2. For a similar but not identical view, see Schmid (1998) 175 n. 29. Our lines of approach thus seem to differ widely from McPherran (2004) 11, who claims that the dialogue 'appears to undermine itself by inviting us to think that such a practice is more quackery than effective medicine.' Cf. also Levine (2016) 56.

17 See e.g. 155d4–5.

18 οὐκέτ' ἐν ἐμαυτοῦ ἦν, 155d4; cf. Pl. *Ion* 535b–c.

in judgment, whereby Socrates' earlier criticism of the unilateral exaltation of beauty is intensified. In addition, it raises suspicions about whether Charmides' evaluation of the ailment he suffers might be in itself poorly grounded. A similar line of thought seems to underlie Socrates' proposed treatment:

> **T2**: 'And I said that it (viz. the remedy) was a certain leaf, and that there was a charm (ἐπῳδή) to go with it. If one sang the charm while applying the leaf, the remedy (φάρμακον) would bring about a complete cure (παντάπασιν ὑγιᾶ ποιοῖ), but without the charm the leaf was useless (οὐδὲν ὄφελος εἴη)' (155e5–8).

This treatment can be summed up in three key points: (a) the remedy for the ailment of the head is a certain leaf; (b) to attain complete well-being, a certain charm must be uttered at the time the leaf is applied; and (c) without the charm, the leaf proves useless. These three statements seem carefully tailored to articulate what we would call the idea of 'indispensability of complementariness'; not only is complete well-being entirely dependent upon that additional charm, which has a great deal to do with the soul and its attachment to the body, but it is also of decisive importance for the attainment of partial well-being. Put differently, the text itself urges us to de-localise an ailment affecting a certain bodily part, and to think of a whole whose parts can be cured only if the whole itself is. It may be that the leaf, if applied, will treat the headache, even if no charm is uttered; but its usefulness will still not be proved, unless it is accompanied by that very charm.[19] Thus ὄφελος ('advantage' or 'benefit') is – and must be – defined solely by reference to complete well-being, in other words, by reference to a certain whole. But what exactly is the whole alluded to here?

2.3 *The Power of the Charm and the Good Practitioner*

Socrates' description of the power (δύναμις, 156b2) of the proposed charm rests upon two main pillars: (a) the charm's non-restrictive, de-isolating therapeutic nature, and (b) its apparently all-embracing acceptance of the holistic medical practice followed by doctors who deem it necessary to simultaneously treat both a bodily part and the whole to which this part belongs, if the part is to be in good order:

> **T3**: 'Its nature, Charmides, is not such as to be able to cure the head alone. You have probably heard this about good doctors (τῶν ἀγαθῶν ἰατρῶν),

19 Cf. Schmid (1998) 17–19; Tuozzo (2001) 327; Levine (2016) 65.

> that if you go to them with a pain in the eyes, they are likely to say that they cannot undertake to cure the eyes by themselves, but that it will be necessary to treat the head at the same time (ἅμα), if things are also to go well with the eyes. And again it would be very foolish to suppose that one could ever treat the head by itself without treating the whole body (ὅλου τοῦ σώματος). In keeping with this principle, they plan a regime for the whole body (ἐπὶ πᾶν τὸ σῶμα) with the idea of treating and curing the part along with the whole' (156b3–c5).

The text makes it clear that this medical practice is founded on a core belief that the well-being of the parts is contingent on the treatment of the whole. What is even more interesting, however, is that all those engaged in this appear to be described as 'good'[20] *precisely because* they hold such a belief. This assumption seems further buttressed by the emphasis Socrates places on the folly permeating the views of those who claim to treat the part by itself, apart from the whole. This transition, from practical performance to the cognitive state of a doctor, takes us one step further: to judge whether a doctor is good or not is to assess him in respect to his wisdom, which is of course reflected in the medical practice he adopts. The deciphering of the intimate connection between goodness and wisdom thus appears to construct a powerful interpretative framework: good medical practice is guided by knowledge of the dependence of the parts' well-being on the health of the whole, and hence by awareness of the need to prescribe a regimen to be applied to the body as a whole in order for the part to be cured along with it.

The above clarification proves salutary for the effort to dispel any perplexity about the nature of the proposed charm. We thus arrive at the following bipartite conclusion: (a) Socrates' charm is unable to cure a particular part without treating the whole to which that part belongs, and (b) its δύναμις consists in

20 The expression τῶν ἀγαθῶν ἰατρῶν has been reasonably taken to draw a contrast between doctors of the Hippocratic school, most likely those who used diet as a means of treating the whole body, and the magico-religious healers found in mystery cults; see e.g. Tuozzo (2001) 325 n. 12. In Plato's *Phaedrus* 270c1, a more expansive holism is attributed to Hippocrates, one that requires doctors to study 'the nature of the whole' – the whole probably referring to the natural environment of which human beings form parts. (As examples of this type of 'environmental medicine', see esp. the Hippocratic *De aere, aquis, locis, Epidemiarum* I and III, and *Prognosticum*). For detailed discussion, see Mansfeld (1980); Gill (2003); Tuozzo (2011) 113–14. Although the peculiar type of holism Socrates offers in the *Chrm.* is not attested in the surviving corpus of Hippocratic writings, we clearly align ourselves with Tuozzo, who claims that this conception could easily have formed part of the Hippocratic environmental holism mentioned above. See also (from different angles), Bartoš and Craik in this volume.

being used by a good/wise 'doctor' to treat that whole and, as a consequence, its part. In other words, the dynamics of such a charm, as the text emphasises, can be defined strictly with reference to the whole, not one of its parts. Charmides is now witnessing a significant dialectical advance: in order to attain complete well-being, he must undergo a treatment whose effectiveness depends on being referred to the whole. Nevertheless, although Socrates' attempts to establish the idea of a whole composed of parts whose well-being is entirely dependent on the whole seem to have been crowned with success, there remains an urgent need to clarify the nature of that whole.

3 True Holistic Dietetics. Socrates' Philosophical Practice

3.1 *Reworking the Notion of the Whole*

There seems no denying that the fundamental qualities of the proposed charm would have been misconceived or incompletely defined, had Socrates not proceeded to clear up the nature of the whole to which that charm refers. What is especially remarkable, however, is that this dialectical move is presented as divinely sanctioned. Specifically, the need to elucidate the nature of the whole that must be placed at the centre of any therapeutic process appears perfectly aligned with the dictates of the Thracian god Zalmoxis, who, although acknowledging the rightness of the statement (καλῶς λέγοιεν, 156d7) that the part is healed through the treatment of the whole, identifies a crucial flaw in the Greek doctors' diagnostic reasoning and practice: neglect of the nature of the true whole.[21] The reference to the divine origin of the charm in fact focuses Socrates' argument on offering a comprehensive approach to human nature as a whole in which the soul is assigned pride of place. τοῦ ὅλου (156e4) thus means not the body and its parts, as suggested so far, but another type of whole, one that renders impossible any attempt to cure the body apart from the soul (156e2).

To clarify the exact nature of that whole and the parts that comprise it, we must address a crucial question: how is the soul understood? As (a) the whole whose part is the body? (b) an integral part of the whole, whose cure needs to be temporally or causally prioritised for the sake of that whole? or (c) perhaps

21 [...] ὅτι τοῦ ὅλου ἀμελοῖεν οὗ δέοι τὴν ἐπιμέλειαν ποιεῖσθαι, οὗ μὴ καλῶς ἔχοντος ἀδύνατον εἴη τὸ μέρος εὖ ἔχειν, 156e4–6 ('[...] that they do not pay attention to the whole as they ought to do, since if the whole is not in good condition, it is impossible that the part should be'). Reading τὸ ὅλον ἀγνοοῖεν with BT and Croiset (1921), rather than Burnet's (1903) τοῦ ὅλου ἀμελοῖεν, has no effect on the meaning of the text. For discussion of the variant readings, see Van der Ben (1985) 15 n. 13; Coolidge (1993) 23–36; Tuozzo (2001) 325 n. 14.

both? It is true that option (a) sounds rather unrealistic, given that there seems to be no evidence in the extant Platonic corpus of a soul-body relationship that could be likened to the one pertaining between the head (the whole) and the eyes (a part of that whole), or between the body (the whole) and the head (a part of that whole).[22] On the other hand, it seems quite reasonable, at least at first glance, to choose the second option (b), the soul-body composite, since Socrates appears to be taking care to accurately report Zalmoxis' words:

> **T4**: 'Because, he said, the soul is the source (ὡρμῆσθαι) of all good and evil in the body and in the whole person (παντὶ τῷ ἀνθρώπῳ), and these flow (ἐπιρρεῖν) from the soul in the same way that the eyes are affected by the head' (156e6–57a1).
>
> trans. SPRAGUE, modified

In this account, therefore, the soul must be emphasized as the determining factor, not only in physical health, but in human health as a whole. At any rate, both options (a and b) appear to call for an adaptation of the holistic program of regimen proposed at T3 to meet the new demands. That is to say, in lieu of 'the whole body' (ἐπὶ πᾶν τὸ σῶμα, 156c4), which was treated as the relevant whole within that regimen, in T4 we are faced with the dilemma of whether we should take Socrates to be proposing the soul (a whole of which the body is a part) *or* the whole person (the soul-body composite, of which both body and soul are parts). How can we reach a clear conclusion? In fact, the key to the interpretation of our passage is supplied by the analogy between the eyes-head connection, on the one hand, and our two most likely candidates, on the other: the body (part)-soul (whole) relationship *or* the soul (part)-person (whole) relationship.[23] What is the point of this 'thought experiment', whereby Socrates wants us to imagine that the soul is a constant source of good and evil of which the head stands as a paradigm (in its relationship to the eyes)?

A closer reading of the text offers a way out of this dilemma by revealing that two mutually inclusive notions of whole are in question: (a) the soul as whole and (b) the soul-body compound as whole.

3.1.1 Unhealthy Psychic State: the Soul as Whole

The analogy in T4 invites us to suspect that a peculiar kind of wholeness (and partiality) is at work here, one that manifests itself primarily in conditions

22 See e.g. 156e1–2.

23 156e8–7a1. Cf. Bloch (1973) 38. For a different interpretation, see Van der Ben (1985) 17, 19 n. 5.

of disruption of psychic health. This kind of wholeness refers to a relation *of beneficial dependency*, according to which something is a part insofar as its being benefitted or harmed depends upon the well-being of something else, and something is a whole insofar as it determines the well-being of something else. In this sense, not just the body, but the whole person should be seen as parts, insofar as their health depends on the health of the soul. This explains why the health of the soul is at the centre of Socrates' holistic medicine. In such a relationship of dependency, the soul as a whole assumes the role of the regulator of the health and order of the body and person overall. The soul is a whole in the sense that its integrity is wholly responsible for maintaining the integrity of the parts.[24] It is also a whole in the sense that its health may be said to represent a projection of the cosmic order as this affects humankind[25] – a whole whose parts have been allotted the position of being conditional upon it.

3.1.2 Restoration of Psychic Health: the Soul-Body Compound as Whole

When we turn to examination of what happens after the soul is restored to a state of health, some crucial questions arise, particularly concerning the treatment of the physical ailment at hand. For example: why does the soul, although it is the source of bodily health and disease, not manage, once it has been healed and has acquired σωφροσύνη, to effect the cure of the headache? Why is the body still subject to sickness, and why does the leaf still need to be applied to the head? And how are we to take Socrates' comment about the ease of procuring health for the head and the rest of the body after σωφροσύνη has been engendered in the soul by means of 'beautiful words'? Let us quote the text:

> T5: 'So it is necessary first and foremost to cure the soul if the parts of the head and of the rest of the body are to be healthy. And the soul, he said, my dear friend, is cured by means of certain charms, and these charms consist of beautiful words (λόγους). It is a result of such words that temperance (σωφροσύνην) arises (ἐγγίγνεσθαι) in the soul, and when the soul acquires and possesses temperance, it is easy to provide health both for the head and for the rest of the body' (157a1–b1).

From this assignment of functional significance to the leaf *per se*, it seems reasonable to infer that, upon restoration of psychic health, a slightly different

24 For a slightly different view, see Tuozzo (2001) 328.

25 *Grg.* 508a3, to be interpreted in its larger textual context 507e–508a4; cf. 504b–d; Friedländer (1964) 63.

notion of the whole comes into play, one that brings to the fore the importance of the soul-body composite, in which the soul is singled out as the central regulatory principle, yet still allows for the possibility that the body needs its own separate treatment. The presence of σωφροσύνη in a healthy soul thus seems to provide a person with a clear awareness not only of the health of his soul, but of the emergence of a particular ailment affecting a bodily part. In addition, although the healthy soul does not claim knowledge of the treatment needed, it alerts a person to the need to be rid of that ailment, in order that both the body and the whole body-soul composite can benefit from the proper functioning of that whole.

This reasoning makes it even more difficult to endorse the suggestion that this text implies that headache, as an ailment of the head, a physical ailment, has its origin in the soul, which has also been acknowledged as the source of bodily disease. This conclusion may appear to some to follow naturally from the thrust of the discussion. But the argument seems to be a *figurative vehicle* for highlighting the harmful effects of being unaware, due to lack of σωφροσύνη, of the care the soul must enjoy, if the whole body-soul composite is to be healthy. Inevitably, therefore, we are faced with the suggestion of a hierarchy of evils which keeps us from accepting that the focus of this text is on the physiological etiology of the ailment at hand.[26] This also renders it virtually impossible to argue that Socrates, in saying that 'the soul is the source of all good and evil in the body and in the whole man' (T3), has in mind physical ailments such as the one discussed here. This is not to say that a physical ailment does not constitute something bad,[27] but rather that it occupies a lower position in Socrates' hierarchy of evils than vice in the soul.

3.2 *How to Care for the Whole: Philosophy as Holistic Medical Practice*

Now that we have seen that two notions of whole are at work, depending on whether we speak of the soul's bad or good condition, we can turn to the logical consequence of this, that there must be two ways of caring for the whole. This brings us back to Socrates' charm, whose nature and power may have been cleared up, while still leaving important questions open. At 157a4–5 (T5) we find Socrates pointedly identifying the charm as a 'beautiful word/speech': τὰς δ' ἐπῳδὰς ταύτας τοὺς λόγους εἶναι τοὺς καλούς.

---

26 As opposed, for example, to the focus of Plato's *Timaeus* 81e6–82b7, where disease is attributed to some disruption of stability in the interaction between the elements out of which the body has been constructed.

27 Cf. 165d1–2 τὴν γὰρ ὑγίειαν καλὸν ἡμῖν ἔργον ('Because health is a fine result for us'); for disease as a defect of the body, e.g. *Grg*. 464c1–66a3. Cf. 214 n. 35.

Yet Socrates' (Zalmoxis') acknowledgement of the beauty characterising the Greek doctors' speech (156d7) a few minutes before he replaces it with a new, holistic one, suggests that this charm, which engenders σωφροσύνη in the soul, refers to a process which admits of different levels of 'beautifully-speaking' and presupposes an argumentative ascent to a certain summit. This 'philosophical' character of Socrates' charm seems further confirmed by the fact that what started as an engagement in philosophical, dialectical inquiry (oriented towards stripping Charmides' soul in order to inspect its well-orderedness) is now further qualified as a philosophical examination of whether or not Charmides partakes sufficiently in σωφροσύνη.[28] One can hardly fail to notice here Plato moving towards equating psychic well-orderedness with possession of σωφροσύνη, or to miss the hint of dropping the idea that σωφροσύνη in the soul could be produced in any way other than through Socratic truth-seeking inquiry.[29]

The identification of the proposed charm with Socrates' philosophical inquiry provides the missing piece required for a deeper understanding of Socrates' self-referential intentions in the *Charmides*. Let us therefore look more closely at the motivation and target-setting agenda behind such an enterprise. Socratic-Zalmoxian philosophical practice, it now seems clear, takes over the mantle of medicine on the grounds that current medical practitioners habitually commit the error of treating physical health and psychic well-being as entirely different things.[30] Accordingly, it sets out to establish the person as a body-soul composite in which the soul plays the most prominent role,[31] and to stress the urgency and priority of treatment of it.[32] On a practical level, this philosophical practice manifests itself, at an initial stage, as a diagnostic tool for measuring a person's degree of σωφροσύνη. Diagnosis of psychic health, in which both soul and body, as parts of the whole soul-body composite, are in harmony with each other and enjoy the benefits of the whole's

28 εἰ δὲ δὴ καὶ πρὸς σωφροσύνην καὶ πρὸς τἆλλα κατὰ τὸν τοῦδε λόγον ἱκανῶς πέφυκας, 158b2–3 ('But if, in addition, you have a sufficient share of temperance and the other attributes mentioned by your friend here'); cf. 158c3–4.

29 Cf. Pl. *Symp.* 198e4. Van der Ben (1985) 13–14, argues for the Platonic character of a passage actually based on Herodotus 4.94–95; cf. Tuozzo (2001) 323 n. 6, and especially Tuozzo (2011) 115–18, for detailed discussion of the Herodotus passage. On the identification of καλοὶ λόγοι with Socrates' elenctic inquiry, see also Reece (1998) 74. Studies casting doubt on whether such an identification can be clearly derived from the text include Schmid (1998) 15; McPherran (2004) 23–26.

30 Cf. 158e2 and 157b5–7.

31 Cf. 157b and 157c2.

32 See in particular 154e6, 157a1, 157b4, 157c3, 158c2. On the idea that psychosomatic unity is Socrates' principal educational goal, see Friedländer (1964) 64.

well-being, renders the practice no longer useful. If correctly applied, however, medical practice takes the form of a philosophical regimen which treats the soul as a source/whole from which all good and evil flow. This practice is oriented towards attaining health through the patient's dialectical ascent to the summit of the most beautiful *logos*. Upon critical inspection, therefore, the Socratic-Zalmoxian charm proves to have served a twofold central purpose: (a) to lay the foundations of a new form of holistic medical practice which rests upon the idea that the essence of a doctor's job is granting equal consideration to σωφροσύνη and physical health; and (b) to establish itself as the only way to diagnose whether or not someone has σωφροσύνη (and subsequently to produce it), thus superseding traditional criteria such as noble birth or high social standing.[33]

3.3 *Decoding Holisms: Further Explorations of the Analogy between Philosophy and Medicine*

Although Socrates' holistic practice attempts to invalidate the current medical one because it rests on a less beautiful λόγος, the very fact that its nature is chiefly medical[34] and not e.g. architectural (along with the frequency with which the *Charmides* appeals to medicine) makes clear that Plato wants us to dwell on the analogy between philosophical inquiry and medicine. That the dialogue fails to arrive at an unassailable definition of σωφροσύνη creates no problem, especially since, before the investigation of σωφροσύνη begins, readers have been repeatedly alerted to the medical nature of Socrates' inquiry. The various references to the medical art in the course of the inquiry into σωφροσύνη indicate the nature of medicine *per se*, yet at the same time clarify Socrates' holistic activity. An interesting example is offered at 164a–c, where Socrates stresses that a doctor's knowledge enables him to bring about health, which is further defined as acting beneficially both for himself and his patient, that is as making his σωφροσύνη manifest in a practical form. This knowledge is elsewhere qualified as knowledge of health, whose benefit consists in producing a 'fine result.'[35] It also renders the doctor capable of distinguishing pretensions to knowledge in this particular area of expertise from true possession of it.[36]

---

33 See e.g. 157e–58c. Santas (1973) 107 n. 3, emphasises in particular that just as in his other early dialogues, so too in the *Chrm.* Plato takes on a venerable tradition, concentrating his efforts on revealing the inadequacy of the traditional definitions of virtue; cf. Mouzala (2016) 183.

34 *Pace* Tuozzo (2001) 327 n. 17.

35 [...] οὐ σμικρὰν ὠφελίαν· τὴν γὰρ ὑγίειαν καλὸν ἡμῖν ἔργον ἀπεργάζεται, 165d1–2. Cf. 170b3–6.

36 170e–71c.

The question then arises: what implications do such evocations of the 'medical' analogy suggest for Socratic philosophical inquiry? If our analysis is correct, Socratic holistic inquiry has a threefold orientation, which is distinctly medical in nature:

3.3.1 Orientation to Prophylaxis

Socratic inquiry must be itself a practical manifestation of σωφροσύνη, one that stems from a kind of knowledge that guides the person initiating it in such a way as to make him aware of the benefits he confers, in initiating it, upon himself and the 'patients' subjected to philosophical examination.[37] Accordingly, knowledge of what benefits oneself can only be construed as pointing to some sort of self-knowledge.[38]

3.3.2 Orientation to Therapy

Socratic inquiry must be founded on knowledge of the health of the whole person and how it can be generated in the human soul.[39] Knowing how to bring about that kind of health, σωφροσύνη, means knowing how to produce the finest and most beneficial result. A practical manifestation of σωφροσύνη, such as Socrates' holism, thus amounts to a practical manifestation of the knowledge of how to produce σωφροσύνη. We may therefore reasonably conclude that Socrates' holism is assigned the role of exemplifying σωφροσύνη's knowledge of (how to produce) itself.[40]

3.3.3 Orientation to Diagnosis

Socratic inquiry must be able, in light of (3.3.1) and (3.3.2 prooem.), to diagnose whether or not one possesses σωφροσύνη. The implication of this admission is initially twofold: Socratic medical inquiry claims to be able to distinguish those who (i) pretend to be 'physicians of the soul' from real such physicians;

---

37 Cf. Tuozzo (2011) 112.

38 Cf. 169e1. On self-knoweldge and its place in the *Chrm.*, see e.g. Tuckey (1968) 4, 25–26; Schmid (1998) 40–60. Cf. Friedländer (1964) 73–74; Bruell (1977); Hyland (1981); Schmid (1983) 344, 348; Mouzala (2016).

39 *Pace* Schmid (1998) 16; cf. Friedländer (1964) 63. We thus cannot agree with West and West (1986), Coolidge (1993) and McAvoy (1996), who claim that Zalmoxian medicine in the *Chrm.* should be treated as avowing its own ignorance of the whole. See also Tuozzo (2001) 326 n. 14. Generally, for discussions of whether Plato's Socrates appears to possess a τέχνη of moral virtue, see e.g. Versenyi (1972); Irwin (1977); Klosko (1981); Roochnik (1981); Schmid (1998) 15–19.

40 Cf. 165e2, 166b5–6, 168a5–9, 169c–e. Carone (1998) contains a useful discussion of the idea that such a kind of knowledge can survive the challenges presented by Socrates in the *Chrm.*

(ii) pretend to have σωφροσύνη from true possessors of this virtue.[41] This is not to say that it also claims to be able to distinguish those possessing expertise in a particular art or science from those who do not; nowhere in the *Charmides*, for instance, does Socratic medical inquiry avow knowledge of what physical health and disease are.[42] Nor do we in any case expect it to be competent to diagnose and treat physical ailments. It is nonetheless also expected[43] to be able to identify σωφροσύνη within the activities involved in any area of expertise, that is, to diagnose whether or not an expert's act is an act of σωφροσύνη. This kind of inquiry can sometimes go as far as to call into question the expertise itself, as with those holistic physicians who, leaving σωφροσύνη out of account, base their practice on a less beautiful, eventually erroneous conception of the whole.

4 Conclusion: Holistic Inquiry, *eudaimonia* and Divine Assimilation

The introduction to this paper outlined the main issue to be addressed, followed by some preliminary remarks (Section 2) regarding the importance of the soul for the person as a whole, and hence the need to de-localise a disease affecting a part of the body. Section 3 then explored in depth what Socrates considers the true whole – the object of his proposed holistic inquiry. Our suggestion was that the nature of that whole must be twofold, manifesting itself in either unhealthy or healthy psychic states, and as a consequence requiring the respective types of care. Whether one approach or the other is to take place proved a matter of whether one must subject oneself to philosophical examination, or whether one already possesses σωφροσύνη and is thus able to care for one's own soul and the souls of others. Finally, further exploration of the analogy with the medical art revealed more conspicuously the medical orientation of Socratic inquiry.

By looking behind the façade of the discussion's conclusion[44] and its apparent implication that no benefit is derived from the presence of σωφροσύνη[45] – a conclusion that seems deliberately at odds with what those who read between the lines are supposed to draw from the *Charmides* – one can form an even more complete picture of the nature of the knowledge upon which Socratic

41 Cf. Dyson (1974) 111.
42 Cf. 170b–e.
43 Partly contrary to the apparent conclusion of the dialogue (cf. 172a, 174d).
44 171d.
45 175d7–e2.

holistic inquiry is founded. Previously identified as knowledge of the soul's health, this knowledge seems now to be qualified as knowledge of good and evil,[46] an inference perfectly aligned with the statement at T4, which acknowledges the soul as the source of all good and evil for the whole person. Knowing the soul's health must therefore mean knowing what good and evil is, a cognitive state that comes to be regarded as ensuring *eudaimonia*.[47] Socratic inquiry, in guaranteeing human beings' epistemic status, thus emerges as the only holistic practice that cares for the true whole, the person as soul-body composite, and hence as the only way to attain real benefit and *eudaimonia*. Even more interesting, this reconceptualised notion of holism is portrayed by Plato as both divine in its origin and enjoying godly sanction. This literary device, it seems clear now, draws our attention to two principal aspects of the nature of the newly-introduced holistic practice. First, this is a sort of divine mission assigned to Socrates to convey a particular message to human beings.[48] Second, by passing on that message, namely by treating the person as a whole in which the soul is given prominence, it brings human beings closer to possessing divine knowledge,[49] allowing them to attain some sort of divinity.[50]

Acknowledgments

We would like to thank Chiara Thumiger for her constructive feedback and suggestions, as well as Prof. Paul Kalligas and the anonymous reviewer for reading and commenting on an earlier version of this paper.

Bibliography

Anagnastopoulos, G. 'Review of T. M. Robinson, *Plato's Psychology*.' *Journal for the History of Philosophy*, 10 (1972) 217–21.

Bloch, G. *Platons* Charmides. *Die Erscheinung des Seins im Gespräch*. Braunschweig: Eberhard-Karls-Universität Tübingen (1973).

46 Cf. 174c3.

47 Cf. 173d, 174c, 176a4–5.

48 Cf. Pl. *Ap*. 28e, 33c. A similar connection is drawn by Dieterle (1966) 147; cf. Tuozzo (2001) 323 n. 5.

49 Cf. Tuozzo (2001) 330; Tuozzo (2011) 118.

50 Cf. Pl. *Tht*. 176a–c, *Phdr*. 246a–53c, *Ti*. 90c–d. Cf. also *Symp*. 207c–209e, 212a; *Lysis* 214a–b; *Ap*. 41c–d; *Resp*. 613a.

Bruell, C. 'Socratic Politics and Self-Knowledge: An Interpretation of Plato's *Charmides*.' *Interpretation*, 6 (1977) 141–203.

Carone, G. 'Socrates' Human Wisdom and *Sophrosune* in *Charmides* 146c ff.' *Ancient Philosophy*, 18 (1998) 267–86.

Coolidge Jr., F. 'The Relation of Philosophy to *Σωφροσύνη*. Zalmoxian Medicine in Plato's *Charmides*.' *Ancient Philosophy*, 13 (1993) 23–36.

Dieterle, R. *Platons* Laches *und* Charmides. *Untersuchungen zur elenktisch-aporetischen Struktur der platonischen Frühdialoge*. Freiburg: Albert–Ludwigs Universität (1966).

Dyson, M. 'Some Problems Concerning Knowledge in Plato's "*Charmides*".' *Phronesis*, 19 (1974) 102–11.

Friedländer, P. *Platon. Vol. II. Die Platonischen Schriften. Erste Periode*. 3rd edition. Berlin: De Gruyter (1964).

Gill, M. L. 'Plato's *Phaedrus* and the Method of Hippocrates.' *Modern Schoolman*, 80 (2003) 295–314.

Hazebroucq, M. *La Folie Humaine et ses Remèdes. Platon*. Charmide *ou de la moderation*. Paris: Vrin (1997).

Hogan, R. 'Soul in the *Charmides*: An Examination of T. M. Robinson's Interpretation.' *Philosophy Research Archives*, 2 (1976) 635–45.

Hyland, D. *The Virtue of Philosophy. An Interpretation of Plato's* Charmides. Athens OH: Ohio University Press (1981).

Irwin, T. *Plato's Moral Theory*. Oxford: Oxford University Press (1977).

Klosko, G. 'The Technical Conception of Virtue.' *Journal of the History of Philosophy*, 19 (1981) 95–102.

Lampert, L. *How Philosophy Became Socratic: A Study of Plato's* Protagoras, Charmides, *and* Republic. Chicago: University of Chicago Press (2010).

Levine, D. *Profound Ignorance: Plato's* Charmides *and the Saving of Wisdom*. Lanham, Boulder, New York and London: Lexington Books (2016).

Mansfeld, J. 'Plato and the Method of Hippocrates.' *Greek, Roman and Byzantine Studies*, 21 (1980) 341–62.

McAvoy, M. 'Carnal Knowledge in the *Charmides*.' *Apeiron*, 24 (1996) 63–103.

McPherran, M. 'Socrates and Zalmoxis on Drugs, Charms and Purification.' *Apeiron*, 37 (2004) 11–33.

Mouzala, M. 'Διαλεκτική, Δραματουργία, και Αυτογνωσία στον *Χαρμίδη* του Πλάτωνος.' *Studia Gilsoniana*, 5 (2016) 179–94.

Reece, A. 'Drama, Narrative, and Socratic *Erōs* in Plato's *Charmides*.' *Interpretation*, 26 (1998) 65–76.

Robinson, T. *Plato's Psychology*. 2nd edition. Toronto: University of Toronto Press (1995).

Roochnik, D. 'Plato's Use of the Techne-Analogy.' *Journal of the History of Philosophy*, 24 (1986) 295–310.

Rowe, C. 'Review of M.-F. Hazebroucq, *La Folie humaine et ses remèdes.*' *Phronesis*, 43 (1998) 87–88.

Santas, G. 'Socrates at Work on Virtue and Knowledge in Plato's *Charmides.*' in *Exegesis and Argument*, ed. E. Lee, A. Mourelatos and R. Rorty. Assen: Van Gorcum (1973) 105–32.

Schmid, W. 'Socratic Moderation and Self-Knowledge.' *Journal of the History of Philosophy*, 21 (1983) 339–48.

Schmid, W. *Plato's* Charmides *and the Socratic Ideal of Rationality*. Albany: State University of New York Press (1998).

Steiner, P. *Psyche bei Platon*. Göttingen: Vandenhoeck & Ruprecht (1992).

Tuckey, T. *Plato's* Charmides. Amsterdam: Adolf M. Hakkert (1968).

Tuozzo, T. 'What's Wrong with These Cities? The Social Dimension of *Sophrosune* in Plato's *Charmides.*' *Journal of the History of Philosophy*, 39 (2001) 321–50.

Tuozzo, T. *Plato's* Charmides*: Positive Elenchus in a 'Socratic' Dialogue*. Cambridge: Cambridge University Press (2011).

Van der Ben, N. *The* Charmides *of Plato. Problems and Interpretations*. Amsterdam: B. R. Grüner (1985).

Versenyi, L. 'Virtue as a Self-Directed Art.' *Personalist*, 53 (1972) 274–89.

West, T., and G. West. *Plato's* Charmides. Indianapolis: Hackett (1986).

Primary Texts: Editions and Translations Used

Platonis Opera. Vol. III. Ed. J. Burnet. Oxford: Oxford University Press (1903).

Platon. Oeuvres completes. Vol. II. Ed. A. Croiset. Paris: Société d'Édition 'Les Belles Lettres' (1921).

Plato. *Charmides*. Trans. R. Sprague in *Plato. Complete Works*. Edited by J. Cooper. Indianapolis: Hackett (1997) 630–63.

CHAPTER 9

A Woman in Flux: Fluidity in Hippocratic Gynaecology

Laurence M. V. Totelin

Abstract

In this chapter, I analyse passages that refer to water features, such as rivers and wells, in the Hippocratic gynaecological treatises. I suggest that the Hippocratic authors drew analogies between the vessels of the female body and riverbeds, thereby pointing to a form of holism in which the female body was a microcosm of the earth, furrowed by watery channels. A young woman's vessels were narrow and prone to blockages, but they widened and became more easy-flowing as a woman gave birth. The transition from *parthenos* to *gynē*, then, was one associated with fluidity. To understand better the context of the Hippocratic texts, I discuss ancient rituals involving water that marked a woman's transition into adulthood. These rituals often involved the Nymphs who resided in rivers and wells.

Any reader of the Hippocratic gynaecological treatises will notice that bodily fluids are there given – rather unsurprisingly – great prominence.[1] A woman's life is marked by fluxes, healthy or otherwise: menstruation, lochial discharge (the blood discharge after birth), fluxes that are symptomatic of illnesses, and lactation.[2] In this chapter, I suggest that the authors of these treatises had a

1 For an overview of women's physiology and the importance of fluids therein in ancient Greek medicine, see most prominently Dean-Jones (1994); King (1998). See also Carson (1990); Andò (2012).

2 The organisation of the Hippocratic gynaecological treatise *On Diseases of Women* I reflects this preoccupation with fluxes. The treatise follows a woman's reproductive cycle, starting with menstruation (chapters 1–9), followed by conception (chapters 10–24), pregnancy (chapters 24–34), and birth and the post-partum period (chapters 35–73); the treatise ends with catalogues of recipes (chapters 74–109). The treatise *On Diseases of Women* II devotes a significant section to morbid fluxes: chapters 1 (110 L.) and 2–13 (112–122 L.). In this chapter, I adopt Paul Potter's numbering of chapters in his new Loeb Classical Library editions of *On Generation* and *On the Nature of the Child* (2012) and *Diseases of Women* II (2018), but I will indicate the Littré numbering in brackets. English titles and abbreviated Latin titles are those found in Craik (2015).

 | DOI:10.1163/9789004443143_011

form of ecological holism in mind, one where the body of a woman was like an earth – or perhaps simply was an earth – furrowed by vessels carrying bodily fluids. To reach this conclusion, I conduct a close analysis of the vocabulary of fluidity and of references to water features in selected passages of these treatises, starting with the famous opening statement of *On Diseases of Women* I, a discussion of flows and discharges:

> Matters regarding the diseases of women. I maintain that a woman who has not given birth suffers more severely and faster from her menses than one who has borne a child. Indeed, when she gives birth, the small vessels become **more easy-flowing** for the menses. What makes them **easy-flowing** is the lochial purgation. If there has been a **liquefaction** of the body, [the flesh] near the belly and the breasts **liquefy** the most, but the rest of the body also **liquefies**. As the body **liquefies**, of necessity, the vessels open themselves and become more **easy-flowing** for the menses, and the womb opens more because the baby has moved through them and caused both pressure and strain.
>
> τὰ δὲ ἀμφὶ γυναικείων νούσων· φημὶ γυναῖκα ἄτοκον ἐοῦσαν ἢ τετοκυῖαν χαλεπώτερον καὶ θᾶσσον ἀπὸ καταμηνίων νοσέειν· ὅταν γὰρ τέκῃ, **εὐροώτερά** οἱ τὰ φλέβιά ἐστιν ἐς τὰ καταμήνια· **εὔροα** δέ σφε ποιέει ἡ λοχείη κάθαρσις. καὶ ἢν **καταρραγῇ** <ἦ> τοῦ σώματος, τὰ πλησιάζοντα μάλιστα τῆς τε κοιλίης καὶ τῶν μαζῶν **καταρρήγνυται**· **καταρρήγνυται** δὲ καὶ τὸ ἄλλο σῶμα· ὑφ' ὅτευ δὲ γίνεται, εἴρηταί μοι ἐν τῇ Φύσει τοῦ Παιδίου τοῦ ἐν Τόκῳ. **καταρραγέντος** δὲ τοῦ σώματος, ἀνάγκη τὰς φλέβας μᾶλλον στομοῦσθαι καὶ **εὐροωτέρας** γίνεσθαι ἐς τὰ καταμήνια, καὶ τὰς μήτρας μᾶλλον στομοῦσθαι, οἷα τοῦ παιδίου χωρήσαντος διὰ σφέων καὶ βίην καὶ τόνον παρασχόντος.[3]

The author then suggested that a woman who has borne a child might still suffer when she has her periods, but she would do so less than one who has not, because she has open space in her body:

> At the same time, there is **more open space** for blood in her body when she has given birth (that is, since her body **has liquefied**); and the blood, since it is **in an open space**, becomes less painful unless the vessels overfill and overstrain.

3 *Mul.* 1.1 (VIII.10 L. = 8 Potter). On this chapter of *On Diseases of Women* I, see Hanson (1975). Unless stated otherwise, all translations in this chapter are mine.

> καὶ ἅμα **εὐρυχωρίη** ἐστὶν ἐν τῷ σώματι πλείων τῷ αἵματι, ἐπὴν τέκῃ, οἷα τοῦ σώματος **καταρραγέντος**, καὶ ἐν εὐρυχωρίῃ ἐὸν τὸ αἷμα ἀπονώτερον γίνεται, ἢν μὴ ὑπερπιμπλῶνται αἱ φλέβες καὶ ὑπερτονέωσιν.[4]

The body of a woman who has not experienced a lochial purgation, the author continued, is harder, firmer, and denser than one who has not. Both women's bodies, however, are spongier and softer than that of a man.[5] The author set to prove this with an analogy: if one were to place a piece of wool and a piece of thickly-woven cloth over water for a couple of days, one would find that the looser fleece has absorbed more water than the thickly-woven cloth. The flesh of women can be compared to fleece, a soft material that absorbs much liquid.

The version of *On Diseases of Women* I that has come down to us is the work of a compiler (author C in Hermann Grensemann's classification), who expressed himself quite regularly in the first person.[6] Through these authorial interventions, which often take the form of cross-references, we gather that this compiler also authored the treatises *On Generation* and *On the Nature of the Child*, where he explained in more detail what happens to the body when it goes through puberty, using the same vocabulary as in the passages of *On Diseases of Women* quoted above:

> But when the young girl and boy grow up, the vessels that lead to the penis in the boy and to the womb in the girl stretch out and become **liquefied** because of their growth, and they [the vessels] open up, and a passage is created through the narrow spaces, and the moisture then can be agitated, for there now is **an open space** in which there can be agitation. Thus, the boy emits seed when he becomes a man, and the girl produces the menses.

> ἐπὴν δὲ αὔξωνται καὶ παρθένος καὶ παῖς, αἱ φλέβες αἱ ἐς τὸ αἰδοῖον τείνουσαι τοῦ παιδὸς καὶ τῆς παρθένου ἐπὶ τὰς μήτρας **εὔροαι** γίνονται ὑπὸ τῆς αὔξης καὶ στομοῦνται, καὶ δίοδος διὰ στενῶν γίνεται, καὶ τὸ ὑγρὸν κλόνησιν τότε ἴσχει, **εὐρυχωρίη** γάρ οἱ τότε γίνεται ἔνθα κλονήσεται· καὶ χωρέει τῷ παιδὶ, ἐπὴν ἁδρὸς ἔῃ, διὰ τόδε, καὶ τῇ παρθένῳ τὰ καταμήνια.[7]

4 *Mul.* 1.1 (VIII.10 L. = 10 Potter).

5 On women's flesh as spongy, see Andò (2012) and below.

6 See Grensemann (1975), (1982). See also Lonie (1981) 51–54.

7 *Gen.* 2 (VII.472–474 L. = 10 Potter).

In children, both male and female, the vessels that lead to the penis in boys and to the uterus in girls are narrow and do not allow for the secretion of fluids. When children grow, their vessels become wider, and fluids can now be secreted. It is only with childbirth, however, that the maturation of the female body becomes complete, and that the vessels become wide enough. In *On the Nature of the Child*, the author gave an account of what happens in childbirth that is very similar to that of *On the Disease of Women* I. He employed the verb *katarrēgnymi* twice, and specified that the process affects mostly the breasts and the moist parts of the body:

> After these events [sc. the birth], a watery discharge tainted with blood comes from the head and the rest of her body, created as a result of the pressure, pain, and heat [of labour], and this leads the way for the lochial purgation. After expulsion of a serous discharge, the purgation occurs for the time mentioned above. Then the breasts and the other moist parts of a woman's body **liquefy**, most poorly with the first birth, but then, as they experience further births, they **liquefy more**, as the vessels are fully emptied by the lochial purgation. That is what I have to say on the topic.
>
> μετὰ δὲ ταῦτα ὕδρωψ ἔρχεται αἱματώδης ἀπό τε τῆς κεφαλῆς καὶ τοῦ ἄλλου σώματος, ἀποκριθεὶς ὑπὸ βίης τε καὶ πόνου καὶ θέρμης, καὶ ὁδὸν ἀφηγήσατο τῶν λοχίων τῇ καθάρσει· μετὰ δὲ τὴν ἔξοδον τοῦ ἰχῶρος ἡ κάθαρσις γίνεται χρόνον τὸν πρόσθεν εἰρημένον. καὶ οἵ τε μαζοὶ καὶ τἆλλα μέλεα ὁκόσα ὑγρότερά ἐστι, **καταρρήγνυται** τῶν γυναικῶν, ἥκιστα μὲν ἐν τῷ πρώτῳ τόκῳ, ἔπειτα δὲ, ὡς ἂν πλειόνων πειρέωνται τόκων, ἔτι μᾶλλον **καταρρήγνυται** διακενουμένων τῶν φλεβῶν ὑπὸ τῆς καθάρσιος τῶν λοχίων. ταῦτα δέ μοι ἐς τοῦτο εἴρηται.[8]

I have opted for the translation 'liquefy' for the verb *katarrēgnymi*, but previous translators have rendered it in various other ways. In the remainder of this chapter, I reflect on the meaning of this term, and its connotations, especially when used in conjunction with the adjective *euroos* (easy-flowing) and the noun *eurychōriē* (open space). I suggest that the author was thinking about water features when he selected the verb *katarrēgnymi*, thereby pointing to a form of ecological holism, where the female body is a microcosm of the environment. I then turn to a famous, yet neglected, reference to water in the Hippocratic text *On Diseases of Girls*: the allusion to wells in which sick young girls wish to jump. I analyse this passage in relation to ancient rituals involving water that marked the transition from *parthenos* to *gynē* in the classical Greek

8 *Nat. Puer.* 19 (30 L.) (VII.538 L. = 90 Potter).

world. This reassessment of water/fluxes in Hippocratic gynaecology will allow us to reflect further on the ambivalent position of women in ancient societies, between wilderness and culture.

1 The Body Liquefies

The verb *katarrēgnymi* and noun *katarragē* are by no means easy to translate in the passages under consideration. The Liddell-Scott-Jones Greek-English dictionary lists those specific passages under meaning 2.6 of the verb, and translates 'of parts of the body, *fall in, collapse*'. That translation, however, is not ideal, as it implies that the process which the female body undergoes is damaging, ruining, when the author considers it to be positive. Paul Potter in his Loeb translations of *On the Nature of the Child* and *On Diseases of Women* opts for 'to involute' and 'involution'.[9] 'Involution' is a medical term referring to the process whereby an organ (and in particular the uterus) returns to its normal condition after pregnancy. There are two issues with this translation choice. First, breasts certainly do not involute soon after birth in a woman who breastfeeds, and as we will see below, the Hippocratic author made provision for breastfeeding women. Second, modern involution is, simply put, a narrowing process, whereas the Hippocratic author considered the *katarrēgnymi* process to be a widening one.

Ann Ellis Hanson, for her part, followed by Lesley Dean-Jones and Helen King, opts to translate *katarrēgnymi* as 'to break down', which is the main meaning of the verb.[10] Although that translation may sound a little negative, it is that the action of breaking (in English) can have positive outcomes (or at least, outcomes that are perceived as positive). Thus, one 'breaks' an animal (especially a horse or an ox) to tame it; and one breaks the soil when they first plough a land.[11] In our passages, the lochial purgation 'breaks down' the woman's flesh, making it even more fertile. While this translation of *katarrēgnymi* is entirely

9 Potter (2012) 91 'Then women's breasts and other moist parts involute, although least in their first delivery; but then after they have experienced more births, they involute more as the vessels are emptied out during the cleaning of the lochia'; Potter (2018) 9 'Also, if there has been an involution of her body, it is the parts nearest to the cavity and breasts that involute, although the rest of the body involutes too.'

10 Hanson (1975) 570 'The lochia and the breaking down of the body make them easy-flowing. The small vessels – especially those near the belly and the breasts – are broken down; the rest of the body is also broken down.' See also Dean-Jones (1994) 63; King (1998) 32.

11 In Greek culture, young women were regularly compared to wild animals to be tamed or land to be ploughed. For analogies with fields, see in particular DuBois (1988); King (1994); Totelin (2017a). See also below for further botanical analogies. For analogies with animals,

accurate, I have chosen to opt for one that refers more openly to liquids. In his translation of *On Diseases of Women*, Emile Littré rendered *katarrēgnymi* as '*fondre*', to melt.[12] It is impossible to tell what melting matter Littré had in mind when he chose that translation – was it wax or was it ice – but I find the notion of melting ice, which starts as a trickle (first birth), then as rush (subsequent births) good to think with. In any case, a translation that refers to fluidity generally, and meteorological fluidity particularly, seems most appropriate. Indeed, the verb is often used in relation to watery natural phenomena in Greek literature: storms, waterfalls, rivers that throw themselves into the sea rush down and burst out. The verb in this sense occurs in the Hippocratic Corpus in chapter 8 of the treatise *On Airs, Waters and Places*, where clouds burst out under the weight of rain.[13] The more frequent use of the verb in the Hippocratic Corpus (it occurs 63 times in total), however, is in relation to a bodily fluid that bursts out. It appears most commonly in combination with the noun *koiliē* (cavity of the body) in phrases such as *koiliē katarēgnytai* and *koiliē katerragē*, which can both be translated as 'suffer from diarrhoea'.[14] Here, the belly bursts out under the pressure of a bodily fluid, faeces. The verb also occurs in combination with the nouns *gynaikeia* and *epimēnia*, both meaning 'menses'.[15] As Antoine Thivel noted, some Hippocratic authors might have been influenced in their thinking about bodily fluids by the meteorological theories of some pre-Socratic philosophers.[16] The pre-Socratics conceived of the cycle of water as positive, but it could be perturbed, stormy, thereby becoming threatening. In the same way, the Hippocratic authors saw the flow of humours and bodily fluids as normal, unless it was disrupted by disease. Our gynaecological author had a good knowledge of the water cycle, which he described in chapter 14 (25 in Littré's edition) of *On the Nature of the Child*, in a long botanical excursus where he compared the growth of the embryo and that of a plant.[17]

---

so perfectly summarised in Semonides fr. 7, see Morgan (2005); for women as bitches in particular, see King (1998) 24–25 (more on dogs below).

12 Littré (1853) 11 'Ce qui les fait devenir coulantes, c'est le flux lochial et la fonte du corps; les parties voisines du ventre et des mamelles se fondent le plus, mais le reste du corps se fond aussi.'

13 *Aer.* 8 (II.34–36 L. = 205–08 Jouanna).

14 The words occur thirty times in combination in the Hippocratic Corpus. The combination is particularly common in *Coan Prognoses*.

15 γυναικεῖα: *Coac.* 530 (V.706 L. = 238 Potter); 537 (V.706 L. = 240 Potter); ἐπιμήνια: *Nat. Mul.* 8 (VII.324 L. = 204 Potter); *Mul.* 2.1 (110 L.) (VIII.234 L. = 262 Potter); 2.24 (133 L.) (VIII.302 L. = 336 Potter).

16 Thivel (1990).

17 See Lonie (1969).

The choice of a translation of *katarrēgnymi* that refers to watery fluidity is further justified by the fact that, in our passages of *On Diseases of Women* I and *On Generation* and *On Nature of the Child*, the verb appears in conjunction with two words that evoke the environment: *euroos* and *eurychōriē*. The adjective *euroos*, easy-flowing, which in our passages qualifies vessels (*phlebia*), commonly qualified rivers: for instance, in the *Iliad*, the River Skamandros is described as *euroos*.[18] A more implicit analogy between rivers and vessels is to be found in another Hippocratic treatise, *On Regimen* IV, where dreams about abnormal rivers signal blood troubles.[19] The noun *eurychōriē*, for its part, referred to large expanses of space, such as the Athenian Acropolis in Demosthenes' *On the False Embassy* (19.272).

I therefore choose the translation 'liquefy', as it retains the sense of breaking, but makes it clear that this breaking occurs under the pressure of a fluid. The liquefaction of the flesh in childbirth, caused by the violent lochial purgation, enables the menses to flow better. The image that comes to my mind is that of a river bursting its banks, pouring out into alluvial plains (the open spaces in our passages) and causing a helpful flood, one that nourishes. A potentially dangerous event, one that appears wild – the birth/river-flood – allows for better future cultivation.[20] The liquefaction of the body does not only affect the vessels near the womb, it also affects those near the breasts. That is, it also facilitates lactation. The Hippocratic author did not mention milk in the passages we have examined so far, but he did in various other places, and in particular in the following passage of *On the Nature of the Child*, where he also used the comparative form of adjective *euroos* three times:

> When the woman gives birth, when the motion of the milk has first started, the milk moves into her breasts, as long as she breastfeeds. For it is thus: when the breasts are suckled, the small vessels leading to the breasts become more easy-flowing. As they become more easy-flowing, they draw the fat from the cavity and pass it to the breasts. Similarly, if a man has regular sexual intercourse, his small vessels become more easy-flowing and lead to more intercourse.

18 *Il.* 7.329.

19 *Vict.* 4.90 (VI.654 L. = 226 Joly) 'Abnormal rivers signal a passage of blood: flowing higher, an excess of blood; flowing lower, a deficiency' (ποταμοὶ δὲ μὴ κατὰ τρόπον γινόμενοι αἵματος περίοδου σημαίνουσι, πλέον μὲν ῥέοντες ὑπερβολὴν, ἔλασσον δὲ ῥέοντες ἔλλειψιν). For analogies between rivers and blood vessels in Latin literature, particularly in Seneca's writings, see Goyette (forthcoming).

20 It is interesting to note that in some Egyptian medical papyri dating to the New Kingdom, menstruation is compared to the Nile flood, which harbours fertility. See Rawlandson (1998) 354.

> καὶ ὁκόταν τέκῃ, ἀρχῆς κινήσιος ὑπογενομένης, χωρέει τὸ γάλα ἐς τοὺς μαζοὺς τούτους, ἢν θηλάζῃ. ἔχει γὰρ οὕτω· θηλαζομένοιν τοῖν μαζοῖν εὐροώτερα γίνεται τὰ φλέβια ἐς τοὺς μαζούς· εὐροώτερα δὲ γενόμενα, ἀπὸ τῆς κοιλίης ἕλκοντα τὸ πιαρὸν, τοῖν μαζοῖν διαδιδόασι. καὶ γὰρ ἀνὴρ ἢν λαγνεύῃ πολλά, εὐροώτερα γινόμενα τὰ φλέβια μᾶλλον ἐπάγει τὴν λαγνείην.[21]

Here the author draws an equivalence between breastfeeding (emission of milk) in women and sexual intercourse (emission of semen) in men: a human being can survive without either processes.[22] Hippocratic doctors might have looked after mothers who did not breastfeed because they could afford wet-nurses.[23] However, they would have known that babies could not survive without breastmilk (there was no safe alternative to breastmilk in the ancient world; very few infants fed on animal milk from birth would have survived), and that poor breastmilk could lead to infant death (see below). I would argue that the Hippocratic authors saw the emission of milk as the final step in the transition from *parthenos* to *gynē*, that which would maintain the life of a child.

To sum up, the transition that a woman experienced from her *parthenos* stage to her *gynē* stage is one that is associated with fluidity: with better flowing of the menses and flowing of the milk. With childbirth, the lochial discharge causes the body to liquify, thereby widening the channels, and rendering the flow of menses and milk easier. In this holistic physiological model, what happens to the flesh is comparable to what happens to an alluvial plain when it is flooded by a river which has burst its banks. The ploughing that is sexual intercourse and the fruit bearing that is pregnancy have transformed the narrow channels of the earth-woman into broader, easy-flowing ones which will be better be able to carry food to the infant, and to future foetuses.

2 Water and the Disease of Young Girls

Before childbirth and the beneficial 'liquefaction' that it causes, the body of a girl is dense and has narrow channels. In addition, before she loses her virginity, the body of a girl might have a closed 'mouth of the uterus' (vagina). In the short text *On Diseases of Girls*, we find a poignant description of the sickness that affects girls of marriageable age when blood accumulates in their uterus but does not find an easy exit because their body is closed up. This extraneous blood rushes – the author uses the verb *anaissei*, which evokes spring

21 *Nat. Puer.* 10 (21 L.) (VII.512–514 L. = 60 Potter).
22 On the physiology of breastmilk in antiquity, see Pedrucci (2013).
23 On breastfeeding and ancient medicine, see Laskaris (2008).

water – to the heart, where it causes numbness.[24] The psychological effects of the disease, however, are the worst: the girl wishes to die by leaping into wells or by hanging herself:

> Their spirit, distraught and sorely troubled by the foulness of their blood, attracts bad things, but names something else even fearful things. They command the young girl to wander about, to cast herself into wells, and to hang herself, as if these actions were preferable and completely useful. Even when without visions, a certain pleasure exists, as a result of which she longs for death, as if something good.
>
> ὑπὸ δὲ τῆς κακίης τοῦ αἵματος ἀλύων καὶ ἀδημονέων ὁ θυμὸς κακὸν ἐφέλκεται· ἕτερον δὲ καὶ φοβερὰ ὀνομάζει, καὶ κελεύουσιν ἅλλεσθαι καὶ καταπίπτειν ἐς φρέατα ἢ ἄγχεσθαι, καὶ ἀμείνονά τε ἐόντα καὶ χρείην ἔχοντα παντοίην· ὁκότε δὲ ἄνευ φασμάτων, ἡδονή τις, ἀφ᾽ ἧς ἐρᾷ τοῦ θανάτου ὥσπέρ τινος ἀγαθοῦ.[25]

The Hippocratic author specified that girls wished to leap into wells, *es phreata*. The word *phrear* refers to an artificial well, one that girls would have visited to fetch water in the ancient world, making it an opportune place to take one's life. Not all sick girls acted upon their suicide ideations, fortunately. According to the Hippocratic author, when they came back to their senses, girls dedicated many items, including expensive cloaks to the goddess Artemis, deceived as they were by seers (*manteis*).

While Helen King has examined the symbolic significance of hanging as a mode of suicide, that of drowning has been more neglected.[26] In her article 'Bound to bleed' and in her book *Hippocrates' Woman*, King has shown that girls whose blood could not flow opted for hanging, a bloodless type of death that linked them to Artemis, the goddess who presided over the transition from *parthenos* and *gynē*, and who bore the epithet *Apankhomenē* (hanged) at Kaphyae in Arcadia.[27] In relation to drowning, King noted that in ancient myths and history, 'a bloodless suicide is … a particularly appropriate way of avoiding the bloodshed of unwanted defloration … Like hanging, jumping down wells is presented as a culturally appropriate response to unwanted sex.'[28] Geneviève Hoffmann, for her part, argued that by choosing death by drowning, the young girl 'dissolves her body, oversaturated with moisture, in the night of its troubled

24 *Virg.* (VIII.466 L. = 248 Flemming and Hanson).
25 *Virg.* (VIII.468 L. = 249 Flemming and Hanson). Translation by Flemming and Hanson.
26 Suicide by means of hanging for virgins has been frequently discussed. See most prominently Loraux (1985); Cantarella (2018) 79 (for the Hippocratic text).
27 King (2002 [1983]); (1998) 80–85.
28 King (1998) 83.

waters.'[29] Valeria Andò, finally, stressed that the Hippocratic author gave prominence to drowning by listing it before hanging.[30] She suggested that the girl may have jumped in the water in the hope of healing her *mania*, and links this leaping into the water to ritual 'deaths' that accompany some transition rituals around the time of puberty, especially rituals in honour of Dionysus. I would like to build on Andò's hypothesis, by exploring links between healing, drowning and the Nymphs, those deities who inhabited rivers, wells, and brooks and who were often associated with Dionysus and Artemis.[31]

The belief that some waters are healing was common in the ancient world. In particular, some waters were thought to be fertilising: there are several examples reported for instance by Pliny the Elder.[32] Conversely, waters in some locations were thought to make women infertile, as in a passage from the Hippocratic treatise *On Airs, Waters and Places*, where waters in places facing cold winds affect women's menses, their ability to bear children, and milk production.[33] As is usual in the Hippocratic Corpus, the explanation given for the effect of the water is mechanistic: hard water causes drying up in the body, and hence infertility. Treatments against sterility in the Corpus often involved bathing, as this was thought irrigate the hard, dry female body and make it fertile again.[34]

The patient of the Hippocratic doctor and the bride on the eve of her marriage, however, may have thought about water as more than a moistening and emollient substance. She would have known of water rituals that accompanied

29 Hoffmann (1992) 307.

30 Andò (1990).

31 On Nymphs, see Larson (2001).

32 Pliny (*HN* 31.10) reports 'The spring at Thespiae causes women to conceive, as does the river Elatum in Arcadia, and the spring Linus, also in Arcadia, guards the embryo and prevents miscarriage. The river in Pyrrha, on the contrary, that is called Aphrodisium, causes barrenness' (trans. W. H. J. Jones).

33 *Aer.* 4 (II.22 L. = 194–95 Jouanna): 'As for the women, first many become barren because the waters are hard, non-concocted, and cold. For the necessary purgation of the menses does not occur, or it is scanty and poor. Then they give birth with difficulty, although miscarriage is rare. When they have given birth, they are unable to feed their children, for the milk dries out because of the hardness and lack of concoction of the waters' (τῇσι δὲ γυναιξί· πρῶτον μὲν στέριφαι πολλαὶ γίνονται διὰ τὰ ὕδατα ἐόντα σκληρά τε καὶ ἀτέραμνα καὶ ψυχρά· αἱ γὰρ καθάρσιες οὐκ ἐπιγίνονται τῶν ἐπιμηνίων ἐπιτήδειαι, ἀλλὰ ὀλίγαι καὶ πονηραί. ἔπειτα τίκτουσι χαλεπῶς τιτρώσκουσί τε οὐ σφόδρα. ὁκόταν δὲ τέκωσι, τὰ παιδία ἀδύνατοι τρέφειν εἰσίν· τὸ γὰρ γάλα ἀποσβέννυται ἀπὸ τῶν ὑδάτων τῆς σκληρότητος καὶ ἀτεραμνίης).

34 See for instance *Mul.* 2.52 (162 L.) (VIII.342 L. = 379 Potter) where, at the end of a long treatment for a closed mouth of the uterus, the woman must bathe in cold water, drink an unsalted cyceon, and sleep with her husband in the hope of becoming pregnant. On this recipe, see Totelin (2009) 92 n. 60.

the transition from *parthenos* to *gynē*, rituals which evoked the Nymphs.[35] Indeed, in numerous Greek *poleis*, spouses-to-be, and especially brides-to-be, took ritual cleansing baths. The best-known example is that of Athens, where the bath was taken in water that had been carried in special vases, the *loutrophoroi*, from the Callirhoe Spring, named after the Nymph, the beautifully flowing one.[36] Nuptial baths would have served a cleansing function, as well as a fertilising one, as a scholion to Euripides' *Phoenicians* suggests:

> The spouses-to-be of old used to cleanse themselves in nearby rivers and besprinkle themselves, taking symbolically the water from rivers and springs, while praying for the procreation of children. For water is prone to create life and to generation.
>
> εἰώθεσαν δὲ οἱ νυμφίοι τὸ παλαιὸν ἀπολούεσθαι ἐπὶ τοῖς ἐγχωρίοις ποταμοῖς καὶ περιρραίνεσθαι λαμβάνοντες ὕδωρ τῶν ποταμῶν καὶ πηγῶν συμβολικῶς παιδοποιίαν εὐχόμενοι, ἐπεὶ ζῳοποιὸν τὸ ὕδωρ καὶ γόνιμον.[37]

The bride-to-be would have felt an affinity with the Nymphs, those divinities whose name – *nymphē* – she shared.[38]

The Nymphs involved in wedding rituals did so in a benevolent manner; but Nymphs were ambivalent deities who were known at times to pull characters, usually male, into the water: water nymphs abducted Hylas as he was drawing water; and the Nymph Salmacis pulled Hermaphroditus into the water of her pool.[39] In Menander's *Dyscolus*, the fall of the irascible Cnemon down a well is attributed to the Nymphs.[40] Conversely, the Nymphs had the power to save drowning mythical characters. For instance, in the *Iliad*, Thetis, one of the Nereids (sea Nymphs) welcomed Dionysus into her *kolpos*, her watery bosom, when he was chased by Lycurgus, son of Dryas.[41] In the Homeric *Hymn*

35 On those rituals, See Håland (2009); Dalmon (2011); Totelin (2017b).

36 See Larson (2001) 112; see also Pirenne-Delforge (1994).

37 Scholion to Euripides, *Phoenician Women* 347.

38 The Greek word *nymphē* was very polyvalent, and in addition to being applied to divinities and brides-to-be, also referred to the clitoris, rose buds about to open, and the larvae of insects. See King (1983) 112; Andò (1996) 61.

39 For references, see Larson (2001) 66–69. See also Sourvinou-Inwood (2005).

40 *Dysc.* 643–44. Stories of drowning in wells are quite rare in the ancient world. One could also note the story of Thales, who fell in a well, as recorded by Plato (*Theaetetus* 174a). Thales was allegedly mocked by a Thracian girl for paying too much attention to what was in the stars, but not enough to what was under his feet. See also the Aesopic Fable of the Fox and the Billy-Goat (Fable 40), where the fox falls into a well.

41 *Il.* 6.130–37.

to Apollo, Thetis also saved Hephaestus, whom Hera had thrown off Olympus into the sea.[42] There too, she took the god into her watery bosom (*kolpōi*).

In later antiquity, children departed too early were said to have been taken by the Nymphs, as in the beautiful second-century CE epigram in honour of Isidora, the human nymph turned goddess in death.[43] When fathers chose to drown deformed children, as we learn from Seneca, they may have done so with the hope that the Nymphs would welcome them.[44] A well (hopefully a disused one) would have been an easily-accessible place where to dispose of a weak or already dead new-born. We know of one well used for such a purpose: the remains of at least four hundred and forty-nine foetuses, infants, and children were excavated in a Hellenistic well on the Athenian Agora. In their recent study of the well, Maria Liston and Susan Rotroff note that the well also contained remains of over one hundred and fifty dogs, animals which were sacrificed to goddesses of childbirth, and in particular to Hecate and Artemis.[45]

While some of the evidence linking Nymphs to the death of children is a little late for our purpose, it remains that, in literary representations from the classical period, suicide by drowning was fitting for a desperate girl on the cusp of womanhood. The girl who could not bleed leapt to her death in a well where the water cleansed her at the same time as it obliterated her: her nuptial and funeral baths merged into one. The narrowness of the well recalled that of the young girl's body channels, which do not allow for the healthy flow of menstrual blood.[46] Eternally a *nymphē*, she joined the Nymphs. We could go further and suggest that the Nymphs encouraged the sick girl to take the leap. Indeed, the author of *On Diseases of Girls* noted that, in their *mania*, some girls' spirit (*ho thymos*) exhorted them (*keleuousin*) to die by suicide; he also referred to these visions as *phasmata*, phantoms, and indicated that suicide ideation was accompanied by a form of erotic pleasure (*hēdonē tis*). This almost erotic experience calls to mind that particular form of inspiration for which Nymphs were responsible: nympholepsy.[47] In the *Phaedrus*, for instance Socrates jokingly – and with sexual hints – stated that he was on the verge of being possessed

42 *Hymn to Apollo* 316–22.

43 *I.Métr.* 87. See Rawlandson (1998) 54–55 for translation and commentary. For other children 'taken by the Nymphs', see Fabiano (2014).

44 Seneca, *On Anger* 1.15. The passage also mentions the killing of mad dogs.

45 Liston and Rotroff (2013) 67–68.

46 In *Regimen* 4.90, mentioned above, dreaming of wells is also mentioned as signifying the internal workings of the body.

47 Jennifer Larson (2001, 13) defines nympholepsy as 'a heightening of awareness and elevated verbal skills believed to result from the nymphs' influence on a susceptible individual.' On nympholepsy, see Connor (1998), Pache (2011, esp. pp. 37–70 for the evidence from classical Greece).

by the Nymphs.[48] More serious in his belief to be taken by the Nymphs was Archedamus the Theran, who in the fifth century BCE, established himself in a cave in the Attic town of Vari for several years.[49] According to inscriptions in the cave, he cultivated a garden in honour of the Nymphs.[50] In that cave were also found *loutrophoroi* vases dating from the fifth century BCE to the first century CE, indicating that the place was visited by brides-to-be wishing to draw water for their nuptial ablutions and/or by the families of girls departed before marriage.[51]

Known ancient nympholepts are male, but one could suggest that the girls described in *On Diseases of Girls* believed that they were possessed by the Nymphs. Their *phasmata* might have been Nymphs, enjoining them to leap into the watery depths of the well, promising to welcome in their bosom girls who could not grow up. The girls who resisted the *phasmata*, the Hippocratic author noted, made offerings to Artemis. Having escaped the lure of the phantoms/Nymphs, the girls dedicated to Artemis, that goddess who presided over a band of Nymphs, items that symbolised civilisation: the fruits of women's labour, woven cloth.[52] The Hippocratic author, however, deplored this religious practice. His advice to the girl affected by the disease of virgins is that she must marry, and hopefully get pregnant, for barren women are vulnerable to the disease throughout their lives.

3 Conclusions

Scholars have often noted the analogy between the ancient female body and the earth in need of ploughing, but the analogy goes much further; the environmental holism in Greek thought about the female body – and especially in Greek medical thought – is much more prominent. Women's vessels are like riverbeds, narrow and prone to blockages in youth, broader and easy-flowing after childbirth; the blood carried by those vessels is like river water, beneficial or damaging depending on the circumstances. The transition from *parthenos* to *gynē* is a fluid one, one that is marked by the flowing of several bodily fluids (menstrual blood, lochial blood, milk). During that fluid phase, the woman is a *nymphē*, sharing a name with those deities who inhabited the interstices

48 Plato, *Phaedrus* 241e.
49 See Connor (1988); Larson (2001) 14–16.
50 *IG* I³ 977 and *IG* I³ 980.
51 See King (1903) for an inventory.
52 On the links between Artemis and Nymphs, see Larson (2001) 107–10.

between wilderness and cultivation. The Hippocratic authors, keen as they were to establish their art as independent from other forms of healing, passed under silence the rituals that accompanied the transition from *parthenos* to *gynē*, rituals that involved water and the Nymphs. They did not, however, distance themselves from a holistic view of the female body as a microcosm of the earth, furrowed by water channels.

The transition from *parthenos* to *gynē* was, in essence, one from wilderness to cultivation: Greek marriage was ploughing, Greek marriage was taming. However, for all its civilising effect, marriage never completely destroyed the wilderness within the female body. In fact, that body distanced itself from the male standard and could be said to become wilder. When the Hippocratic author describes what happens to the body in childbirth, he employs analogies that refer to the natural world: the easy-flowing river and the fleece. The porous body of a mature woman is not like a tightly-woven cloth, a product that requires numerous stages of manufacture; it is like a clean fleece, a product in a relatively 'raw' state. The channels of the mature woman are not like human-built irrigation channels, cisterns, or wells; they are like easy-flowing rivers. Those rivers may bring nourishment when they burst their banks, but they remain mysterious phenomena, which are difficult to control. The nourishing flood may fail to occur: the woman's body may not purge itself of the lochia, an affliction which leads to an almost certain death; her body may not produce milk, a failure, which may cause the infant's death. A woman can never fully be tamed; instead, she must be managed so that the wilderness within remains benevolent and not manifest itself as *mania* or some other disease. In being both wild and cultivated, the woman keeps throughout her life something of the Nymph.

Bibliography

Andò, V. 'La Verginità Come Follia: il 'Peri Parthenion' Ippocratico.' *Quaderni Storici*, 3 (1990) 715–37.

Andò, V. '"Nymphe": la Sposa e le Ninfe.' *Quaderni Urbinati di Cultura Classica*, 52 (1996) 47–79.

Andò, V. 'Come una Spugna: Umidità del Femminile nel Pensiero Medico e Biologico della Grecia Classica.' In *Cultura e Religione delle Acque. Atti del Convegno Interdisciplinare "Qui Fresca l'Acqua Mormora …" (S. Quasimodo, Sapph. Fr. 2,5), Messina, 29–30 Marzo 2011*, ed. A. Calderone. Rome: Giorgio Bretschneider editore (2012) 17–26.

Cantarella, E. *I Supplizi Capitali: Origine e Funzioni delle Pene di Morte in Grecia e a Roma*. Nuova edizione rivista. Milan: Feltrinelli Editore (2018).

Carson, A. 'Putting her in her Place: Woman, Dirt, and Desire.' In *Before Sexuality: The Construction of Erotic Experience in the Ancient World*, ed. D. M. Halperin, J. J. Winkler and F. I. Zeitlin. Princeton: Princeton University Press (1990) 135–67.

Connor, W. R. 'Seized by the Nymphs: Nympholepsy and Symbolic Expression in Classical Greece.' *Classical Antiquity*, 7 (1988) 155–89.

Craik, E. *The 'Hippocratic' Corpus: Content and Context*. London: Routledge (2015).

Dalmon, S. 'Les nymphes dans les rites du mariage.' *Cahiers « mondes anciens »* 2 [online] 2011 (accessed May 2020).

Dean-Jones, L. A. *Women's Bodies in Ancient Greek Science*. Oxford: Clarendon Press (1994).

DuBois, P. *Sowing the Body: Psychoanalysis and Ancient Representations of Women*. Chicago: University of Chicago Press (1988).

Fabiano, D. 'Raptus a Nymphis. Emozioni e Gender nelle Epigrafi Funerarie di Bambini.' In *La Presenza dei Bambini nelle Religioni del Mediterraneo Antico: la Vita e la Morte, i Rituali e i Culti tra Archeologia, Antropologia e Storia delle Religioni*, ed. C. Terranova. Rome: Aracne (2014) 111–40.

Goyette, M. 'Seneca's Corpus: A Sympathy of Fluids and Fluctuations.' In *Bodily Fluids in Antiquity*, ed. M. Bradley, V. Leonard and L. Totelin. London: Routledge (forthcoming).

Grensemann, H. *Knidische Medizin. Teil I. Die Testimonien zur ältesten knidischen Lehre und Analysen knidischer Schriften im Corpus Hippocraticum*. Berlin: De Gruyter (1975).

Grensemann, H. *Die gynäkologischen Texte des Autors C nach den pseudohippokratischen Schriften* De Muliebribus *I, II und* De Sterilibus. Wiesbaden: Steiner (1982).

Håland, E. J. '"Take, Skamandros, my Virginity": Ideas of Water in Connection with Rites of Passage in Greece, Modern and Ancient.' In *The Nature and Function of Water, Baths, Bathing and Hygiene from Antiquity through the Renaissance*, ed. C. Kosso and A. Scott. Leiden: Brill (2009) 109–48.

Hanson, A. E. 'Hippocrates: Diseases of Women 1. Translated and with a Headnote by Ann E. Hanson.' *Signs*, 1 (1975) 567–84.

Hoffmann, G. *La jeune fille et la mort dans l'Athènes classique*. Paris: De Boccard (1992).

King, H. 'Bound to Bleed: Artemis and Greek Women.' In *Images of Women in Antiquity*, ed. A. Cameron and A. Kuhrt. London: Routledge (1983) 77–97. Reprinted in *Sexuality and Gender in the Classical World: Readings and Sources*, ed. L. K. McClure. Oxford: Blackwell Publishers (2002) 109–27.

King, H. 'Sowing the Field: Greek and Roman Sexology.' In *Sexual Knowledge, Sexual Science: The History of Attitudes to Sexuality*, ed. R. Porter and M. Teich. Cambridge: Cambridge University Press (1994) 29–46.

King, H. *Hippocrates' Woman. Reading the Female Body in Ancient Greece*. London: Routledge (1998).

King, L. S. 'The Cave at Vari. IV. Vases, Terra-cotta Statuettes, Bronzes, and Miscellaneous Objects.' *American Journal of Archaeology*, 7 (1903) 320–34.

Larson, J. *Greek Nymphs: Myth, Cult, Lore*. Oxford: Oxford University Press (2001).

Laskaris, J. 'Nursing Mothers in Greek and Roman Medicine.' *American Journal of Archaeology*, 112 (2008) 459–64.

Liddell, H. G., R. Scott and H. S. Jones. *A Greek-English Lexicon. Compiled by H. G. Liddell and R. Scott. Revised and Augmented throughout by Sir H. S. Jones, with the Assistance of R. McKenzie and with the Cooperation of many Scholars. With a Revised Supplement*. Oxford: Clarendon Press (1996).

Liston, M. A., and S. I. Rotroff. 'Babies in the Well: Archaeological Evidence for Newborn Disposal in Hellenistic Greece.' In *The Oxford Handbook of Childhood and Education in the Classical World*, ed. J. E. Grubbs, T. Parkin and R. Bell. Oxford: Oxford University Press (2013) 62–82.

Lonie, I. M. 'On the Botanical Excursus in De Natura Pueri 22–27.' *Hermes*, 97 (1969) 391–411.

Lonie, I. M. *The Hippocratic Treatises* 'On Generation', 'On the Nature of the Child', 'Diseases IV': *A Commentary by Iain M. Lonie*. Berlin: De Gruyter (1981).

Loraux, N. *Façons tragiques de tuer une femme*. Hachette: Paris (1985).

Morgan, T. 'The Wisdom of Semonides fr. 7.' *The Cambridge Classical Journal*, 51 (2005) 72–85.

Pache, C. O. *A Moment's Ornament: The Poetics of Nympholepsy in Ancient Greece*. Oxford: Oxford University Press (2011).

Pedrucci, G. 'Sangue Mestruale e Latte Materno: Riflessioni e Nuove Proposte Intorno all'Allattamento nella Grecia Antica.' *Gesnerus*, 70 (2013) 260–91.

Pirenne-Delforge, V. 'La loutrophorie et la "prêtresse-loutrophore" de Sicyone.' In *L'eau, la santé, la maladie dans le monde grec*. Actes du colloque de Paris (novembre 1992), ed. R. Ginouvès. Paris: de Boccard (1994) 147–55.

Rawlandson, J. *Women and Society in Greek and Roman Egypt*. A Sourcebook. Cambridge: Cambridge University Press (1998).

Sourvinou-Inwood, C. *Hylas, the Nymphs, Dionysos and Others: Myth, Ritual, Ethnicity: Martin P. Nilsson Lecture on Greek Religion, Delivered 1997 at the Swedish Institute at Athens*. Stockholm: Paul Åströms Förlag (2005).

Thivel, A. 'Flux d'humeurs et cycle de l'eau chez les présocratiques et Hippocrate.' In *La maladie et les maladies dans la collection hippocratique. Actes du VI*[e] *colloque international hippocratique* (Québec, 28 sept.–3 oct. 1987), ed. P. Potter, G. Maloney, and J. Desautels. Quebec: Editions du Sphinx (1990) 279–302.

Totelin, L. M. V. *Hippocratic Recipes: Oral and Written Transmission of Pharmacological Knowledge in Fifth- and Fourth-Century Greece*. Leiden: Brill (2009).

Totelin, L. M. V. 'Whose Fault is it anyway? Plant Infertility in Antiquity.' In *The Palgrave Handbook of Infertility in History: Approaches, Contexts and Perspectives*, ed. G. Davies and T. Loughran. London: Palgrave (2017a) 57–75.

Totelin, L. M. V. 'Motherhood in Flux: Greek Nymphs, Breastfeeding, and Ancient Gynaecology.' In *Maternità e Politeismi. Motherhood(s) and Polytheisms*, ed. F. P. Guignard, G. Pedrucci and M. Scapini. Bologna: Patron Editore (2017b) 359–70.

Primary Texts: Editions and Translations Used

Hippocrates. *Coan Prognoses.* (*Coac.*). Ed. P. Potter. Cambridge MA and London: Harvard University Press (2010).

Hippocrates. *On Airs, Waters and Places.* (*Aer.*). Ed. J. Jouanna. Paris: Les Belles Lettres (1996).

Hippocrates. *On Diseases of Girls.* (*Virg.*). Ed. R. Flemming and A. E. Hanson, 'Hippocrates' Peri Partheniôn ('Diseases of Young Girls'): Text and translation.' *Early Science and Medicine*, 3 (1998) 241–52.

Hippocrates. *On Diseases of Women.* (*Mul.*). Ed. P. Potter. Cambridge MA and London: Harvard University Press (2018).

Hippocrates. *On Generation* and *On Nature of the Child.* (*Genit.* and *Nat. Puer.*). Ed. P. Potter. Cambridge MA and London: Harvard University Press (2012).

Hippocrates. *On Regimen.* (*Vict.*). Ed. R. Joly and S. Byl. Berlin: Akademie Verlag (2003).

Hippocrates *On the Nature of Women.* (*Nat. Mul.*). Ed. P. Potter. Cambridge MA and London: Harvard University Press (2012).

Homer. *Hymn to Apollo*. Ed. T. W. Allen et al. Oxford: Clarendon Press (1936).

Homer. *Iliad.* (*Il.*). Ed. T. W. Allen. Oxford: Clarendon Press (1931).

Menander. *Dyscolus.* (*Dysc.*). Ed. F. H. Sandbach. Oxford: Clarendon Press (1972).

Plato. *Phaedrus*. Ed. J. Burnet. Oxford: Clarendon Press (1901).

Plato. *Theaetetus*. Ed. J. Burnet. Oxford: Clarendon Press (1900).

Pliny. *Natural History, Book 31*. Trans. W. H. S. Jones. Cambridge MA and London: Harvard University Press (1963).

Scholia in Euripidem. Scholia in Phoenissas. Ed. E. Schwartz. Berlin: Reimer (1887).

Seneca. *On Anger*. Trans. J. W. Basore. Cambridge MA and London: Harvard University Press (1928).

Inscriptiones Graecae. 3rd edition. (*IG I*[3]). Ed. D. Lewis and L. Jeffery. Berlin: De Gruyter (1994).

Metrical Inscriptions of Graeco-Roman Egypt. (*I.Métr.*). Ed. E. Bernand, *Inscriptions métriques de l'Egypte gréco-romaine*. Paris (1969).

CHAPTER 10

Cohesive Causes in Ancient Greek Philosophy and Medicine

Sean Coughlin

Abstract

This paper is about the history of a question in ancient Greek philosophy and medicine: what holds the parts of a whole together? The idea that there is a single cause responsible for cohesion is usually associated with the Stoics. They refer to it as the *synectic cause* (αἴτιον συνεκτικόν), a term variously translated as 'cohesive cause,' 'containing cause' or 'sustaining cause.' The Stoics, however, are neither the first nor the only thinkers to raise this question or to propose a single answer. Many earlier thinkers offer their own candidates for what actively binds parts together, with differing implications not only for why we are wholes rather than heaps, but also why our bodies inevitably become diseased and fall apart. This paper assembles, up to the time of the Stoics, one part of the history of such a cause: what is called 'the *synechon*' (τὸ συνέχον) – that which holds things together. Starting with our earliest evidence from Anaximenes (sixth century BCE), the paper looks at different candidates and especially the models and metaphors for thinking about causes of cohesion which were proposed by different philosophers and doctors including Empedocles, early Greek doctors, Diogenes of Apollonia, Plato and Aristotle. My goal is to explore why these candidates and models were proposed and how later philosophical objections to them led to changes in how causes of cohesion were understood.

1 Parts and Wholes

Aristotle is often credited with the phrase, 'the whole is greater than the sum of its parts.' He may never have said it (it does not appear in any of the writings we have), but that has not stopped it from being quoted, almost always without a reference, in order to suggest an ancient pedigree for certain twentieth-century topics like holism, synergy, systems theory and emergence – topics at whose core is some kind of anti-reductive stance.[1] This is not a coincidence. There

1 The attribution to Aristotle is remarkably common across disciplines. A sample: Vallero (2011) 80 on engineering and bioethics; Scalambrino (2018) 56–57 on psychology; Hanson

DOI:10.1163/9789004443143_012

is something Aristotelian about the phrase. After all, Aristotle is the ancient Greek philosopher most associated with the idea that some kinds of things in the world require explanations that go beyond the enumeration of their parts. If Aristotle asked you what a house is, you would not get away with telling him that it is the bricks and beams that went into building it, even if you managed to mention every one of them; and you certainly would not get away with telling him that bread is simply flour, salt, water and yeast.[2] This is because, for Aristotle, if what we are talking about is not a heap of random things, but a whole, then citing only a list of ingredients misses something essential about the whole the ingredients are meant to explain. They fail to tell us how and why the parts are arranged the way they are and so why those parts form a unified thing. Not just any arrangement of materials, even of the appropriate materials, counts as a barn or a bagel, and Aristotle thinks the same goes for natural things as well.[3] To understand what a horse is, it is not enough to give a list of every hair and hoof. Something more needs to be added, something about the overall form and arrangement of those parts for it to count as an explanation of a horse. People who study Aristotle today tend to refer to this as his *hylomorphism*: the idea that unified things, especially natural and living things, are composed of matter and form and that both need to be mentioned

(1995) 1 and Forrest (2018) 3 on systems theory; Hanson (2014) 84 on social theory; Elliott (2004) 454 on business; Marks et al. (2008) 599 on molecular biology. Schuster (2007) claims it is in Aristotle's *Metaphysics*, but does not cite a passage. It is also associated with Gestalt psychology, although no Gestalt theorist seems to have said it either, on which see Fuller (1990) 101–2. For a discussion of instances found on the internet (where it pops up quite often as well), see the blog, Sententiae Antiquae, 'No, Aristotle didn't write "a whole is greater than the sum of its parts."' Last accessed at sententiaeantiquae.com/2018/07/06/no-aristotle-didnt-write-a-whole-is-greater-than-the-sum-of-its-parts/ on 02-04-19.

2 The view is first stated in Plato's *Phaedo* (Pl. *Phd.*) 98b–e, but Plato develops it extensively in the *Theaetetus*, particularly the discussion of Hesiod's wheel at 206e4–208b9. It is worth noting that this is not always the case. If someone asked me to explain the things on my desk, it would be fine to say that they are two books, a computer, a lamp; and it is perfectly fine (in North America anyway) to say that a quarter is twenty-five cents. These, according to Aristotle, are not wholes (τὰ ὅλα), but totals (τὰ πάντα). The total / whole distinction first shows up, as far as I know, also in Plato's *Theaetetus* (Pl. *Tht.*) at 204a11–b1: 'Do you in fact call 'total' (τὸ πᾶν) and 'whole' (τὸ ὅλον) the same thing or something else?' Aristotle takes up Plato's distinction in *Metaphysics* (Arist. *Metaph.*) 8.6, 1045a8–12, quoted below. On *Theaetetus*, see Harte (2002), especially chapter 1.

3 For the house example, see Aristotle, *De partibus animalium* (Arist. *Part. an.*) 1.1, 639b5–30. See also Aristotle, *Topics* 6.13, 150b22–26. The extension of the analogy to natural objects is found in many works, but the point is made most explicitly at Aristotle, *Meteorologica* (Arist. *Mete.*) 4.12, 390b2–14.

in any explanation of what those things are.[4] If, like Aristotle, we think the parts of a thing count as its matter,[5] then it is not too far off to say he thinks 'the whole is more than the sum of its parts.' Some things are not identical to their parts alone: they are also their arrangement. As Aristotle would say, they are also their forms.

Now, while Aristotle never said, 'the whole is greater than the sum of the parts,' he does come close to saying it over a few pages in books 7 and 8 of his *Metaphysics*. At *Metaphysics* 8.6 he comes especially close. There he says that *if* something with parts is also a whole, then there must be some cause – some reason – that explains why those parts form a whole in the first place. He writes:

> What is the cause (αἴτιον) of something being one? For, for everything that has a plurality of parts (πλείω μέρη) and the totality (τὸ πᾶν) is not like a heap (οἷον σωρός), but the whole (τὸ ὅλον) is something besides the parts (παρὰ τὰ μόρια), there is some cause, since even in the case of bodies, the cause of their being one is sometimes contact, other times stickiness (γλισχρότης) or some other such property.
>
> ARISTOTLE, *Metaphysics* 8.6, 1045a8–12[6]

One thing worth pointing out about this passage is that Aristotle does not say that the whole is *greater* (μεῖζον) than the sum of its parts; rather, he says that there are cases (presumably self-evident ones) where the whole is something *besides* (παρά) or *in addition to* the parts. The difference between 'greater' and 'besides' is not merely grammatical. Aristotle, like some early Gestalt theorists, thinks the difference is ontological.[7] Wholes are different kinds of things from the parts that make them up, just as syllables are different from (but not in any straightforward sense *more than*) the letters that make them up. This is

---

4 'Hylo-' from *hylē* (Aristotle's neologism for matter) and '-morphism' from *morphē* (or form). There is substantial literature on Aristotle's hylomorphism (a word Aristotle himself never uses) and its more recent revivals. Good surveys of the idea and issues surrounding it can be found in Peramatzis (2018), and the Stanford Encyclopedia articles by Ainsworth (2016), Cohen (2016) and Shields (2016). For contemporary defences, see Scaltas (1994), Koslicki (1998, 2006, 2018), Marmodoro (2013).

5 Aristotle, *Physics* (Arist. *Phys.*) 2.3, 195a15–21; *Metaph.* 5.2, 1013b17–23.

6 τί αἴτιον τοῦ ἓν εἶναι; πάντων γὰρ ὅσα πλείω μέρη ἔχει καὶ μὴ ἔστιν οἷον σωρὸς τὸ πᾶν ἀλλ᾽ ἔστι τι τὸ ὅλον παρὰ τὰ μόρια, ἔστι τι αἴτιον, ἐπεὶ καὶ ἐν τοῖς σώμασι τοῖς μὲν ἁφὴ αἰτία τοῦ ἓν εἶναι τοῖς δὲ γλισχρότης ἤ τι πάθος ἕτερον τοιοῦτον. (All translations are my own unless noted otherwise.)

7 Heider (1977) 383.

something Aristotle argues for explicitly at *Metaphysics* 7.17, 1041b11–42a2.[8] He believes that if we were to think that wholes are greater than their parts (or greater than their 'elements', as Aristotle refers to them here), then we run into a problem. If, for example, the syllable BA were *greater* than the sum of its parts, B and A, then something would need to have been added to make it greater. The whole, therefore, is presumably B + A + X. Now, however, we need something else to explain why B, A and X form a whole, and so we would need to posit another part to get B + A + X + Y, a process that would go on *ad infinitum*. Aristotle thinks such a regress is hopeless and so he argues that wholes are not created by adding something.[9] Instead, there must be some other kind of thing (ἕτερόν τι) that makes a syllable a syllable, or a whole a whole. In the example of the syllable BA, this other kind of thing will be whatever it is that causes the elements B and A to be the syllable BA and Aristotle indicates two causes that fit the bill: one, the arrangement of the letter B (or the sound 'B') before the letter A (or the sound 'A') – what he calls the formal cause; the other, the person or agent who places the B before the A, what he calls the efficient cause. The form and the agent which causes the elements to take on that form are different kinds of thing altogether. The form is a cause to the parts of their *being* a whole rather than a heap; while the agent is a cause to the parts of their *becoming* a particular thing and so of the form and the matter becoming one.[10]

---

8 Arist. *Metaph.* 7.17, 1041b11–42a2: 'Since what is compounded out of something in such a way that the totality is one, not like a heap, but like the syllable – the syllable is not the letters, nor are B and A identical to BA, nor is flesh fire and earth (…); the syllable therefore is something, not only the letters (the vowel and the consonant), but also something else; and flesh is not only fire and earth or hot and cold, but also something else.' (ἐπεὶ δὲ τὸ ἔκ τινος σύνθετον οὕτως ὥστε ἓν εἶναι τὸ πᾶν, [ἂν] μὴ ὡς σωρὸς ἀλλ' ὡς ἡ συλλαβή – ἡ δὲ συλλαβὴ οὐκ ἔστι τὰ στοιχεῖα, οὐδὲ τῷ « βα » ταὐτὸ τὸ « β » καὶ « α », οὐδ' ἡ σὰρξ πῦρ καὶ γῆ (…)· ἔστιν ἄρα τι ἡ συλλαβή, οὐ μόνον τὰ στοιχεῖα τὸ φωνῆεν καὶ ἄφωνον ἀλλὰ καὶ ἕτερόν τι, καὶ ἡ σὰρξ οὐ μόνον πῦρ καὶ γῆ ἢ τὸ θερμὸν καὶ ψυχρὸν ἀλλὰ καὶ ἕτερόν τι). The passage is incorrectly interpreted as stating the whole is more than the sum of its parts in the translation by Adolf Lasson (1907) 129: 'Das was aus Bestandteilen so zusammengesetzt ist, dass es ein einheitliches Ganzes bildet, nicht nach Art eines Haufens, sondern wie eine Silbe, das ist offenbar mehr als bloß die Summe seiner Bestandteile.' Again, Aristotle seems to be taking up themes from the *Theaetetus*. See n. 2 above.

9 On this, see Menn (2001) 125–34. I avoid for the purposes of this paper the question – equally perplexing to Scotus and Ockham as to contemporary metaphysicians – of how matter and form, conceived as parts of the form-matter composite (the 'hylomorphic compound' or σύνολον), comprise a unified whole. On this issue, see the seminal paper by Ackrill (1972/3); for contemporary philosophical approaches, see Fine (1999) and (2010), Johnston (2006), Koslicki (2008); on Medieval approaches, e.g. Cross (1999) and Ward (2014); on its relevance to holism and the notion of sympathy, see Holmes in this volume.

10 Cf. Arist. *Metaph.* 8.6, 1045b20–23; *Phys.* 2.3, 194b16–32 (where they are called causes of generation and corruption, not being and becoming – thanks to David Ebrey for pointing

The account I have just sketched – or something close to it – is what people normally have in mind when they think about Aristotle's relationship to holism. Wholes are not just their parts, they are also their forms, and while we might think things are composed of matter and form, forms are not, at least in any straightforward sense, another part of a thing. Rather, they are a special kind of cause, which confers to the parts their being and unity. Aristotle famously refers to this kind of cause as *ousia* or substance. The story I wish to tell in the paper is about a different name he gives it: the *synechon* (τὸ συνέχον) – that which holds things together.

The idea that there is a kind of cause responsible for holding things together and whose weakening or dissolution brings with it disease and decay appears often in ancient philosophy and medicine. The cause itself goes by many different names.[11] It is, however, perhaps most commonly associated with the Stoics. The Stoics refer to it as the *synectic cause* (αἴτιον συνεκτικόν), a term variously translated as 'cohesive cause,' 'containing cause' or 'sustaining cause,' although none of these intuitively express in English what the Stoics meant (I will use 'cohesive'). For the Stoics, the cohesive cause is a body, namely *pneuma* (πνεῦμα), a mixture of fire and air, which is active within all things as a kind of binding movement or force.[12] Now, Galen claims that 'the first philosophers of [his]

---

this out to me). Typically, this is expressed by saying that some agent causes what is potentially F (the matter) to be actually F. B and A are potentially BA, but they are also potentially AB or perhaps even ABBA. Aristotle thinks that the cause of the letters being actually BA, instead of just being able to be BA, is their substance or formal cause, while the cause of the letters taking on the form, of actually becoming BA, is the agent or efficient cause. While it is an understatement to say the distinction between being potentially and being actually is important for Aristotle's metaphysics, it does not have much of a place in the story I tell here.

11 Galen gives a good summary of synonyms for the term: 'the cause that holds together [συνέχον], or the cohesive cause [συνεκτικόν], or proximate cause [προσεχές] or however one might wish to call it …' (Galen, *De symptomatum causis* 1.5, VII.109.7–10 K.). Philip van der Eijk points out to me that the author of the treatise *Fevers*, attributed to Alexander of Aphrodisias (c. second century CE), uses the term 'coupling cause' (συνεζευγμένον αἴτιον) (ps.-Alexander, *De febribus* 27.1–12, 22,8–24,24 Tassinari). I discuss other terms in what follows.

12 For writers after Galen, 'cohesive' (συνεκτικός) comes to mean simply 'primary,' e.g. Simplicius: '(Aristotle) says 'highest cause' in the sense of 'what is most properly (a cause),' which others call 'cohesive' (« ἀκρότατον » μὲν λέγει « αἴτιον » τὸ κυριώτατον λεγόμενον, ὃ ἄλλοι συνεκτικὸν ὀνομάζουσιν)' (Simplicius, *In Aristotelis physicorum libros commentaria* (Simpl. *in Arist. Phys.*) 9.326,13–21 Diels, *ad* Arist. *Phys.* 2.3, 195b21). It is important to note that by calling it a force, I do not imply that it is non-bodily or immaterial. For the Stoics, forces were bodies, insofar as anything that acts or is acted upon must, for them, be a body; this is not so foreign, as forces continue to be conceived of as bodies, e.g. gluons, photons and bosons more generally.

acquaintance to speak of a cohesive cause were the Stoics,' and something like Galen's view of the history of the concept continues to be held today.[13] The consensus among scholars today is roughly that the Stoics introduce the cohesive cause as an active, corporeal analogue of the Aristotelian form: Aristotelian forms and Stoic cohesive causes explain what something is, why it acts the way it does and why it persists as that thing, while the Stoic innovation is to understand this cause as a kind of bodily (but perhaps non-material) force binding things together as a whole.[14] I think, however, that Galen's claim that this is a Stoic innovation is potentially misleading. Once we see that Aristotle's *synechon* and the Stoic cohesive cause are both answers to the question, 'what actively holds the parts of a whole together?,' then it becomes clear that they are more than analogues. In fact, the Aristotelian *synechon* and the Stoic cohesive cause refer to the same thing: the nature or soul (the Stoics also add 'cohesion' (ἕξις), which is more or less an Aristotelian inanimate nature) understood as an internal principle of motion and rest. Aristotle believes this nature or soul is an immaterial yet substantial unmoved mover – an agent that always acts in the same way to produce the same kind of activity in the parts that make what it is. The Stoics believe that this (cohesion or) nature or soul is *pneuma*, an active, self-moving corporeal cause which interpenetrates and binds the passive material into a whole through what the Stoics call its 'tensional movement.' The Stoics' answer to the question 'what holds things together' might, therefore, more closely resemble Plato's self-moving world-soul in the *Timaeus* than the unmoved souls of Aristotle's *De anima*. Nevertheless, Aristotle and the Stoics both believe that a thing's parts are bound together by a kind of internal, active cause that is not an additional part.

Plato, Aristotle and the Stoics offer refined notions of the *synechon* in response to what they see as inadequacies in earlier attempts to explain how parts might form a whole. Their responses, however, were not the only ones possible. Democritus seems simply to have rejected the idea of wholes altogether, suggesting they are figments of the imagination.[15] Alcmaeon of Croton

13 Galen, *De causis contentivis* (Gal. *CC*) 1.1 (52,1–2 Lyons); *Adversus Iulianum* 6.13 (XVIIIA.279–80 K. = 57,15–58,6 Wenkebach); *Synopsis librorum suorum de pulsibus* (IX.458.8–14 K.). Cf. Frede (1987) 145. Susan Bobzien (1999) 228 argues (more precisely) that the term is a later Stoic invention and not found in Chrysippus.

14 See e.g. Frede (1987) 145; Long and Sedley (1987) 340–41; Hankinson (1998) 240–41; Bobzien (1999) 229. These authors all seem to rely on the same testimony of Galen. I return to this below. On cohesive causes as things other than agents, but still causes of effects, see Hankinson (1987) 81–85.

15 Simplicius, *In Aristotelis De caelo commentaria* (Simpl. *in Airst. De cael.*) 295,1–14 Heiberg = Democritus 68 A 37 DK.

believed cohesion resulted from an equipollence of opposing powers among the parts, and a similar view is found in Galen's criticism of the Stoic notion of a cohesive cause. The first thinker, however, who is reported to have talked about something like a cohesive cause is not a Hellenistic Stoic, but the sixth-century BCE Ionian physicist Anaximenes. After him, different candidates for the *synechon* are proposed by different philosophers and doctors, including Empedocles, some early Greek (i.e. Hippocratic) medical writers, and Diogenes of Apollonia. In what follows, I proceed by looking at these various thinkers' proposals – the early Greek philosophers and doctors, and also Plato, Aristotle and the Stoics –, how they think they bind the parts of a thing into a whole and the problems these proposals raised. I think there is something important gained by examining this history, even though it means I have to leave aside many details and that, given the nature of some of our evidence, the account I give will at times be speculative. The views of the Stoics in particular need more careful treatment than what I can provide here (the school was hardly united on this issue).[16] Still, I think this approach offers a productive way of thinking about the history of wholes, active causes and cohesion, of which Aristotle is a part.

2 Early Greek Philosophers and Physicians

I begin this story with the earliest accounts of bodily cohesion in Greek philosophy. Many philosophers and doctors before Aristotle explain how the parts of something are bound together into a whole, and one of their common strategies is to posit some special kind of part, a *synechon* (or related term), which holds the other parts together. The idea is intuitive. Glue, nails, fasteners, thread, etc., are all what we might call 'binding parts': bodies that hold something together, while at the same time being a part of it. Early Greek philosophers posited such binding parts to explain the unity of things, from simple solid bodies to the cosmos itself.

A familiar example of this kind of thinking is Empedocles' Love (Φιλότης). Love in Empedocles' cosmology is a hypostatized notion of a unifier – that which 'brings everything together into one' (συνερχόμεν' εἰς ἓν ἅπαντα).[17] Love

16 Frede (1987) remains the best entry point to these issues in Stoic philosophy. In this paper, I avoid discussions of determinism and responsibility as motivations for the Stoic theory of causes. I also will not be discussing Cicero's report of Chrysippus' causal distinctions at *De fato* 41–43, which I think raises more questions than it answers.

17 Simpl. *in Arist. Phys.* 9.158,7 Diels = Empedocles 31 B 17 DK. An anonymous reviewer points out to me that unity is not the same as holism: both Love and Strife result in wholes, either

works in opposition to the great cosmic 'Strife' (Νεῖκος), which Empedocles thinks is responsible for separating the cosmic elements out into different kinds, fire, air, water and earth. This cosmogonic requirement of difference and sameness, narrated as separation and unification, is already anticipated in early Greek mythology. In the *Theogony*, for example, Hesiod describes the birth of the cosmos as an act of divine separation: Kronos, son of Gaia (earth) and Ouranos (sky), separated the primordial gods by castrating Ouranos, who had forced himself on Gaia in perpetual sexual union, with an adamantine sickle. When Kronos later tossed Ouranos' genitals into the sea, Aphrodite, the personification of union (Φιλότης) was born from them (Hesiod, *Theogony* 190–206; on Empedocles' identification of Love with Aphrodite, see Simpl. *in Arist. Phys.* 158,24 Diels = Emped. 31 B 17 DK). The difference for Empedocles is that, like other physicists of the sixth and fifth centuries, he begins to think of the unifier as an element: something equiprimordial, bodily and able to extend throughout the cosmos (Arist. *Metaph.* 14.4, 1091b28), and which is able to determine what things are by becoming a part of them.[18] Empedocles' Love does this by spreading out from the centre of the cosmos to its limits, becoming integrated into the mixtures of things it unifies (Simpl. *in Arist. De cael.* 529,1–15 = Emped. 31 B 35 DK, cf. Arist. *Metaph.* 1.4, 985a27–28). Other thinkers posit different cosmogonic elements and narratives. The pattern, however, at least in its general details, is the same.

When the *synechon*, like Empedocles' Love, is conceived of as a binding part, we find that it shows up at different levels of the cosmic hierarchy (in inanimate objects, in living things, in the cosmos as a whole); at all levels, however, binding parts share three general characteristics. First, they are conceived of as parts of the whole they compose; second, the whole depends on them in a different way than it depends on the other parts; and third, perhaps most important, they bring about wholeness by preventing the other parts from acting according to their own impulse. In other words, to form a whole or unity, a

---

by Love's uniting all the elements into one whole, or by Strife's uniting the elements into separate wholes; *holism*, however, arises somewhere in the middle, when the little wholes differentiated by Strife can work together to function as parts of a larger whole. The issue here is not whether Love is a *synechon* but whether it is the only one, since one could consider Strife to be what unifies the elements into separate wholes, a point already made by Aristotle in his criticism of Empedocles (Arist. *Metaph.* 1.4, 985a23–29), and who thinks Empedocles is confused. And it is interesting to note that, for Empedocles, cosmogony occurs *between* the complete rules of Love or Strife, and therefore holism results from *both* causes. Love, however, is still the cause of *different* things being unified, and so a more plausible candidate for the history of the *synechon* I am sketching here, even if Strife is the cause of the parts maintaining their distinctness *as parts*.

18 Menn (1995) treats many related issues here. My story is guided by his study.

binding part needs to somehow overpower the other parts in order to compel them to maintain their arrangement.

The first characteristic of early theories of *synechon* is that what holds a whole together is a part of that thing. In the passage from *Metaphysics* 8.6 quoted earlier, Aristotle mentions stickiness (γλισχρότης) as a cause of bodily parts being a whole. This is not an idle example, but something Aristotle actually believes. As far as I can tell, the abstract noun 'stickiness' is first found in the writings of Aristotle and his student Theophrastus. Aristotle often, however, slips back into an earlier paradigm and simply calls it 'the sticky' (τὸ γλίσχρον). The difference is that 'the sticky' need not be an abstract entity, and Aristotle sometimes speaks of it as itself a part of the body (rather than as a quality of some part). At *Generation of Animals* 2.1, 737a36–b1, for instance, he emphasizes that 'the sticky' (τὸ γλίσχρον) is that which 'holds all bodies together (πάντα δὲ τὰ σώματα συνέχει).'[19] And in the Aristotelian *Problemata* 21.6, 927b6–14, the sticky moisture within loaves of bread (τὸ ἐν αὐτοῖς γλίσχρον ὑγρόν) is thought to be the reason why hot loaves of bread placed next to one another cohere (συνέχονται) or become glued together (κολλῶνται).[20] The *Problemata* comes either from the time of Aristotle or not too long after, and it too continues to conceive of some *synechonta* as kinds of parts. The characteristic of parthood can also be inferred in thinkers earlier than Aristotle. Aristotle suggests that bodies that bring about cohesion were part of Empedocles' physics, and he emphasizes the similarities between Empedocles' views and his own. In the *Meteorology*, he writes, 'the moist (τὸ ὑγρόν) is a cause to the dry of it being determined (ὁρίζεσθαι), and one is like a glue (κόλλα) for the other – as Empedocles wrote in his poem on Nature: 'gluing meal together with water' (ἄλφιτον ὕδατι κολλήσας)' (Arist. *Mete.* 4.4, 381b29–82a8 = Emped. fr. 31 B 34 DK). Empedocles is using glue as a metaphor here, but (at least according to Aristotle) the metaphor implies that he thinks the cohesion of a whole results from the composition of earth and water, where water is given the role of binding part. Aristotle agrees with Empedocles and he himself adopts this view in *Generation and Corruption*: 'the moist is what holds it (sc. the dry) together (τὸ συνέχον).'[21] The point of all this, however, is not to make a porridge. Empedocles and Aristotle are both saying that water or wetness is responsible

19 πάντα δὲ τὰ σώματα συνέχει τὸ γλίσχρον. Cf. Arist. *Phys.* 5.3, 227a16–17, 'and however the *synechon* happens to be one (τὸ συνέχον ἕν), in this way, too, the whole will be one, e.g. either by a bolt, glue, contact or adhesion' (καὶ ὥς ποτε γίγνεται τὸ συνέχον ἕν, οὕτω καὶ τὸ ὅλον ἔσται ἕν, οἷον ἢ γόμφῳ ἢ κόλλῃ ἢ ἁφῇ ἢ προσφύσει).

20 The sticky moisture is also referred to as 'the gluey' (τὸ κολλῶδες) in the same passage.

21 Cf. Aristotle, *Generation and Corruption* (Arist. *Gen. corr.*) 2.8, 334b30–35a3: 'earth has no ability to remain together (συμμένειν) without the moist (ἄνευ τοῦ ὑγροῦ). On the contrary,

for the fact that solid bodies cohere, while the different proportions of water and earth, or wet and dry, will determine the different levels of cohesion. Too much fluid and a body will no longer be solid; too little fluid and the parts will not form a whole. There still remains the question of what determines these proportions. For Empedocles, it seems they are determined by a different kind of glue, the 'glue of Harmonia' ('Ἁρμονίης κόλλησιν ἀρηρότα,' Simpl. *in Arist. Phys.* 300,24 Diels = Emped. fr. 31 B 96 DK), where Harmonia is, at least according to Simplicius, another of Empedocles' names for Love conceived, as before, as something actively binding things together.[22] I will come back in the next section to what Aristotle thinks determines these proportions. For now, it is enough to say that water causes the cohesion of solid bodies by becoming, along with earth or the dry, a part of them.

The second characteristic of the *synechon* conceived of as a binding part is that, so long as it remains present in a thing and maintains its own cohesion, then the whole which it causes to cohere will remain coherent. If, however, the *synechon* leaves or loses cohesion, the parts will cease to form a whole. This is the case with Empedocles' cosmos, which, when Love retreats from that which it had been mixed with previously, results in the parts dissociating. Similarly, when wood is completely burned and the water expelled from it, what is left behind is uncohesive ash. Or when there is a loss of cohesion in the sinews that hold a joint together, then the joint loses cohesion as well and can no longer function – an obvious point perhaps, but worth making nonetheless. It appears often among early Greek medical writers. For instance, the author of *Instruments of Reduction* writes that, among other bones, 'the vertebrae are held together by sinew (σπόνδυλοι ... νεύρῳ συνεχόμενοι)' (Hippocrates, *Leverage* (*Mochl.*) 1, IV.342 L. = 246,9–11 Kühlewein); and the author of the second *Prorrhetics* writes about lameness caused by injuries that sever the 'sinews that hold the internal joints together (τὰ νεῦρα τὰ συνέχοντα)' (Hippocrates, *Prorrheticus II* 15, IX.40 L. = 254,26–28 Potter). The idea that there are bodily tissues like cords that hold us together is obvious enough, and like the earlier example of 'the sticky,' the *synechon* as a bodily tissue is also adopted by Aristotle: 'the nature of sinew (ἡ τοῦ νεύρου φύσις) holds together the parts of animals (συνέχει τὰ μόρια τῶν ζῴων)' (Aristotle, *Generation of Animals* 2.1, 737a34–b7).[23] Reflection on this aspect of the *synechon* may have led later

the moist is what holds it together (τὸ συνέχον); for it (sc. earth) would fall to pieces if the moist were eliminated from it completely.'

22 Many thanks to Gábor Betegh for pointing me to this passage.

23 Some scholars excise this passage. The passage shares affinities with the Hippocratic work *Fleshes*: 'that, on the other hand, which happened to be more gluey [κολλωδέστερα] and to contain cold, could not be burnt up on being heated or become dry, [...] for this reason

thinkers to define cohesive causes as causes such that when they are present the effect is present and when they are absent the effect is absent.[24] This aspect will become central to debates about cohesive causes in ancient medicine from Erasistratus (third century BCE) onwards, where the notion of cohesive causes is extended to all causes that are contemporaneous with their effects, but most importantly, from a medical point of view, to causes of disease, e.g. that thing which is, right now, causing disease, like a kidney stone, as opposed to that thing which, at some earlier point in time, did something which later led to disease, like a bite from a dog.[25] In our case, while the parts remain what they are even when the *synechon* and the whole do not exist, the existence of the whole requires the simultaneous existence and presence of the *synechon*.

The last characteristic of the *synechon* I want to look at is its role as a 'preventer' (τὸ κωλῦον): something which checks or hinders the tendencies of the other parts that comprise the whole. Early Greek physicists believed that there are basic, unchanging elements that have (or just are) tendencies or powers, and they needed some story to tell about what it is that prevents the different parts from either separating out or collapsing. Clay may be a mixture of fire and earth, but fire tends to go up, earth to go down, and clay does not routinely fly apart. The sky and the earth may both be made of things that have weight and so tend to fall, but, at least for now, the sky has not fallen. With the products of human craft, one can say, e.g., that the pillars hold up the roof, or the glue holds the joints. Different options were offered for what serves the analogous preventing or hindering function in nature.

It will take a little work to present the evidence, but at least according to Plato and Aristotle, one of the earliest figures to think of the *synechon* along these lines was Diogenes of Apollonia. There is some evidence that before Diogenes, the Ionian physicist Anaximenes did so as well. Some sources report that Anaximenes argued that, as our soul is a kind of air that holds us together (συγκρατεῖ), so there also exists some kind of *pneuma* or air that

it took a form rather different [...] and became cords and vessels [νεῦρα καὶ φλέβες]' (Hippocrates, *De carnibus* (Hipp. *Carn.*) 3, VIII.586 L. = 134.6–18 Potter, tr. Potter, modified). Aristotle, too, thinks the vessels hold the body together. See Arist. *Part. an.* 3.6, 668b20–27. The shell is the analogue of cords and vessels in non-blooded animals. See Arist. *Part. an.* 2.8, 654a3–8.

24 On this, see Frede (1987) 146–47, Bobzien (1999), and the excellent discussions in Hankinson (1998) 376–79 and Havrda (2016) 262–73, 306.

25 For the debate, see Gal. *CC* 2.1 (55,6–11 Lyons); *Adversus Iulianum* 6.13 (XVIIIA.279–80 K. = 57,15–58,6 Wenkebach). For examples, see Ps.-Galen, *Introductio sive Medicus* ([Gal.] *Int.*) 8 (XIV.691–92 K. = 16,9–24 Petit); ps.-Galen, *Definitiones medicae* ([Gal.] *Def.*) 157; XIX.392–93 K.; Sextus, *Pyrrhoniae hypotyposes* (S. E. *PH*) 3.15; Clement, *Stromata* 8.33.1–7 (101,16–102,16 Havrda).

encompasses (περιέχει) the cosmos as a whole (ὅλον τὸν κόσμον) (Ps.-Plutarch, *Placita*, 876a10–12 = Anaximenes 13 B 2 DK).[26] If this fragment is authentic, then it is the earliest explicit reference to the soul being that which holds the body together, as opposed to some other part like sinews or bones. It is also one of the first places where we find parallel cohesive entities mentioned at micro- and macrocosmic levels. Yet the authenticity of the fragment is at best dubious; instead, the earliest point at which we can reliably say the *synechon* becomes an object of philosophical reflection is in response to the works of Diogenes of Apollonia.

Diogenes is an eclectic thinker, who combines ideas from Anaximenes, Heraclitus, Anaxagoras and Leucippus. He attempts to update the theories of an earlier generation, which posited a single material principle from which everything arose, and he is especially fond of Anaximenes, agreeing with him that everything in the cosmos derives from air and is moved by air and that our soul, which animates us and moves us, is also a portion of cosmic air contained within our body. He combines this old-fashioned view with the new physics of Anaxagoras, who posited a special kind of stuff called reason (νοῦς), which he thinks permeates all things and is responsible for moving the other bodies in a rational way to form a cosmos. Anaxagoras believed that νοῦς, which is 'the absolute ruler (αὐτοκρατές)', must be 'unmixed with any of the other stuff (μέμικται οὐδενὶ χρήματι)' of the cosmos, for if it were mixed, 'it would be hindered … so that it could not rule any of the stuff (μηδενὸς χρήματος κρατεῖν) as it now does being alone by itself' (Simpl. *in Arist. Phys.* 156,13–15 = Anaxagoras 48 B 12 DK). Diogenes agrees with Anaxagoras that the fact that the cosmos is intelligible and well-ordered needs to be explained by proposing a rational cause of order – and what better cause of rational order than hypostatized reason itself? He thinks, however, that reason is not independent of all the other stuff, but is instead to be identified with air, which he thinks possesses thinking (νόησις). The air, therefore, is the source of movement in the cosmos, while its thought is the source of the order of that movement.[27] We can speculate that

26 There is a great deal of uncertainty both about the reliability and the interpretation of this fragment. Kirk et al. (1999) 159–61 claim the form συγκρατεῖ is impossible in the sixth century. They are likely correct. A search of the TLG shows no use before the late Hellenistic period. Their suggestion that it is a combination of συνέχειν and κρατεῖν is plausible. It is possibly Stoic: see its uses at [Plut.] *Plac.* 14, 907a8 and [Gal.] *Def.* 96, XIX.372 K., the latter in which συνέχειν and συγκρατεῖν are treated synonymously. πνεῦμα and κόσμον are also unlikely in Anaximenes' time. On this, see also Vlastos (1955) 363–64 and n. 56.

27 This account broadly follows Menn (1995). Cf. Simpl. *in Arist. Phys.* 152,13–22 = Diogenes 64 B 3–4 DK. Intelligence is attributed to air by the author of *The Sacred Disease*, but whether the author identifies them is unclear to me. See e.g. Hippocrates, *De morbo sacro* 19

Diogenes believes the advantage of this kind of account is that rationality in us and the cosmos, as well as life and movement, are explained by the same entity.

In a fragment from his *On Nature* preserved by Simplicius, Diogenes writes that air:

> is great, strong (ἰσχυρόν), eternal (ἀΐδιον) and immortal (ἀθάνατον) and knows many things (πολλὰ εἰδός).
>
> Simpl. *in Arist. Phys.* 153,21–2 = Diogenes of Apollonia 64 B 8 DK

What Diogenes means by claiming air is strong (ἰσχυρόν) is not immediately clear from the fragment, but parallels of this fragment in Plato and Aristotle can at least tell us how they understood him. For Plato and Aristotle, the strength of air refers to its role as a *synechon*, and they took Diogenes to be saying that it exercised its role as a *synechon* by hindering the impulses of other bodies. The first passage is in Plato's *Phaedo*, and although Diogenes is not named, the similarity to the fragment above is suggestive of the fact that Plato has Diogenes' *On Nature* in mind. He writes that the physicists

> believe they will one day discover an Atlas that is stronger (ἰσχυρότερον), more immortal (ἀθανατώτερον) and better able to hold everything together (συνέχοντα) than this (sc. the Good); and they think that that which is truly good and binding (τὸ ἀγαθὸν καὶ δέον) doesn't bind (συνδεῖν) and hold together (συνέχειν) anything.
>
> PLATO, *Phaedo* 99c2–6[28]

If this is a representation of Diogenes' views, then Plato thinks that Diogenes is talking about the *synechon* in *On Nature*. Plato goes so far as to call the *synechon* Atlas: a Titan strong enough to hold the cosmos together.[29]

(VI.390 L.). The author of the Hippocratic *Fleshes*, however, attributes almost an identical set of properties to 'heat' (τὸ θερμόν) at Hipp. *Carn.* 2 (VIII.584 L.).

28 τὴν δὲ τοῦ ὡς οἷόν τε βέλτιστα αὐτὰ τεθῆναι δύναμιν οὕτω νῦν κεῖσθαι, ταύτην οὔτε ζητοῦσιν οὔτε τινὰ οἴονται δαιμονίαν ἰσχὺν ἔχειν, ἀλλὰ ἡγοῦνται τούτου Ἄτλαντα ἄν ποτε ἰσχυρότερον καὶ ἀθανατώτερον καὶ μᾶλλον ἅπαντα συνέχοντα ἐξευρεῖν, καὶ ὡς ἀληθῶς τὸ ἀγαθὸν καὶ δέον συνδεῖν καὶ συνέχειν οὐδὲν οἴονται.

29 Why the Titan Atlas? David Ebrey suggests to me that Plato may be contrasting the earth-born Titan with notions of Olympian divinity. It is possible, moreover, that some physicist used Atlas illustratively, but we do not know which one. See next passage. Also similar is the Hippocratic *Breaths*: Hippocrates, *De flatibus* 4 (VI.96 L. = 93,18–19 Heiberg) and 15 (VI.114 L. = 101,16–23 Heiberg). On Diogenes as a common source for both Plato and the author of *Breaths*, see Menn (1995) 39–41.

The second parallel is from Aristotle's *Metaphysics* 5.23, and this passage makes the connection between the *synechon* and the 'preventer' explicit. Aristotle writes:

> That which prevents (τὸ κωλῦον) something from moving or acting in accordance with its own impulse is said 'to hold it' (ἔχειν), as e.g. pillars 'hold' (ἔχειν) the weights lying upon them and as the poets make Atlas 'hold' (ἔχειν) the sky, since it would fall upon the earth, just as some of the physicists also say. In this way what holds together (τὸ συνέχον) is said to hold (ἔχειν) what it holds together (συνέχει), since each would separate in accordance with their own impulse.
>
> ARIST. *Metaph.* 5.23, 1023a17–23[30]

According to Aristotle, one way of understanding the *synechon* is as that which prevents (τὸ κωλῦον) the parts from acting according to their own impulses. The sky, for instance, left to its own impulses, would fall to the earth;[31] but, as long as it is held up by Atlas and as long as Atlas can overpower the tendency of the sky to fall, the cosmos will be sustained.[32] In the same way, the *synechon* prevents the parts of a thing from separating out. The assumption, then, is that the parts of things have impulses, which on their own would lead them to separate out; since wholes exist, those impulses must somehow be restrained. The *synechon* is the name given to whatever it is that does this.

3 Plato

The model of the *synechon* of the early Greek physicists is, we might say, *tyrannical*, at least as it is understood by Plato and Aristotle. The *synechon* is a distinct kind of part which holds things together, what I have called a binding

---

30 ἔτι τὸ κωλῦον κατὰ τὴν αὑτοῦ ὁρμήν τι κινεῖσθαι ἢ πράττειν ἔχειν λέγεται τοῦτο αὐτό, οἷον καὶ οἱ κίονες τὰ ἐπικείμενα βάρη, καὶ ὡς οἱ ποιηταὶ τὸν Ἄτλαντα ποιοῦσι τὸν οὐρανὸν ἔχειν ὡς συμπεσόντ' ἂν ἐπὶ τὴν γῆν, ὥσπερ καὶ τῶν φυσιολόγων τινές φασιν· τοῦτον δὲ τὸν τρόπον καὶ τὸ συνέχον λέγεται ἃ συνέχει ἔχειν, ὡς διαχωρισθέντα ἂν κατὰ τὴν αὑτοῦ ὁρμὴν ἕκαστον.

31 Diogenes is reported to think it sometimes does fall as meteorites. See Aetius *Placita* 2.13.15 and 9 = no. 608 Kirk et al. (1999) 445.

32 One might object that Atlas is clearly keeping things apart, rather than holding them together, and the variation between Plato's and Aristotle's terminology, where Plato says that Atlas 'holds together' (συνέχειν) all things, while Aristotle says that it 'holds' (ἔχειν), suggests the terminology was not settled. The general agreement, however, is that the *synechon* holds things together by being stronger than the things it holds together and restraining the parts that make up the whole.

part, and it does this by overpowering the tendencies or impulses of the other parts.[33] A whole is made up of competing forces, subdued by the strength of a dominant force, compelling and forcing them to unite as one.

The tyrannical model of the *synechon* we find in Diogenes is adopted and refined by both Plato and Aristotle (I will turn to Aristotle in the next section). In the passage from the *Phaedo* above, Plato complains that they 'think that that which is truly good and binding (τὸ ἀγαθὸν καὶ δέον) does not bind (συνδεῖν) and hold together (συνέχειν) anything.' Plato agrees with Diogenes (and Anaxagoras, Empedocles and the others), that intelligence or the good should be that which holds the cosmos together, but he thinks this needs a different kind of model of cohesion, one that does not unite parts into a whole merely through force and compulsion, but under a common virtue or good. Plato has Socrates make a similar point in the *Gorgias*: 'the wise say that fellowship and friendship, orderliness, self-control and justice hold together (συνέχειν) the heaven and earth, gods and men, and because of these things, my friend, they call this whole (τὸ ὅλον) a cosmos (κόσμος) and not unarranged (ἀκοσμία) or uncontrolled (ἀκολασία)' (Plato, *Gorgias*, 507e6–8a4).[34] At this level of abstraction, the point is not idle. If the parts of a whole share a unity of purpose, such that they are directed towards achieving one good, then Plato thinks such an entity has a better claim to being a whole than if it were merely assembled by force.

Why Plato thinks this is not entirely clear, but there have been some suggestions. In an article on Socrates' objections to the earlier physicists in the *Phaedo*, Stephen Menn points out that one thing Plato might be criticizing is the failure of materialist accounts like Diogenes' to explain why things are

33 So, in Euripides, *Supplices* 311–14:

> ... and all those who confuse the customs of Hellas,
> stop. For what holds together (τὸ συνέχον) the cities of men
> is this: when someone rightly preserves (σῴζῃ) the laws.

Alexander of Aphrodisias thinks Aristotle was trying to avoid this implication, claiming the difference between the way a tyrant 'holds' a city and the *synechon* 'holds' a whole, is that a tyrant imposes his impulse on things, while the *synechon* prevents other things from acting according to their impulse (Alexander, *In Aristotelis Metaphysica commentaria* 421,17–21 Hayduck).

34 φασὶ δ' οἱ σοφοί, ὦ Καλλίκλεις, καὶ οὐρανὸν καὶ γῆν καὶ θεοὺς καὶ ἀνθρώπους τὴν κοινωνίαν συνέχειν καὶ φιλίαν καὶ κοσμιότητα καὶ σωφροσύνην καὶ δικαιότητα, καὶ τὸ ὅλον τοῦτο διὰ ταῦτα κόσμον καλοῦσιν, ὦ ἑταῖρε, οὐκ ἀκοσμίαν οὐδὲ ἀκολασίαν. Xenophon's Socrates also discusses 'the one who coordinates and holds together the whole cosmos (ὁ τὸν ὅλον κόσμον συντάττων τε καὶ συνέχων)' as a cause of everything beautiful and good (πάντα καλὰ καὶ ἀγαθά) (Xenophon, *Memorabilia*, 4.3.13).

wholes at all.[35] A mass of things held together by compulsion may have spatial contiguity, but this would not be enough to get us substantial or conceptual unity, since it leaves unexplained the most important fact about it: that it is a whole, a single subject, with parts that have the arrangement, or cosmos, they have. To explain that there is a single thing, we need a different kind of *synechon*, something unlike air or the other kinds of material things which the tyrannical model assumes.

In addition to this conceptual problem, Plato may also believe that it is implausible to consider the kinds of things Diogenes or Anaxagoras posit to be sources of orderly, rational movement in other things. Plato believes, and thinks his interlocutors believe as well, that all perceptible things share one feature: water, earth, even Diogenes' air, Anaxagoras' Reason, or Empedocles' Love, move by contact: by moving and being moved by other things.[36] This may be why Plato says the physicists are looking for an Atlas stronger than the bodies it compels and also why he thinks these projects are bound to fail. If bodies move by being moved, then when Atlas pushes up against the sky to hold it, the sky will push back against him. For Plato, however, such an arrangement is implausible: no matter how rational Atlas is, as long as he is a body, he will be moved by the things he is moving contrary to his reason. Given a long enough time, perhaps the cosmos might descend into disorder,[37] or perhaps this is too impious a position to attribute to a divine cause of order. But whatever Plato's precise reason, the cosmos is not disorderly, and so he thinks what holds the cosmos together must be an even more absolute ruler than Diogenes' tyrant, one which can hold the cosmos together without its authority being threatened. To do this, it needs to be a different kind of thing altogether, some entity that can bring about an effect in the parts and preserve the whole they compose, without itself being subject to change from the things it is acting upon.

To conclude this section, I think it is useful to compare Plato's revision of Diogenes' tyrannical model (we can call it the monarchic model) with a still earlier one, which appeals to another political metaphor – that of equality or *isonomia*. Its most famous proponent is Alcmaeon of Croton, who (at least according to the report) claimed, 'what is cohesive of health is the equality of powers' (τῆς μὲν ὑγιείας εἶναι συνεκτικὴν <τὴν> ἰσονομίαν τῶν δυνάμεων), while, of diseases and corruption more generally, 'the agent is a monarchy among

35 Menn (2010) 53–61.
36 Plato develops these themes further in *Timaeus* 52a–e and *Laws* X 893b–99d.
37 Menn (1995) 41. This study continues to serve as a foundational introduction to Plato's critique and refinement of early Greek physics.

them, since monarchy is each thing's agent of destruction' (τὴν δ' ἐν αὐτοῖς μοναρχίαν νόσου ποιητικήν· φθοροποιὸν γὰρ ἑκατέρου μοναρχίαν) ([Plutarch], *Placita philosophorum* 30, 911a2–9 = Alcmaeon 14 B 4 DK). As Gregory Vlastos points out in 'Equality and Justice in Early Greek Cosmologies,' for many early Greek physicists and physicians, including Alcmaeon, 'the order of nature is maintained because it is an order of equals.'[38] Rather than assuming there is one body or force which compels unity on parts to form a whole, this model assumes that cohesion is something that emerges from an equality or equipollence among opposing bodily forces. The same model of equality is found in some Hippocratic writers, who see the equal mixture (κρᾶσις) of the powers in the body (e.g. hot cold moist dry) to be equivalent to health. It is also found in Plato's *Phaedo* as the view proposed by Simmias, who claims 'our body is as it were made taut (ἐντεταμένον) and held together (συνεχόμενον) by hot, cold, dry, wet, and things like them, and our soul is a mixture (κρᾶσις) and *harmonia* or attunement (ἁρμονία) of those same things' (Pl. *Phd.* 86b7–c1).[39] The fact that the *isonomia*/mixture model is put forward by Simmias, with his apparent ties to Pythagoreanism, suggests the model may also be at work in theories in which the soul is conceived of as a *harmonia*, where the *harmonia* literally is the mixture or attunement of the constituent elements.[40] The author of the text attributed to Alcmaeon in the *Placita*, of course, is himself stretching when he writes that Alcmaeon calls *isonomia* 'cohesive' of health and monarchy its agent of destruction. Alcmaeon almost certainly did not use the term 'συνεκτικήν' for 'cohesive', which in this quotation has its later, Hellenistic sense of a cause such that when it is present the effect is present. The author's interpretation nevertheless highlights what Alcmaeon and Simmias are suggesting, namely that coherence and unity emerge from an equipollence of opposing parts.

The idea that cohesion arises from an equality of opposing forces is about as far as one can get from Diogenes' tyrannical model of the *synechon* of living bodies and of the cosmos as a whole. Nevertheless, mixture (κρᾶσις), or an equality of forces, remained a productive way of understanding material composition and cohesion. The physician Galen will go so far as to write a treatise in this tradition, *That the Qualities of the Soul follow the Mixtures of the Body* (*QAM*), which sets out to prove that the qualities of the soul depend on, and so emerge from, the mixture of elements in the body, thus suggesting that

38 Vlastos (1996) 58–61.

39 I am grateful to Gábor Betegh and David Ebrey for suggesting a connection with Simmias' claims in the *Phaedo*.

40 On Simmias' Pythagoreanism, see Sedley (1995).

the body is what holds the soul together, rather than the other way around.[41] Aristotle, however, took a different approach to the notion of mixture. He supposed, like Plato, that bodies cannot be causes of their own cohesion. This role must be filled by something else, some cause that is not another part, which Aristotle called nature or soul.

4 Aristotle

So far, I have claimed that the *synechon* of Plato's and Aristotle's predecessors share three characteristics, which I call the 'tyrannical' model of cohesion. The first is that the *synechon* is a part of what it holds together, what I call a binding part. The second, that the whole it holds together only exists so long as the *synechon* exists. And the third is that the *synechon* holds parts together by hindering the impulses of those parts. I have also argued that Plato criticized and refined two of these characteristics. Against the first characteristic, Plato argues that, at least at the level of living things and the cosmos as a whole, the *synechon* cannot be another part of the whole the same as other bodily parts. If it were, it would end up being jostled around too much by the things it is trying to hold together to plausibly maintain the order and integrity of the cosmos we observe.[42] Against the third characteristic, Plato argues that the *synechon*, if it is to produce a whole, cannot merely be what hinders the impulses of the parts, but also needs to be what directs those impulses towards a common purpose. This may involve tempering or hindering the individual impulses, but what unifies them into a whole is not merely their being forced into some kind of contiguity, but the purpose to which they are being aimed.

I have also shown that at the bodily level, Aristotle continues to use the tyrannical model of cohesion presented by his predecessors. He thinks the

41 Galen, *QAM* (IV.767–822 K. = 32,1–79,24 Müller). I cannot here do justice to the complexities around theories of mixture and their rise in Hellenistic and later thought. For an overview, see Singer et al. (2018) 1–46; and Mirrione (2017).

42 Plato does often talk about the soul in ways that make it seem similar to perceptible bodies, e.g. especially in the *Timaeus*, where he says it is something spatially extended and jostled around by the bodies it inhabits. As David Ebrey points out to me, this might imply souls as *synechonta* are subject to the same criticism – and this may be true, and perhaps even desired, since living things, unlike the cosmos, are not immortal, which they would be if what held them together could never be weakened. Plato needs to give other arguments in the *Timaeus* to explain why the cosmos is immortal, namely because there are no bodies outside of it which might impede its activity by acting on it from without. See Pl. *Ti.* 32c–34b.

cohesion of things like chairs or animal bodies can be explained by the presence of binding parts like glue, rivets or sinews. At the same time, he agrees with Plato that if a whole is to be a true unity, then there needs to be some cause that unifies the parts more than spatially or by contact. There needs to be a unity of purpose, what Plato calls the good and Aristotle 'that for the sake of which' something exists. In this section, I want to focus on another model of bodily coherence which Aristotle uses to illustrate this kind of cause, namely the arts.

There are three passages in Aristotle's *De anima* where he addresses the question, what is it that actively holds the parts of the body together? In these passages, Aristotle uses the characteristics of the *synechon* accepted by his predecessors, including Plato, to argue for a different model of the *synechon* that is not based on the relation of a tyrant to what it rules or on an equipollence among opposing powers, but on the relation of an art to its instruments or organs.

In the first passage, Aristotle uses the argument from the *Phaedo* to show that the soul cannot be made up of several different elements, in other words, that the soul cannot arise, like health does for Alcmaeon, from several different elements combining.

> Someone might also raise the problem: (if the soul is composed of different elements), what is it that makes them one (τὸ ἑνοποιοῦν)? For the elements, at any rate, look like matter, while the *synechon* – whatever it is – is most powerful. But it is impossible for anything to be stronger than and rule over (κρεῖττον καὶ ἄρχον) the soul, even more impossible (for something to rule over) reason.
>
> ARIST. *De an.* 1.5, 410b10–14[43]

This argument is similar to the ones from Diogenes and Plato we met earlier, but Aristotle is extending those arguments from macro- to microcosm. Whatever the *synechon* is, whether it is a body or an immaterial substance or something else, it must be 'the most powerful,' i.e., more powerful than any of the things it is meant to hold together. Otherwise, it would not be able to hinder the impulses of the things it binds. And Aristotle, following the *Phaedo*, will argue that this means the *synechon* cannot be material: matter can always be moved, because it is always just as strong as any other matter. The *synechon*

43 ἀπορήσειε δ' ἄν τις καὶ τί ποτ' ἐστὶ τὸ ἑνοποιοῦν αὐτά· ὕλῃ γὰρ ἔοικε τά γε στοιχεῖα, κυριώτατον δ' ἐκεῖνο τὸ συνέχον, ὅ τί ποτ' ἐστίν· τῆς δὲ ψυχῆς εἶναί τι κρεῖττον καὶ ἄρχον ἀδύνατον· ἀδυνατώτερον δ' ἔτι τοῦ νοῦ.

must instead be something that cannot be moved, at least by the things it binds, and so must be something immaterial, i.e. soul or reason.

Aristotle then turns to a slightly different question, namely what holds the parts of the soul together. This argument appeals to the second characteristic of the *synechon*, that the whole exists only so long as the *synechon* exists and is present in it. Aristotle uses it against an opponent who thinks the soul is naturally divided (μεριστὴ πέφυκεν), asking what it is that holds the divided soul together (συνέχει τὴν ψυχήν). Aristotle argues that it is 'surely not the body,' since the opposite is obvious, namely that the soul 'holds (συνέχειν) the body together, since the body evaporates and putrefies when it departs' (Arist. *De an.* 1.5, 411b6–9).[44] Aristotle's target here is almost certainly Plato. In the discussion of different kinds of soul at *Timaeus* 69c–73d, Plato has the lesser gods construct and localize the mortal kinds of soul in different regions of the body. When he goes on to explain how the different kinds of soul are bound together, including the immortal soul, he explains it by their common bond to the body: the god 'bound the kinds of souls together by implanting them in the marrow (φυτεύων ἐν αὐτῷ [sc. τῷ μυελῷ] κατέδει τὰ τῶν ψυχῶν γένη)' (Pl. *Ti.* 73c3–4).[45] Aristotle thinks this explanation cannot succeed. Even if only the immortal, i.e. intellectual, soul departs at death, the body nevertheless rots, and this implies that the other souls (or parts of soul) have departed as well. These souls must, therefore, form a whole and not merely because they are present in the same body.

The third passage contains Aristotle's own solution to the problem of the *synechon* of the body. Aristotle has been discussing Empedocles' explanation of why the roots of plants grow down and their tops grow up (answer: earth naturally tends to go down, fire tends to go up, and the growth of the plant spreads along this axis). After some initial criticisms, Aristotle asks:

> What is the thing that holds together (τὸ συνέχον) fire and earth, which tend to move in opposite directions? For they will be pulled apart if there is nothing preventing it (τὸ κωλῦον). But if there is, then this is the soul and the cause of nutrition and growth. Some people think the nature of fire is the cause of nutrition and growth, especially since it is the only body that seems to be fed and to grow, and for this reason someone might assume, in the case of animals and plants too, this is the agent (τὸ ἐργαζόμενον). Although it is somehow the contributing cause (τὸ συναίτιον), surely the

44 τί οὖν δή ποτε συνέχει τὴν ψυχήν, εἰ μεριστὴ πέφυκεν; οὐ γὰρ δὴ τό γε σῶμα· δοκεῖ γὰρ τοὐναντίον μᾶλλον ἡ ψυχὴ τὸ σῶμα συνέχειν· ἐξελθούσης γοῦν διαπνεῖται καὶ σήπεται.

45 Thanks to Gábor Betegh for pointing me to this passage.

> cause (τὸ αἴτιον) strictly speaking is not (fire), but rather the soul: for fire's growth is unlimited as long as there is something to burn, while of things composed by nature, there is a limit and proportion of both size and growth. These belong to soul rather than fire and to reason (λόγος) rather than matter.
>
> ARIST. *De an.* 2.4, 416a6–18[46]

Aristotle begins this passage by appealing to the *synechon*'s role as that which prevents the parts from separating according to their own impulses. The target is Empedocles and his attempt to explain the growth of plants according to the elements (the parts) that make them up. Aristotle's point is that Empedocles' strategy of trying to explain the activities of a whole in terms of the activities of the parts is hopeless, especially since those parts have opposing impulses, which, rather than leading to a complex activity and arrangement, as we in fact find, should simply lead to the plant being torn apart. Aristotle does not want to deny that the powers of the elements have a role in the growth and maintenance of a living thing; but he wants to reconsider what that role is in light of the fact that the elements cannot explain the arrangement and limit of a thing's growth. So, Aristotle calls fire in this case a co-cause (τὸ συναίτιον), while he reserves the term cause (τὸ αἴτιον) for the soul, since the soul is properly speaking the agent (τὸ ἐργαζόμενον) acting in accordance with a rational principle (λόγος), rather than a chaotic one. But what is the relationship between the two?

Aristotle appeals to a different model of the *synechon* from that of a tyrant or monarch, opting instead for a model based on the arts. In broad strokes, Aristotle thinks that, among living things, what makes them wholes is not a specific material part, but the soul, which actively holds the parts of the body together. The soul does this not by constraint or force, but by producing and maintaining the various parts of the body through nutrition and growth, an activity which uses the body and its components as instruments or *organs* (in Greek, τὰ ὄργανα). What guarantees the cohesion of the body in this instance is the fact that the body is a prerequisite for the soul to do whatever else it does

46 πρὸς δὲ τούτοις τί τὸ συνέχον εἰς τἀναντία φερόμενα τὸ πῦρ καὶ τὴν γῆν; διασπασθήσεται γάρ, εἰ μή τι ἔσται τὸ κωλύον· εἰ δ' ἔσται, τοῦτ' ἔστιν ἡ ψυχή, καὶ τὸ αἴτιον τοῦ αὐξάνεσθαι καὶ τρέφεσθαι. δοκεῖ δέ τισιν ἡ τοῦ πυρὸς φύσις ἁπλῶς αἰτία τῆς τροφῆς καὶ τῆς αὐξήσεως εἶναι· καὶ γὰρ αὐτὸ φαίνεται μόνον τῶν σωμάτων [ἢ τῶν στοιχείων] τρεφόμενον καὶ αὐξόμενον, διὸ καὶ ἐν τοῖς φυτοῖς καὶ ἐν τοῖς ζῴοις ὑπολάβοι τις ἂν τοῦτο εἶναι τὸ ἐργαζόμενον. τὸ δὲ συναίτιον μέν πώς ἐστιν, οὐ μὴν ἁπλῶς γε αἴτιον, ἀλλὰ μᾶλλον ἡ ψυχή· ἡ μὲν γὰρ τοῦ πυρὸς αὔξησις εἰς ἄπειρον, ἕως ἂν ᾖ τὸ καυστόν, τῶν δὲ φύσει συνισταμένων πάντων ἔστι πέρας καὶ λόγος μεγέθους τε καὶ αὐξήσεως· ταῦτα δὲ ψυχῆς, ἀλλ' οὐ πυρός, καὶ λόγου μᾶλλον ἢ ὕλης.

(reproduce, perceive, think). So long as the soul is present in the body, it will actively maintain the arrangement of the body in order that the body continues to serve as its instrument.

Aristotle does not use this model to suggest that the soul is like an artist using instruments; rather, he seems to be thinking of the soul like an *art* using its instruments.[47] The muses may always need a poet, but nature needs no such medium – it can act immediately through bodies. This leads Aristotle to make some bizarre-sounding claims. He says things like, 'if the art of ship-building were in the wood, it would produce the same results by nature' (Arist. *Phys.* 2.8, 199b28–29), i.e. the wood would turn itself into a ship. There is also a thought experiment about an axe as a natural body (φυσικὸν σῶμα), something like a cybernetic hatchet, whose soul is the capacity to cut things (ἡ δύναμις τοῦ ὀργάνου) and whose activity is to get up and cut things on its own, no carpenter required (Arist. *De an.* 2.1, 412b10–13a10). In the world of human craft, an artist is a necessary intermediary between the art and the instruments or organs through which it acts; nature, however, needs no intermediary. It operates like a doctor who cures herself (ὅταν τις ἰατρεύῃ αὐτὸς ἑαυτόν) (Arist. *Phys.* 2.8, 199b31).

That is not to say that outside influences cannot act on the body and threaten its cohesion. The soul may be unaffected or unmoved by the body when it acts, since 'like, the art of medicine … when it produces health, it is in no way affected by the patient who is being healed' (Arist. *Gen. Corr.* 1.7, 324a35–b1).[48] Nevertheless, the matter, i.e. the body, like food or a drug acting as instruments of the agent, is always affected when it carries out the soul's activities: 'the food, *when it produces* (health), *is also affected* in some way: for it is heated or cooled or otherwise affected at the same time as it acts' (Arist. *Gen. Corr.* 1.7, 324b1–3). Over time, the body, like a blunted instrument, will become incapable of carrying out the activities of the soul, including the activity of maintaining its own cohesion.[49]

47 Menn (2002) 95.

48 Cf. Arist. *De an.* 3.5, 430a17–19 'for reason (ὁ νοῦς) is separate, unaffected and unmixed, being substance in actuality. For the agent is always more honourable than the patient, and the principle than the matter.' On the *Gen. Corr.* passage and its relevance, see Menn (2002) 95–99; Falcon (2005) 25.

49 Menn (2002) 113.

5 The Stoics, Pneumatists and Galen

The history of the *synechon* or cohesive cause which I have been tracing leads in the end to the more familiar Stoic notion. The Stoic position on cohesive causes resembles something like an eclectic mix of Diogenes of Apollonia and Aristotle. A comparatively large amount of literature exists on the Stoic theory of cohesive causes, at least much more than on earlier theories.[50] Rather than rehearse this literature, I want to conclude by noting a few aspects of the Stoic notion of cohesive causes that seem to me most closely related to this earlier tradition.

The first is perhaps trivial, but worth mentioning. It is often said that the Stoic cohesive cause is an analogue to the Aristotelian form,[51] but speaking this way tends to obscure how similar the causal role of the Stoic cohesive cause and its Aristotelian equivalents are, whether that equivalent is soul, nature or the notion of actuality more generally – whatever that metaphysical item is which is the immaterial cause to the matter of its having the kind of activity it has: the force, so to speak, existing in the matter, as soul is the cause to a body of its being actually a living body. We may not think of 'being a living body' as a kind of activity, but for Aristotle, being alive or being anything else is to exist in actuality (ἐνεργείᾳ), which is for him a kind of activity without movement. The Stoic view is remarkably close to this except, because they believe only bodies can be causes, they deny there are activities without movement. They do, however, maintain a distinction between the cause and the matter and, as does Aristotle, they believe the cause acts to confer cohesion to the matter. Galen gives the most complete summary of their view in his work on *Cohesive Causes*:

> The first philosophers of my acquaintance to speak of a cohesive cause were the Stoics. Their view is that from the four elements are produced those bodies that Aristotle calls homoiomerous and that are described by Plato as 'the first to be generated,' while all other bodies are simply compounds of these. Of the elements themselves, some they call material and some active and dynamic. They maintain that the material elements are held together by those that are dynamic, fire and air being dynamic and active in their view, while earth and water are material. They say that, when the elements are intermingled, the dynamic wholly penetrate the material, that is to say, air and fire penetrate water and earth. Air is cold

50 See especially Frede (1987), Hankinson (1998), Bobzien (1999), and papers in Coughlin, Leith and Lewis (2020).

51 See n. 14 above.

> and fire is hot. The natural effect of air is to consolidate and thicken a substance, whereas fire naturally causes expansion, loosening and widening. The two active elements have fine parts and the other two thick parts. Every substance with fine parts the Stoics call spirit (sc. *pneuma*), and they think that the function of this spirit is to produce cohesion in natural and in animal bodies. By natural bodies I mean those that are produced by nature and not by human skill, like stones, gold, wood and those parts of the animal body that are called the primary and homoiomerous parts, that is, nerves, arteries, veins, cartilages, bones and everything else of the same sort. Men join bits of wood together with glue, nails, pegs, clay, gypsum and lime. Similarly nature is found connecting all the parts of the body so as to form a united whole by means of cartilage, ligaments and tendons. If you like, you can call the parts of the body that produce this union in the simple members cohesive causes of the compounds, and the same term can be applied to clay, gypsum, lime and the other things that serve the same purpose in externals which are connected by the skill of man and not by nature. It is not these, however, but rather material substance with fine parts that the Stoics call a cohesive cause.
>
> GAL. *CC* 1.1–5, 53,2–55,3 Lyons, trans. LYONS[52]

Galen's summary, that *pneuma* (a mixture of fire and air) is the active element and brings about cohesion in the material elements, earth and water, by producing a two-fold movement outward and inward, is echoed in numerous other ancient sources.[53] Sextus Empiricus tells us that the Stoics also called 'what holds together (τὸ συνέχον) the whole compound' the soul.[54] Galen's other claim that things, like glue and nails, ligaments and tendons, can be called *synechon*, echoes the earlier use of the term, where it meant a binding part, as opposed to an active cause.[55] Galen himself rejects the Stoic cohesive

52 cf. Galen, *De plenitudine liber* 3 (VII.525 K.) '… most of those who propose the cohesive capacity (τὴν συνεκτικὴν δύναμιν), like the Stoics, make what holds together (τὸ συνέχον) one thing and what is held together (τὸ συνεχόμενον) another. For the pneumatic substance (τὴν πνευματικὴν οὐσίαν) is what holds together, while the material (substance) (τὴν ὑλικὴν οὐσίαν) is what is held together, which is why they say air and fire hold together, but earth and water are held together.'

53 [Gal.] *Def.* 96, XIX.372.1–2 K.; Plutarch, *De Stoicorum repugnantiis* 43, 1053f3–7.

54 Sextus Empiricus, *Adversus Mathematicos* 7.234.2–4 '[Some Stoics] assert soul is said in two ways: what holds the whole compound together [τό τε συνέχον τὴν ὅλην σύγκρισιν], and the leading part [τὸ ἡγεμονικόν] on its own.'

55 It is used in a similar way in Plutarch, *Quaestiones Convivales* 8.10, 735e5–f2, where the loss of leaves in autumn is explained in terms of the mixture (κρᾶσις) no longer being able to preserve them because what is glutinous and cohesive (τὸ ἐχέκολλον καὶ συνεκτικόν) no longer remains in it.

cause altogether in his work *On Cohesive Causes*, arguing that either (a) every whole needs a cohesive cause, in which case *pneuma* will also need a cohesive cause and we get a regress; or (b) some things need cohesive causes, while others are self-cohesive, in which case Galen thinks a much better case could be made for something like adamantine to be self-cohesive than hot air, since things like adamantine are solid and less prone to disperse (Gal. *CC* 6.2–5, 61,26–63,16 Lyons).

One of the most remarkable differences between the Aristotelian and Stoic notion of the cohesive cause, however, is what it says about us, or at any rate about how we fall apart. Atlas may be strong and eternal, but our cohesion is limited. Aristotle blames the instrument. The Stoics also blame the soul – at least, the Stoic-influenced Pneumatist physician,[56] Athenaeus of Attalia sees the source of incoherence in the powers of the soul itself:

> Old age requires a more exact regimen and additional aids. For the psychic and physical capacities (ψυχικαί τε καὶ φυσικαὶ δυνάμεις) which hold us together and preserve us (συνέχουσαι καὶ διασῴζουσαι ἡμᾶς) lose their strength, their functions are brought to an end and the body wrinkles and becomes malnourished, loose and dry. And so when the capacity which keeps the body upright (ἡ μὲν διευθύνουσα τὸ σῶμα δύναμις), offers resistance against external things that cause us injury, and resists in accordance with certain spermatic principles (σπερματικοὺς λόγους) and natural necessities (φυσικὰς ἀνάγκας), falls to the floor (ὑπὸ πόδας χωρῇ, i.e. declines in strength), the body is easily affected and easily injured, requiring but a small cause and chance influence for harm. At the start, then, from an early age, one should also take precautions for the time of old age. For as those who wear out their cloak in the summer spend the winter in tatters, so those who in their youth neglect their bodily strength suffer the clothes of old age with great difficulty.
>
> ATHENAEUS OF ATTALIA, quoted in Oribasius, *Collectiones Medicae* (libri incerti 39) 140,13–36 Raeder

I think we must enjoy our summers.

56 On the role of *pneuma* in the Pneumatist school of medicine, see Coughlin and Lewis (2020). On Athenaeus' relationship to thinkers other than the Stoics, see Coughlin (2018) 109–13.

Acknowledgments

The research and writing of this paper were funded by a postdoctoral fellowship from the Deutsche Forschungsgemeinschaft (German Research Foundation) – Exzellenzcluster 264 *Topoi. Die Formation und Transformation von Raum und Wissen in den antiken Kulturen* – Projekt-ID 39235742 held at Humboldt-Universität zu Berlin. Additional funding saw it to completion: fellowships at Einstein Centre Chronoi in Berlin and from the Deutsche Forschungsgemeinschaft (German Research Foundation) – SFB 980 *Episteme in Bewegung. Wissenstransfer von der Alten Welt bis in die Frühe Neuzeit* – Projekt-ID 191249397. The first draft was presented at the conference, *Ancient Holisms*, held in London 11–12 September 2017; the last, at Philip van der Eijk's Ancient Medicine Research Colloquium at the Institut für Klassische Philologie, Humboldt-Universität zu Berlin, on 18 May 2020. I am grateful to audiences at both, with special thanks to Elizabeth Craik, Philip van der Eijk, P. N. Singer, and Chiara Thumiger for helpful comments. Many thanks also to Gábor Betegh, David Ebrey, and three anonymous reviewers for comments on the written draft.

Bibliography

Ackrill, J. L. 'Aristotle's Definitions of Psuche.' *Proceedings of the Aristotelian Society*, 73 (1972) 119–33.

Ainsworth, T. 'Form vs. Matter.' In *The Stanford Encyclopedia of Philosophy*, ed. E. N. Zalta. Metaphysics Research Lab, Stanford University (2016). Available at https://plato.stanford.edu/ archives/spr2016/entries/form-matter/.

Bobzien, S. 'Chrysippus' Theory of Causes.' In *Topics in Stoic Philosophy*, ed. K. Ierodiakonou. Oxford: Oxford University Press (1999).

Choulant, J. L. *Handbuch der Bücherkunde für die ältere Medicin, zur Kenntniss der griechischen, lateinischen und arabischen Schriften im ärztlichen Fache und zur bibliographischen Unterscheidung ihrer verschiedenen Ausgaben, Uebersetzungen und Erläuterungen*. Leipzig: L. Voss (1841).

Choulant, J. L., F. H. Garrison, E. C. Streeter, and M. Frank. *History and Bibliography of Anatomic Illustration in Its Relation to Anatomic Science and the Graphic Arts*. Chicago: University of Chicago Press (1920).

Cohen, S. M. *Aristotle on Nature and Incomplete Substance*. Cambridge and New York: Cambridge University Press (1996).

Cohen, S. M. 'Aristotle's Metaphysics.' In *The Stanford Encyclopedia of Philosophy*, ed. E. N. Zalta. Metaphysics Research Lab, Stanford University (2016). https://plato.stanford.edu/archives/win2016/entries/aristotle-metaphysics/.

Coughlin, S. 'Athenaeus of Attalia on the Psychological Causes of Bodily Health.' In *Mental Illness in Ancient Medicine: From Celsus to Paul of Aegina*, ed. C. Thumiger and P. N. Singer. Leiden: Brill (2018) 109–42.

Coughlin, S., and O. Lewis. 'Pneuma and the Pneumatist School of Medicine.' In *The Concept of Pneuma after Aristotle*, ed. S. Coughlin, D. Leith and O. Lewis. Berlin: Edition Topoi (2020) 203–36.

Coughlin, S., D. Leith and O. Lewis. *The Concept of Pneuma after Aristotle. Berlin Studies in the Ancient World*. Berlin: Edition Topoi (2020).

Cross, R. *Duns Scotus*. Oxford: Oxford University Press (1999).

D'Acquisto, F., G. Piras and L. Rattazzi. 'Pro-Inflammatory and Pathogenic Properties of Annexin-A1: The Whole Is Greater than the Sum of Its Parts.' *Biochemical Pharmacology*, 85.9 (May 1, 2013): 1213–18.

Elliott, G. *Global Business Information Technology: An Integrated Systems Approach*. Harlow and New York: Pearson Addison Wesley (2004).

Falcon, A. *Aristotle and the Science of Nature: Unity Without Uniformity*. Cambridge: Cambridge University Press (2005).

Fine, K. 'Things and Their Parts.' *Midwest Studies in Philosophy*, 23.1 (1999) 61–74.

Fine, K. 'Towards a Theory of Part.' *Journal of Philosophy*, 107.11 (2010) 559–89.

Forrest, J. Y.-L. *General Systems Theory: Foundation, Intuition and Applications in Business Decision Making*. Cham: Springer (2018).

Frede, M. *Essays in Ancient Philosophy*. Minneapolis: University of Minnesota Press (1987).

Frede, M. 'The Original Notion of Cause.' In *Essays in Ancient Philosophy*, ed. M. Frede. Minneapolis: University of Minnesota Press (1987) 125–50. Originally printed in *Doubt and Dogmatism: Studies in Hellenistic Epistemology*, ed. J. Barnes, M. F. Burnyeat and M. Schofield. Oxford: Oxford University Press (1980) 217–49.

Fuller, A. R. *Insight into Value: An Exploration of the Premises of a Phenomenological Psychology*. Albany: SUNY Press (1990).

Graham, D. W. 'Plato and Anaximenes.' *Études Platoniciennes* [Online], 12 (2015). http://journals.openedition.org/etudesplatoniciennes/706.

Hankinson, R. J. 'Evidence, Externality and Antecedence: Inquiries into Later Greek Causal Concepts.' *Phronesis*, 32.1 (1987) 80–100.

Hankinson, R. J. *Cause and Explanation in Ancient Greek Thought*. Oxford: Oxford University Press (1998).

Hanson, B. *What Holism Can Do for Social Theory*. Routledge Studies in Social and Political Thought. New York: Routledge (2014).

Hanson, B. *General Systems Theory. Beginning with Wholes*. London and New York: Routledge (2013).

Harte, V. *Plato on Parts and Wholes: The Metaphysics of Structure*. Oxford: Oxford University Press (2002).

Havrda, M. *The So-Called Eighth Stromateus by Clement of Alexandria: Early Christian Reception of Greek Scientific Methodology*. Leiden: Brill (2016).

Heider, G. M. 'More about Hull and Koffka.' *American Psychologist*, 32.5 (1977) 383.

Johnston, Mark. 'Hylomorphism.' *Journal of Philosophy*, 103.12 (2006) 652–98.

Kirk, G. S., J. E. Raven and M. Schofield. *The Presocratic Philosophers: A Critical History with a Selection of Texts*. Cambridge: Cambridge University Press (1999).

Koslicki, K. *Form, Matter, Substance*. Oxford and New York: Oxford University Press (2018).

Koslicki, K. 'Towards a Hylomorphic Solution to the Grounding Problem.' *Royal Institute of Philosophy Supplements*, 82 (July 2018) 333–64.

Koslicki, K. 'Towards a Neo-Aristotelian Mereology.' *Dialectica*, 61.1 (March 2007) 127–59.

Lasson, A. *Aristoteles Metaphysik*. Jena: E. Diederichs (1907).

Long, A. A., and D. N. Sedley. *The Hellenistic Philosophers: Volume 1, Translations of the Principal Sources with Philosophical Commentary*. Cambridge: Cambridge University Press (1987).

Marks, F., U. Klingmüller and K. Müller-Decker. *Cellular Signal Processing: An Introduction to the Molecular Mechanisms of Signal Transduction*. Heidelberg: Garland Science (2008).

Marmodoro, A. 'Aristotle's Hylomorphism Without Reconditioning.' *Philosophical Inquiry*, 37.1–2 (2013) 5–22.

Menn, S. 'On Socrates' First Objections to the Physicists (Phaedo 95 E 8–97 B 7).' *Oxford Studies in Ancient Philosophy*, 38 (2010) 37–68.

Menn, S. 'Aristotle's Definition of Soul and the Programme of the De Anima.' *Oxford Studies in Ancient Philosophy* 22 (2002) 83–139.

Menn, S. 'Metaphysics Z10–16 and the Argument-Structure of Metaphysics Z.' *Oxford Studies in Ancient Philosophy*, 21 (2001) 83–134.

Menn, S. *Plato on God as Nous*. Carbondale: Southern Illinois University (1995).

Mirrione, C. *Theory and Terminology of Mixture in Galen: the Concepts of* krasis *and* mixis *in Galen's Thought*. Dissertation Humboldt-Universität zu Berlin (2017).

Peramatzis, M. 'Aristotle's Hylomorphism: The Causal-Explanatory Model.' *Metaphysics*, 1.1 (May 21, 2018) 12–32.

Scalambrino, F. *Philosophical Principles of the History and Systems of Psychology: Essential Distinctions*. Cham: Palgrave Macmillan (2018).

Scaltsas, T. *Substances and Universals in Aristotle's Metaphysics*. Ithaca: Cornell University Press (1994).

Schuster, P. 'A Beginning of the End of the Holism versus Reductionism Debate?: Molecular Biology Goes Cellular and Organismic.' *Complexity*, 13.1 (September 2007) 10–13.

Sedley, D. 'The Dramatis Personae of Plato's Phaedo.' In *Philosophical Dialogues: Plato, Hume, Wittgenstein*, ed. T. J. Smiley. Oxford: Oxford University Press (1995) 3–26.

Shields, C. 'Aristotle's Psychology > A Fundamental Problem about Hylomorphism.' In *Stanford Encyclopedia of Philosophy*, ed. E. N. Zalta. Metaphysics Research Lab, Stanford University (2016). Available at https://plato.stanford.edu/entries/aristotle-psychology/suppl1.html.

Singer, P. N., P. J. van der Eijk and P. Tassinari. *Galen. Works on Human Nature.* Volume 1, 'Mixtures (*De temperamentis*).' Cambridge Galen Translations. Cambridge: Cambridge University Press (2018).

Vallero, D. A. *Biomedical Ethics for Engineers: Ethics and Decision Making in Biomedical and Biosystem Engineering.* Amsterdam: Elsevier (2011).

Vlastos, G. *Studies in Greek Philosophy*, Volume I: The Presocratics. Princeton: Princeton University Press (1996).

Ward, T. M. *John Duns Scotus on Parts, Wholes, and Hylomorphism.* Leiden and Boston: Brill (2014).

Witt, C. 'Hylomorphism in Aristotle.' *The Journal of Philosophy*, 84.11 (1987) 673–79.

Primary Texts: Editions and Translations Used

Aëtius, *Placita Philosophorum* (Aët.): *Doxographi Graeci.* Ed. H. Diels. Berlin: Reimer (1879) 273–444.

Alcmaeon of Croton: See DK

Alexander of Aphrodisias, *In Aristotelis Metaphysica Commentaria* (Alex. Aphr. *in Arist. Metaph.*): *Alexandri Aphrodisiensis in Aristotelis Metaphysica commentaria.* Ed. M. Hayduck. *Commentaria in Aristotelem Graeca* 1. Berlin: Reimer (1891).

Anaxagoras (Anax.): See DK

Aristotle, *De anima* (Arist. *De an.*): *Aristotelis De anima.* Ed. W. D. Ross. Oxford Classical Texts. Oxford: Oxford University Press (1956).

Aristotle, *De generatione animalium* (Arist. *Gen. an.*): *Aristotelis De Generatione Animalium.* Ed. H. J. Drossaart Lulofs. Oxford Classical Texts. Oxford: Oxford University Press (1965).

Aristotle, *De Generatione et Corruptione* (Arist. *Gen. corr.*): *Aristote. De la Génération et de la corruption.* Ed. and trans. M. Rashed. Collection des Universités de France. Paris: Les Belles Lettres (2005).

Aristotle, *Partibus Animalium* (Arist. *Part. an.*): Aristote. *Les parties des animaux.* Ed. and trans. P. Louis. Collection des Universités de France. Paris: Les Belles Lettres (1993).

Aristotle, *Metaphysica* (Arist. *Metaph.*): *Aristotelis Metaphysica.* Ed. W. Jaeger. Oxford Classical Texts. Oxford: Oxford University Press (1957).

Aristotle, *Meteorologica* (Arist. *Mete.*): *Aristotelis Meteorologicorum Libri Quattuor.* Ed. F. H. Fobes. Cambridge MA: Harvard University Press (1919).

Aristotle, *Physica* (Arist. *Phys.*): *Aristotelis Physica*. Ed. W. D. Ross. Oxford Classical Texts. Oxford: Oxford University Press (1950).

Aristotle, *Problemata* (sp.) ([Arist.] *Pr.*): *Aristotle*. Volume XVI. *Problems*, Books 20–38. Ed. and trans. R. Mayhew. *Rhetoric to Alexander*. Ed. and trans. D. C. Mirhady. Loeb Classical Library 317. Cambridge MA: Harvard University Press (2011) 1–449.

Clement of Alexandria, *Stromateis* (Clem. *Strom.*): Havrda, Matyáš. *The So-Called Eighth Stromateus by Clement of Alexandria: Early Christian Reception of Greek Scientific Methodology*. Leiden: Brill (2016).

Democritus (Democr.): See DK

Diogenes (Diog.): See DK

DK = Diels Kranz: *Die Fragmente der Vorsokratiker*. Ed. H. Diels and W. Kranz. Sixth Edition. Berlin: Weidmann (1951–1952).

Empedocles (Emped.): See DK

Euripides, *Supplices* (Eur. *Supp.*): *Euripidis Fabulae*. Ed. J. Diggle. Vol. 2. Oxford: Oxford University Press (1981) 3–53.

Galen, *Adversus Iulianum* (Gal. *Adv. Iul.*): *Galeni Adversus Lycum et Adversus Iulianum libelli*. Ed. E. Wenkebach. Corpus Medicorum Graecorum V 10,3. Berlin: Akademie-Verlag (1951) 33–70.

Galen, *Claudii Galeni Opera omnia*. Ed. C. G. Kühn. 22 Vols. Leipzig: Knobloch (1821–1833).

Galen, *De Causis Contentivis* (Gal. *CC*): *Galeni De Partibus Artis Medicativae, De Causis Contentivis, De Diaeta in Morbis Acutis Secundum Hippocratem Libelli Versio Arabica*, edidit et in linguam Anglicam vertit M. Lyons; *De Partibus Artis Medicativae, De Causis Contentivis Libelli Editio* ab H. Schöne alterius a K. Kalbfleisch curata, retractaverunt J. Kollesch, D. Nickel, G. Strohmaier. Corpus Medicorum Graecorum Supplementum Orientale II. Berlin: Akademie-Verlag (1969) 52–73, 133–41.

Galen, *De Plenitudine* (Gal. *Plen.*): *Claudii Galeni opera omnia*. Ed. C. G. Kühn. Vol. 7. Leipzig: Knobloch (1824) 513–83.

Galen, *De Symptomatum Causis* (Gal. *Caus. Symp.*): *Claudii Galeni Opera Omnia*. Ed. C. G. Kühn. Vol. 7. Leipzig: Knobloch (1824) 85–272.

Galen, *Definitiones Medicae* (sp.) ([Gal.] *Def.*): *Claudii Galeni Opera Omnia*. Ed. C. G. Kühn. Vol. 19. Leipzig: Knobloch (1830) 346–462.

Galen, *Introductio sive Medicus* (sp.) ([Gal.] *Int.*): Galien [sp.]. Tome III. *Le Médecin*. Introduction [=Int.]. Ed. and trans. C. Petit. Collection des Universités de France. Paris: Les Belles Lettres (2009).

Galen, *Synopsis Librorum Suorum de Pulsibus* (Gal. *Syn. Puls.*): *Claudii Galeni Opera Omnia*. Ed. C. G. Kühn. Vol. 9. Leipzig: Knobloch (1825) 431–533.

Hesiod, *Theogonia* (Hes. *Theog.*): *Hesiod*. Theogony. Ed. M. L. West. Oxford: Clarendon Press (1966).

Hippocrates, *De Carnibus* (Hp. *Carn.*): Hippocrates. Volume VIII. Ed. and trans. Paul Potter. Loeb Classical Library 482. Cambridge MA: Harvard University Press (1995) 127–166.

Hippocrates, *De Flatibus* (Hp. *Flat.*): *Hippocratis Indices Librorum, Iusiurandum, Lex, De arte, De medico, De Decente Habitu, Praeceptiones, De Prisca Medicina, De Aere Locis Aquis, De Alimento, De Liquidorum Usu, De Flatibus*. Edidit J. L. Heiberg, Corpus Medicorum Graecorum I 1. Leipzig and Berlin: Teubner (1927) 91–101.

Hippocrates, *Mochlicum* (Hp. *Mochl.*): Hippocrates. Volume III. Ed. and trans. E. T. Withington. Loeb Classical Library 149. Cambridge MA: Harvard University Press (1928) 399–450.

Hippocrates, *OEuvres complètes d'Hippocrate*. Ed. and trans. É. Littré. 10 Vols. Paris: J.-B. Ballière (1839–1861).

Hippocrates, *Prorrheticus II* (Hp. *Prorrh. II*): Hippocrates. Volume VIII. Ed. and trans. Paul Potter. Loeb Classical Library 482. Cambridge MA: Harvard University Press (1995) 213–94.

Oribasius, *Collectiones Medicae* (Orib. *Coll. Med.*): *Oribasii Collectionum Medicarum Reliquiae*. Vol. IV, libri XLIX–L, *Libri incerti, Eclogae medicamentorum*. Ed. J. Raeder. Corpus Medicorum Graecorum VI 2,2. Leipzig et Berlin (1933).

Plato, *Phaedo* (Pl. *Phd.*): *Platonis Opera*. Ed. J. Burnet. Vol. 1. Oxford Classical Texts. Oxford: Oxford University Press (1900).

Plato, *Theaetetus* (Pl. *Tht.*): *Platonis Opera*. Ed. J. Burnet. Vol. 2. Oxford Classical Texts. Oxford: Oxford University Press (1900).

Plato, *Timaeus* (Pl. *Ti.*): *Platonis Opera*. Ed. J. Burnet. Vol. 4. Oxford Classical Texts. Oxford: Oxford University Press (1900).

Plutarch, *De Stoicorum Repugnantiis* (Plut. *Stoic. repug.*): *Plutarchi Moralia* VI, 2. Ed. R. Westman and M. Pohlenz. 2nd edn. Bibliotheca scriptorum Graecorum et Romanorum Teubneriana (Scriptores Graeci). Leipzig: Teubner (1959) 2–58.

Plutarch, *Placita philosophorum* (sp.) ([Plut.] *Placit.*): *Plutarchi Moralia* V,2,1. Ed. J. Mau. Bibliotheca Scriptorum Graecorum et Romanorum Teubneriana (Scriptores Graeci). Leipzig: Teubner (1971) 50–153.

Sextus Empiricus, *Adversus Mathematicos* (*S. E. M.*): Sexti Empirici Opera. Ed. H. Mutschmann. Vol. 2. Bibliotheca Scriptorum Graecorum et Romanorum Teubneriana (Scriptores Graeci). Leipzig: Teubner (1914).

Pyrrhoniae hypotyposes (S. E. *PH*): *Sexti Empirici Opera*. Ed. H. Mutschmann. Vol. I. Bibliotheca Scriptorum Graecorum et Romanorum Teubneriana (Scriptores Graeci). Leipzig: Teubner (1912).

Simplicius, *In Aristotelis De Caelo Commentarius* (Simpl. *in Arist. De cael.*): *Simplicii in Aristotelis De caelo commentaria*. Ed. I. L. Heiberg. Commentaria in Aristotelem Graeca 7. Berlin: Reimer (1894).

Simplicius, *In Aristotelis Physicorum Libros Commentaria* (Simpl. *in Arist. Phys.*): *Simplicii in Aristotelis Physicorum libros quattuor priores commentaria*. Ed. H. Diels. Commentaria in Aristotelem Graeca 9. Berlin: Reimer (1882).

Xenophon, *Memorabilia* (Xen. *Mem.*): Xenophon. Volume IV. *Memorabilia, Oeconomicus*. Trans. E. C. Marchant. *Symposium, Apology*. Trans. O. J. Todd. Loeb Classical Library 168. Cambridge MA: Harvard University Press (1923).

CHAPTER 11

Pneuma as a Holistic Concept in Galen

Julius Rocca

Abstract

Galenic physiology is an interconnected system of capacities (*dunameis*) made possible by the coordinated activities of individual structures and organ systems which ensure function (*chreia*). The two principal modalities operating within this milieu are the four humours and *pneuma* in its elaborated vital and psychic forms. Our potential as a rational agent depends on the proper exercise of intellection, of the sense organs, and of voluntary motion. As is well known, Galen incorporates the Platonic conception of the tripartite division of the soul, the Stoic notion of the governing principle (*hēgemonikon*), as well as a syncretic adaption of the Aristotelian and Stoic concept of *pneuma*. For Galen, the brain is the controlling organ of the body, containing the rational soul. This soul is somatised to an appreciable extent, in that it operates through the actions of a first instrument (*prōton organon*), which for Galen is *psychic pneuma*. This form of *pneuma* is elaborated by key organs of the body in a series of stepwise qualitative changes involving air, vital heat and blood. This series of elaborative changes imparts to *pneuma*, in its psychic manifestation, the function of an overall holistic property. Since it is formed as a physiologic whole which is more than the sum of its individual constituents, it enables the potential rational flourishing of *gens humana*. *Psychic pneuma* may also be considered as approaching the definition of an emergent property, although aspects of its function seem to depend on the physical characteristics of some of its parts. As far as pathological conditions are concerned, a completely holistic classification for *pneuma* is less clear. However, there is evidence that certain disease processes, whilst *caused* by humoural imbalance, are nevertheless *symptomatically* interpreted by Galen as being due primarily to blockage of pneumatic flow.

1 Introduction

Timaeus, in his matchless story of creation, tells of the god (θεός) who constructs the cosmos as a living being (τὸ ζῶον), a 'totality of totalities' (ὅλον ὅλων), from the constituent elements of fire, air, earth and water (*Ti.* 32c–33a). Another ζῷον, on a far smaller scale, is the human body, which manifestly is

 | DOI:10.1163/9789004443143_013

more than simply the sum of its component parts.[1] Galenic physiology of the body and soul is an interconnected system of capacities (δυνάμεις) made possible first and foremost by the coordinated activities of precisely delineated anatomical structures that collectively ensure function (χρεία).[2] The two principal modalities that make this system function are the four humours (especially blood, αἷμα) and two types of *pneuma* (πνεῦμα).[3] These *pneumata* are conceptualized as qualitatively and substantially different and represent vital and psychic modalities.[4] It is *psychic pneuma* that this chapter will examine, since its holistic potential is arguably more defined. In its psychic manifestation, *pneuma* is more than the sum of its constituent parts, since it is acting for and on behalf of the rational soul. It is the actions of the rational soul which make human beings more than simply living organisms. Human beings, as rational agents, depend on the proper exercise of intellection, the employment of the sense organs, and the exercise of voluntary motion. Apart from his adaptation of the Platonic soul tripartition, placed in the brain, heart and liver,[5] Galen incorporates the Stoic notion of the controlling principle (*principatus*) or regent part (ἡγεμονικόν)[6] together with a syncretic adaption of Aristotelian and Stoic *pneuma*. For Galen, the brain (ὁ ἐγκέφαλος) is the principal hegemonic organ of the body, the source of the nervous system, and the location of

1 This organization is teleological: 'The parts of the organism, although not temporally prior to the whole, are *for the sake* of the whole. Their combined *telos* is to maintain the whole alive' (Scolnicov 2017, 47; italics in original).

2 This is traditionally translated as 'use' by May (1968) 9 and Wilkie in Furley and Wilkie (1984) 58–59. Hankinson (1989) 217 n. 32 opts for 'function' as 'perhaps ... the least misleading.' If *chreia* is difficult to render precisely into English, this is because it is a placeholder for a number of coordinated, naturally occurring tasks (or fitting actions) that the body, expressed either as the sum of its parts or at the level of a given individual component, must perform to fulfil the requirement of an organism. Sometimes it expresses pure function (the peristaltic actions of the stomach, for example); at other times it seems to convey the wider range of meanings (the complex cascade of movements of the hand in performing a defined task).

3 Galenic humours and *pneuma* are interconnected insofar as one of the humours, blood, is part of the elaborative process that makes vital *pneuma* in the heart. See Part 3 below. Otherwise, it does appear to be the case that the humours and *pneumata* function as quasi-independent systems.

4 Galen flags the possibility that a 'natural *pneuma*' (φυσικὸν πνεῦμα) may exist, housed in the liver. But it is only mentioned once, and its physiological and psychic attributes are never explored. See Rocca (2012). This virtual absence represents a source of considerable tension in Galen's adoption of Platonic soul tripartition as far the liver is concerned. See De Lacy (1988).

5 For a summary, see Schiefsky (2012).

6 For a summary of the hegemonic concept, see Rocca (2003) chapter 1. Galen's espousal of Platonic soul tripartition commits him to endorsing, however tentatively, a triple hegemonic system. As Gill (2007) 108 observes: 'For the Stoics, by contrast, there is a single psychological agency, the *hēgemonikon*, located in the heart and controlling all psychic processes.'

the rational soul. The rational soul's activities are somatised, in that it is said to operate through the actions of a 'first instrument' (πρῶτον ὄργανον), which for Galen is *psychic pneuma* (πνεῦμα ψυχικόν).[7] This is elaborated by key organs of the body in a series of progressive qualitative changes involving the outside air, vital heat and blood. These changes, which occur in lung, heart and brain, impart a recognizably holistic property to *psychic pneuma*, since its psycho-physiological function is far more than the sum of its individual constituents.[8] It is possible to regard *psychic pneuma* as an emergent property, that is, its functions cannot be ascribed to those of its constituent parts, but only in the sense that its activities are not derived from its constituent components. However, as will be shown, key aspects of its function are dependent on the physical characteristics of at least one of those parts. However, not only are aspects of its overall function dependent on the physical characteristics of its parts, but the use of emergentism distorts what Galen has to say in regard to how elements, their qualities and the parts interrelate and function. As far as pathological conditions are concerned, a holistic classification for *pneumata* is less clear. This chapter begins with an overview of key aspects of the concept of *pneuma* before Galen.

2 Some Antecedents

Aristotle, *Metaphysics Theta* 6, 1045a8–10, remarks: 'In the case of all things which have several parts and in which the whole (τὸ πᾶν) is not, as it were, a mere heap, but the totality is something besides the parts (τὸ ὅλον παρὰ τὰ μόρια), there is a cause of unity.' A chief 'cause of unity' which Greek medicine and philosophy deployed to try to account for the phenomenon of life was air or *pneuma*. It 'lies at the heart of several Greek attempts to bridge the gap that they themselves opened up between mind and body.'[9] The association of air with both life form and life force has a long pedigree. In this respect, *pneuma*

7 Galen's refusal to commit himself to stating what he considers the soul to be, much less its precise relationship to *psychic pneuma* (beyond the tag 'first instrument') is notorious. See Hankinson (1991), (2006); Von Staden (2000) 111–16. That Galen at times (almost) equates soul with *pneuma*, is to acknowledge, albeit implicitly, the corporeality of both in the absolute Stoic sense.

8 I do not discuss *vital pneuma* here, except in passing. It does have a physiological life of its own, apart from being the immediate precursor to *psychic pneuma*. It can also be said to participate in the elaboration of the latter, in the sense that *vital pneuma* via the arteries enters both the retiform and the choroid plexuses.

9 Lloyd (2007) 135.

'originates as a concept in physiology.'[10] The Hippocratic text *Breaths* (*De flatibus*) states that *pneuma* is not only a source of nourishment for the body, but 'within bodies it is called breath (φῦσα), and outside bodies it is called air (ἀήρ). It is the most powerful of all and in all (πᾶσι τῶν πάντων δυνάστης ἐστίν), and it is worthwhile examining its power.'[11] Although Galen's notion of *pneuma* is different from that of *Breaths*, he picks up the crucial notion of *pneuma*'s primal active power. In *On Semen* (*De semine*), for example, Galen describes *pneuma* as actively pushing the body parts it has moulded.[12] This is Nature using air – differentiated nominally but not ontologically – as its perforating instrument to actively mould the developing embryo.

Galen's broad claims for what *pneuma* is able to accomplish are not in themselves novel, but are rooted in both general and specific assertions made for and about it by a number of his predecessors.[13] Take two representative Presocratic examples. Anaximenes maintained that air (ἀήρ, πνεῦμα) is soul, and that it controls us (συγκρατεῖ ἡμᾶς).[14] Diogenes of Apollonia explicitly equated the air we breathe with soul (life) and intelligence.[15] This life-giving air is described in a holistic way, as the 'nature of the totality' (τὴν δὲ τοῦ παντὸς φύσιν ἀέρα).[16] Diogenes gives as his opinion that air, which contains or holds intelligence (τὸ τὴν νόησιν ἔχον εἶναι), both steers (κυβερνᾶσθαι) and controls (κρατεῖν) all things.[17] Air is also responsible for sensation (or is somehow connected with it).[18] Air is presented as a noetic, hegemonic, holistic conception. Further, it is distributed about the body in a carrier system, the blood vessels.[19]

10 Rist (1985) 27.

11 τὰ σώματα καὶ τὰ τῶν ἄλλων ζῴων καὶ τὰ τῶν ἀνθρώπων ὑπὸ τρισσῶν τροφέων τρέφεται· τῇσι δὲ τροφῇσι τάδε ὀνόματά ἐστι· σῖτα, ποτά, πνεῦμα. πνεῦμα δὲ τὸ μὲν ἐν τοῖσι σώμασιν φῦσα καλεῖται, τὸ δὲ ἔξω τῶν σωμάτων ἀήρ. οὗτος δὲ μέγιστος ἐν τοῖσι πᾶσι τῶν πάντων δυνάστης ἐστίν. ἄξιον δὲ αὐτοῦ θεήσασθαι τὴν δύναμιν (*Flat.* 3, VI.92–4 L. = 105,12–16 Jouanna, tr. Jones, slightly modified).

12 ὅταν δ' ὑπογράψηται τὸ τῶν δημιουργουμένων εἶδος, ἀθροωτέρᾳ φορᾷ χρησαμένη τοῦ πνεύματος ἅμα μὲν ἔξω προωθεῖ τὸ διαπλασθέν, ἅμα δὲ ῥηγνύει τὸ περιέχον (*Sem.* 2.5, IV.638 K. = 192,12–14 De Lacy). A similar view of *pneuma* acting under pressure is seen in the Hippocratic text *Nature of the Child* (*Nat. Puer.*) 1 (VII.486, 488 L.); see the discussion in Hankinson (2017) 245–46.

13 Singer (2020) provides an excellent overview.

14 Aetius, [Plutarch] *Placita* 1.3.4, S1.10.12 (DKB2, TEGP 8).

15 Simplicius, *Physics* 152.16(18)–21 (DKB4, TEGP 7). See the discussion in Pinto (2018), who takes a slightly divergent tack.

16 Simplicius, *Physics* 25.1–13 (DKA5, TEGP 8).

17 Simplicius, *Physics* 152.21(22)–153.13 (DKB5, TEGP 9). Cf. Arist. *On the Soul* 405a21–25 (DKA20, TEGP 31).

18 Theophrastus *On the Senses* 39–45 (DKA9, TEGP 30).

19 Simplicius *Physics* 153.13–17 (TEGP 33).

The author of the Hippocratic text *Sacred Disease* (*De Morbo Sacro*) holds that certain blood vessels take in most of the outside air, distributing it through the body. This breath cools the body, and some also goes straight to the brain, where it is responsible for intelligence and motion.[20]

Aristotle distinguished between external air and connate (inborn) *pneuma*, which was located in the heart.[21] He further established the notion that the incorporeal soul could somehow 'move' the material body through instruments, the most important of which was inborn *pneuma* (*GA* 5, 789b9; *de An.* 433b18).[22] In [Aristotle] *On Breath* (*De Spiritu*), in comments on the difference between outside air and *pneuma*, while the external air is at rest, air within the body is referred to as *pneuma*, defined as 'being condensed and distributed in a certain way' (καθάπερ πυκνωθεὶς καὶ διαδοθείς πως).[23]

Stoicism adapted *pneuma* as a compound of fire and air; it was the body's animating principle, explicitly identified as the soul itself.[24] Moreover, this *pneuma*, we are told, suffuses and sustains the entire cosmos (Chrysippus *ap.* Alexander, *Mixt.* 3 = *SVF* 2.473), and owing to its different degrees of tensional capacity it is the principle of coherence of our bodies (Seneca, *Nat.* 2.6.6). *Pneuma* in Stoic hands is thus readily understood as forming a complete holistic system.[25] The Hellenistic physicians Herophilus and Erasistratus are noteworthy for their respective groundbreaking anatomical and physiological studies, carried out within a broad Aristotelian framework. Herophilus' use of *pneuma* seems to explain nervous action, but is remarkably lacking in details.[26] In *On the Doctrines of Hippocrates and Plato* (*De Placitis Hippocratis et Platonis*), Galen states that the distinction between *vital pneuma* (located in the heart) and *psychic pneuma* (located in the brain) was known to Erasistratus.[27] Acting together with blood and the body's structural *triplokia* of artery, vein and nerve, *pneuma* (however qualified) was for Erasistratus one of the proximate elements of the body in the Aristotelian sense, and also represented the limits of investigation into the function of the body appropriate to a physician.[28]

20 *Morb.Sacr.* 10, VI.372 L. = p. 72 Grensemann.

21 See Peck (1942) Appendix B, 580–81, 593.

22 See Rist (1985) 28.

23 483b2–8 = 102 Roselli. See Sharples (2006) 174–76.

24 The literature is extensive. See for example Hahm (1977) 158–74.

25 'Stoic thought expresses, in a consistent way, a holistic or 'structure' approach …' (Gill 2010, 15). See also Gill (2006). For an analysis of the contrast between Stoic unified or holistic psychology and Galen's part-based Platonic one, see Gill (2007) 108–18.

26 See Rocca (2003) 38.

27 *PHP* 2.8, V.281 K. = 164,14–16 De Lacy = fr. 112B Garofalo.

28 See Leith (2015) 470–71.

This brief survey has highlighted several influences[29] and themes capable of lending themselves to further manipulation: inspired air as the source of *pneuma*, vasculature as its carrier system, and, most significantly, the use of air or *pneuma* to account for sensation and voluntary motion. Galen's contribution to the developmental concept of *pneuma* is based absolutely on it being subject to a series of qualitative changes, which in part highlight the functional capacities of the key organs of the body. His specific achievement is to further elaborate an animating principle (*psychic pneuma*) into an entity which allows the brain and nerves, from its motor and sensory components to the cognitive apparatus, to act as a coordinated whole. The following examines the formation of *psychic pneuma* and its functional attributes.

3 Galen's Pneumatic Physiology

Sensation, voluntary motion and intellection are made possible, according to Galen, by the brain and nervous system of the body working together as an aggregate entity. *Pneuma* (in its ultimate transformation into a psychic form) is described as the soul's 'first instrument' (πρῶτον ὄργανον). In *On the Elements according to Hippocrates* (*De elementis ex Hippocratis sententia*), the nature (φύσις) of *pneuma* is composed mostly of air (ἀήρ), but also of fire (πῦρ):

> Do not then look for anything unmixed (ἄμικτον) in the bodies of animals either. But be content, when you see this part cold and dry and solid, to call earth to mind, and when you see that part rarefied and wet and fluid, to think of water. Let the considerable heat in the body of the animal remind you of fire; and let the nature of the *pneuma*, without which the animal cannot exist, remind you especially of air (ἀέρος μὲν μάλιστα), but also of fire (πυρός) together with it.[30]

29 The influence of the Pneumatist school on Galen's use of *pneuma* should not be discounted. It is arguably more pervasive than previously thought. See the discussion in Kupreeva (2014) 172–78. See also Mirrione (2017).

30 μὴ τοίνυν μηδ' ἐν τοῖς τῶν ζῴων σώμασιν τι ζήτει, ἀλλ' ἀρκείτω σοι τουτὶ μὲν ψυχρὸν καὶ ξηρὸν καὶ πυκνὸν ἰδόντι τὸ μόριον ἀναμνησθῆναι γῆς, τουτὶ δὲ ἀραιὸν καὶ ὑγρὸν καὶ ῥυτὸν εἰς ἔννοιαν ὕδατος ἀφικέσθαι. ἀναμιμνησκέτω δέ σε καὶ ἡ πολλὴ θερμασία κατὰ τὸ σῶμα τοῦ ζῴου πυρός. ἥ τε τοῦ πνεύματος φύσις, ἧς χωρὶς οὐχ οἷόν τε συστῆναι ζῷον, , σὺν αὐτῷ δὲ καὶ ἀναμιμνησκέτω σε. *Hipp. Elem.* 5, I.454 K = 98,12–17 De Lacy (tr. De Lacy, slightly modified). Here the elements are to be identified as the bodies that manifest the qualities.

Note that it is *pneuma*'s *nature* (φύσις) to be made up of two elemental qualities: air and fire. This recalls on one level the creation of vital *pneuma* in the heart (see below), where vital heat, air and blood are the ingredients in its elaboration. But fundamentally, Galen's statement here that *pneuma* should remind one *especially* (μάλιστα) of air, carries the implication that *pneuma* can operate physiologically in a way one can understand as residing in the elemental property of air. As will be discussed below, this particular quality of air helps account for the visual process.

Galen's pneumatic elaboration begins in the lung (a singular term for Galen, as the left and right lung form an anatomic and physiologic unity). *Pneuma* is derived from 'the outside air' (ὁ ἔξωθεν ἀήρ) and, in a series of progressive steps, is finally elaborated as *psychic pneuma*.[31] In one of several comparisons Galen makes with the processing of nutriment,[32] the outer air is referred to as the τροφή of the *pneuma*, and such a process, like the elaboration of nutriment to blood, is a gradual one, as the following from *On the Function of the Parts* (*De usu partium*) attests:

> For it is reasonable (εὔλογον) that the outer air does not become the nutriment of the *pneuma* (πνεύματος γίγνεσθαι τροφήν) in the animal's body suddenly and all at once; rather, it is altered gradually (ἀλλὰ κατὰ βραχὺ μὲν ἀλλοιούμενον), just as the food is too, and over a period of time acquires the quality proper to the innate *pneuma* (τῷ συμφύτῳ πνεύματι), the principal instrument of this alteration being the flesh of the lung, just as I have shown the flesh of the liver to be responsible for changing (μεταβολῆς) the nutriment into blood.[33]

The unique physical property of the lung makes this preliminary pneumatic elaboration possible:

> And we are right to admire [Nature] also because she made the flesh of the lung soft, loose-textured and foamy in order to perform the preliminary concoction of the outer air, for so she provided suitable nutriment (τροφὴν οἰκείαν) for the *psychic pneuma*.[34]

31 For more details, see Rocca (2003) 59–66.
32 The Aristotelian antecedents (from which Galen draws) are explored in Lloyd (1996) chapter 4.
33 *UP* 7.8, III.539–40 K. = I,392 Helmreich (tr. May).
34 *UP*, 7.9, III.545 K. = I,396 Helmreich (tr. May, slightly modified). I discuss the lung as an instrument of pneumatic elaboration in detail in Rocca (2020).

The product of the alteration of air by the lung is the '*pneuma*-like' (πνευματῶδες) entity, and Galen now sets the scene for a series of remarkable physiological transformations. This *pneuma*-like material is presented to the left ventricle of the heart (ἡ ἀριστέρα κοιλία τῆς καρδίας) via the pulmonary vein (ἀρτηρία φλεβώδης: the vein-like artery). The left ventricle is a pneumatic *ergasterion*, where the *pneuma*-like material, innate heat[35] and blood combine to manufacture *vital pneuma* (ζωτικὸν πνεῦμα).[36] Following its elaboration in the heart, *vital pneuma* now has access to all parts of the body via the arteries – for Galen the heart is the source or origin (ἀρχή) of this part of the vascular system – and is able to enter the brain, where it infuses two vascular structures critical for its final elaboration into *psychic pneuma*: the *retiform plexus* (δικτυοειδὲς πλέγμα), a network of fine arteries at the base of the brain, and the *choroid plexuses* (χοριοειδῆ πλέγματα), a cluster of arteries and veins situated within the ventricles of the brain. In *On the Function of the Parts*, Galen summarises his pneumatic elaborative system as follows:

> The outer air drawn in by the rough arteries (ἐκ τῶν τραχειῶν ἀρτηριῶν, sc. trachea and bronchii) receives its first elaboration in the flesh of the lung, its second in the heart and the arteries, especially those of the retiform plexus, and then a final (τελεωτάτην) elaboration in the ventricles of the brain, which completes its transformation into *psychic pneuma*. This is not the right place to speak of the function (χρεία) of this *pneuma* or to say how it is that we who confess that we are still completely ignorant (ἀγνοεῖν ἔτι τὸ ἀκριβέστατον ὁμολογοῦντες) of the nature of the soul nevertheless dare to call this *pneuma* psychic.[37]

These vascular structures complete the transformation of *vital pneuma* into *psychic pneuma*. However, Galen also allows the ventricles to elaborate a certain amount of outside air through the nasal passages, especially if there is an interruption to the supply of *vital pneuma* via the carotid arteries.[38] The ventricles of the brain are the final repositories of *psychic pneuma*, and by virtue of the fact that the cranial nerves and spinal cord arise from the brain, *psychic pneuma* can provide sensation and voluntary motion.

35 On the vital heat in Galen, see Durling (1988).

36 Cf. Aetius 1.7.33; *SVF* 2.1027 = LS 46A, where *pneuma*, according to Stoic theory, acquires different names due to the changes of the matter through which its passes.

37 *UP* 7.8, III.541–42 K. = I,393–94 Helmreich (tr. May, modified).

38 See Rocca (2003) 224–34.

Blood in the left ventricle of the heart has been noted above as forming part of the process of pneumatic elaboration. Galen also seeks to establish a further linkage of blood with *pneuma*, as the following from *On the Function of the Parts* illustrates:

> Indeed, the notion is not impossible that the *psychic pneuma* is a sort of exhalation of useful blood (ἀναθυμίασίς τίς ἐστιν αἵματος χρηστοῦ). I have explained this as well in more detail in my other works.[39] For the present, it is enough simply to tell the reason why the arteries need to contain blood that is pure and thin, namely that such blood is intended to provide nourishment to the *psychic pneuma*.[40]

The relation of (arterial) blood to *pneuma* is an interesting one. Blood should be regarded as far more than simply a pneumatic carrier of *pneuma*, and is instead essential for its existence within the body. As the citation from *On the Elements according to Hippocrates* discussed above shows, Galen regards it as an elemental part of the structure of *pneuma*. Galen bolsters this notion by referring to the nature of the blood supplying nutriment to *psychic pneuma*. Note the shift in his qualification from it being 'not impossible' (οὐδ' ἀδύνατος) in the citation above, to being considered 'plausible' (πιθανόν), a stronger yet nevertheless qualified philosophical construction:[41]

> Now, if the *psychic pneuma* should also need the vapour arising from the blood (αἵματος ἀναθυμιάσεως) as nourishment (for this too is plausible), then animals would have this very great use for heat in due proportion. For how could the blood that is cold be resolved into vapour? On the other hand, that which is unduly hot easily disperses into vapour, only it is a dark and smoky vapour. Such a character, of course, cannot suit the *psychic pneuma*: it above all other things must be most pure and excellent (καθαρωτάτῳ τε καὶ χρηστοτάτῳ). After all, when the blood is carrying either black or yellow bile, being resolved into nasty vapours it leads in the former case to melancholy, in the latter, to phrenitis.[42]

---

39 Cf. *On the Use of Breathing* 5, IV.502 K. = 120,23–122,1 Furley-Wilkie. Here Galen states that the assertion is 'not improbable' (οὐκ ἀπεικός), and indeed seemed true to many 'excellent physicians and philosophers' (ἐλλογίμων ἰατρῶν τε καὶ φιλοσόφων).

40 *UP* 6.17, III.496 K. = I,361 Helmreich (tr. May, modified).

41 See Chiaradonna (2014), esp. 73–80.

42 *Usu Resp.* 5, IV.506–507 K. = 126,18–128,7 Furley-Wilkie (tr. Furley-Wilkie).

The humours black and yellow bile are introduced at the end of this citation as blood *pollutants*, which can lead to (nervous) disorders such as melancholy and phrenitis (as shall be discussed in Part 4 below). Galen, in *On the Causes of Symptoms* (*De Symptomatum Causis*), gives a further boost to blood's importance by coupling it to *pneuma* and the innate heat, while at the same time flagging the possibility that one or more, or a combination of them, may function as the soul's first instrument:

> Perhaps I shall have the audacity to give an opinion about the soul itself in some other work, but for what is now at hand, apart from being audacious, this is also superfluous. It seems, then, that whatever this might be, it is one of two things: either it uses the first instruments for all activities (πρώτοις ὀργάνοις εἰς ἁπάσας τὰς ἐνεργείας) by the *pneuma* or the blood, or the heat in one or both together, or it is in these themselves.[43]

Raising the question of the nature of the soul here is an excellent rhetorical device to highlight the critical interdependence of the three physiological agents that account for the function of the body: heat, blood and *pneuma*, which in turn requires the participation of the first two for its existence.

Turning now to Galen's rather vexed relationship of *psychic pneuma* to the rational soul, it is telling that he is apparently so confident in the existence of *psychic pneuma* based on his experiments with the ventricles of the brain, that he promotes it to the status of the soul's first instrument, as the following records. Here, in a remarkable passage from *On the Doctrines of Hippocrates and Plato*, Galen has already opened the ventricles of the brain in a living animal:

> From these phenomena you might suppose either of two things about the *pneuma* in the ventricles of the brain: if the soul is incorporeal, the *pneuma* there is, so to speak, its first home; or if the soul is corporeal, this very thing is the soul. But when presently, after the ventricles have been closed up, the animal regains sensation and motion, it is no longer possible to accept either alternative. It is better, then, to assume[44] that the soul dwells in the actual body of the brain, whatever its substance may be – for the inquiry has not yet reached this question – and that the soul's first instrument for all the sensations of the animal and for its voluntary motions as well is this *pneuma*; and therefore, when the *pneuma*

43 *Caus. Symp.* 2, 5, VII.191 K. (tr. Johnston, slightly modified).

44 The soul's physical location is presented here only as a supposition (ὑπολαβεῖν) for the sake of the argument.

> has escaped, and until it is collected again, it does not deprive the animal of its life, but renders it incapable of sensation and motion. Yet if the *pneuma* were itself the substance of the soul, the animal would immediately die along with the escape of the *pneuma*. Thus it is reasonable that this *pneuma* is produced at the ventricles of the brain, and that for this reason no small number of arteries and veins terminate there, forming the choroid plexuses as they are called, and that the *pneuma* is, as I said, the first instrument of the soul.[45]

Experimental procedures such as these testify to Galen's extraordinary level of proficiency and successful manipulation of a number of variables. *Psychic pneuma* is claimed to be the first instrument of the rational soul, which, as noted above, resides in the 'actual body of the brain' (ἐν αὐτῷ μὲν τῷ σώματι τοῦ ἐγκεφάλου τὴν ψυχὴν οἰκεῖν). It is necessary that this particular *pneuma* be of the best or highest quality in order to properly fulfill the noetic, sensory and motor capacities on behalf of the rational soul. This is picked up in the following from *On the Function of the Parts*, where Galen notes that not only is there a 'very large quantity' of psychic *pneuma* in the *encephalon*, but also that it receives its own special quality:

> I was right, then, when I showed (ἀπεδείκνυτο) in those commentaries that the vital *pneuma* passing up through the arteries is used as the proper material for the generation of *psychic pneuma* in the brain ... In those commentaries [*PHP*] I have given the demonstrations (ἀποδείξεις) proving that the rational soul (τὴν λογιστικὴν ψυχήν) is lodged in the brain; that this is the part with which we reason (ἡμᾶς τὸ μόριον λογίζεσθαι); that a very large quantity (πάμπολυ) of *psychic pneuma* is contained in it; that this *pneuma* acquires its own special quality (ἰδιότητα τῆς ποιότητος) from elaboration (κατεργασίας) in the brain.[46]

A more specific reference to the importance of *psychic pneuma's* quality is the following, where, in the course of discussion of the parts of the brain (*encephalon*)[47] and its convolutions, Galen introduces the notion of the perfection of the intellect, and that this depends not on the quantity but on the quality of the psychic *pneuma*:

---

45 *PHP* 7.3, V.605–609 K. = 442,36–444,15 De Lacy (tr. De Lacy, slightly modified).

46 *UP* 9.4, III.700 K. = II,12–13 Helmreich (tr. May).

47 The Greek for 'brain' is *encephalos*. The neuter, *encephalon*, is here employed purely as convention since this is the form it takes in the OED and in medical texts.

> Now since much *psychic pneuma* is contained throughout the body of the brain and not just in its ventricles, as shown in other works of mine, we ought to think that the *parencephalis*[48] too, which must be the source of the nerves for the whole body, contains a very large quantity of this *pneuma*, and that the intervening regions that connect the parts of it are its pathways. Erasistratus was correct when he stated that the *epencranis* – which is what he terms the *parencephalis* – has a more intricate structure than the *encephalon*. On the other hand, when he says that the *epencranis* itself together with the *encephalon* are more complex in man than in the other animals, since man's intelligence is greater than theirs, it seems to me that his understanding is no longer as correct; for even donkeys possess an extremely complex *encephalon*, whereas, to judge by their stupidity, it should be completely simple and uncomplicated. Hence it would be better to think that intelligence depends on the well-blending of the substance of the thinking body (τῆς οὐσίας εὐκρασίᾳ τοῦ νοοῦντος σώματος), whatever it may be, and not on intricacy of structure. Indeed, it seems to me that perfection of the intellect (τὴν ἀκρίβειαν τῆς νοήσεως) should be ascribed not to the quantity (πλήθει τοῦ πνεύματος) but rather the quality (ποιότητι) of psychic *pneuma*. Now, however, unless we restrain this discourse with a curb, so to speak, it will run off the course and lay hold on greater subjects than my proposed theme warrants. And yet to avoid altogether saying something about the substance of the soul if one is explaining the structure of the body containing it is impossible (ἀδύνατον).[49]

The significance of this passage lies in the fact that it is the only place, as far as I am aware, where Galen makes such an association between intellect and *psychic pneuma*. Linking intellection with the level of quality of *psychic pneuma* is perhaps the ultimate expression of Galen's overall insistence on the importance of the qualitative changes undergone by *pneuma* in its elaborative pathway to its ultimate transformation to *psychic pneuma*, as well as underlining its relationship to the rational soul. Also to be noted here is a reference to the dependence of the intellect itself: on the 'well-blending of the substance of the intelligent body' (τῆς οὐσίας εὐκρασίᾳ τοῦ νοοῦντος σώματος). What that particular body might be is never spelt out, but it is possible to regard it as a reference either to the rational soul or to where it resides, the brain itself.

48 The cerebellum.
49 *UP* 8.13, III.673–74 K. = I,488–89 Helmreich (tr. May, slightly modified).

If Galen offers no details as to how *psychic pneuma* facilitates intelligence, we are on slightly better ground when it comes to visual capacity, expressed in pneumatic terms. Of all the body's sensory instruments, the most important are the organs of sight; moreover, the instrument of vision has *pneuma* linked to it in an explicitly teleological way. *On the Function of the Parts* states this as follows:

> You cannot admire (θαυμάσαι) Nature as she deserves for her construction (τῇ κατασκευῇ) of these nerves if you do not know how we see. Accordingly, if you are willing to employ a good amount of your leisure in testing the demonstrations I have given in Book 13 of my *On Demonstration* and in certain other places to show that the instrument of vision (ὄψεως ὄργανον) has a luminous *pneuma* (αὐγοειδὲς πνεῦμα) always flowing to it from the brain, you will admire (θαυμάσεις) the structure of the optic nerves which have been made hollow (τὴν κατασκευὴν κοίλων) within in order to receive the *pneuma*, and which proceed up as far as the ventricle of the brain itself for the same reason. For they grow out from the place where the two anterior ventricles come to an end toward the side, and this thalamus, as it were (ἡ οἷον θαλάμη), of the ventricles was made for the sake of these nerves (δι' ἐκεῖνα τὰ νεῦρα γέγονεν). The anatomists have not recognized this marvellous work of Nature (ἔργον τοῦτο θαυμαστὸν τῆς φύσεως) since they have not followed the ventricles to their terminations, or considered for what purpose these have been formed, or seen that the upper origins of the optic nerves are attached to the ends of the ventricles.[50]

In his experiments on the ventricles in living animals, Galen notes that when pressure is applied to the anterior ventricle, the pupil of the eye ceases to react.[51] In *On the Doctrines of Hippocrates and Plato*, Galen interprets this in pneumatic terms: the flow of *psychic pneuma* from optic nerve to eye is impeded.[52] The processing of what is perceived presupposes that the body possesses discrimination and hence cognition.[53] Exactly how *psychic pneuma* mediates the

50 *UP* 16.3, IV.275–76 K. = II,384–85 Helmreich (tr. May, slightly modified).

51 On these experiments, see Rocca (2003) chapter 5.

52 *PHP* 7.4, V.614–16 K. = 450,10–452,7 De Lacy. Cf. 7.5, V.624 K. = 458,19–22 De Lacy, where the psychic (qua luminous) *pneuma* mixes with that of the vitreous humour of the eye.

53 'It is in virtue of this psychic *pneuma* that we have the ability to see. Quite generally it seems to be his view that cognition presupposes psychic *pneuma*' (Frede 2003, 120).

entire visual process is a complex problem Galen never entirely resolves,[54] although the key parts are the eye as the instrumental modality of sight, the concept of *continuity* (συνέχεια), the divine power of sunlight (a capacity used both metaphorically and literally), the fact that light and *psychic pneuma* both possess a quality of luminosity,[55] and the presence of a substantial amount of a *pneuma*-like substance (πνευματικὴ οὐσία) which flows from the ventricles to the eye.[56] Very briefly, the visual process is as follows. When the surrounding air is lit by the sun, 'it is already an instrument of vision of the same description as the *pneuma* coming from the brain; but until it is illuminated it does not turn into a sympathetic instrument (ὁμοιοπαθὲς ὄργανον) by virtue of the change effected in it by the outflow of the *pneuma*.'[57] Just as sunlight is sensitive, so too is the *pneuma* in the eye itself. The notion of sympathetic continuity is part of a seamless whole that involves brain, optic nerve and *psychic pneuma*: 'We must say, then, that this (*pneuma*) itself extends through all the brain, and that by partnership with it the optical *pneuma* becomes luminous.'[58] Is *pneuma* here to be considered an emergent property? The classic definition of emergentism, that of Hempel and Oppenheim, is as follows: 'Generally speaking, the concept of emergence has been used to characterize certain phenomena as 'novel', and this not merely in the psychological sense of being unexpected, but in the theoretical sense of being unexplainable, or unpredictable, on the basis of information concerning the spatial parts or other constituents of the systems in which the phenomena occur, and which in this context are often referred to as wholes.'[59] By this definition, vision is explicable according to the conjoined properties of the external air and the air-like nature of *psychic pneuma*. There is therefore the important fact that *psychic pneuma*, at the end of the day, is an elemental compound and as such, according to Galen's system,

54 '[I]t is not entirely clear what exactly is … the function of the psychic *pneuma* that makes it indispensable for visual perception' (Ierodiakonou 2014, 247).

55 Aristotle is correct in the notion of a quality emitted from the visual object to the eye via an alteration in the surrounding air, but errs, says Galen, in not making the air between object and eye sensitive. *PHP* 7.7, V.643 K. = 474,15–22 De Lacy. On Galen's acknowledgement of the sun's divine power, see Singer, this volume, 177–78.

56 *PHP* 7.5, V.623 K. = 458,3 De Lacy.

57 πεφωτισμένος γὰρ ὑφ' ἡλίου τοιοῦτόν ἐστιν ἤδη [τὸ] τῆς ὄψεως ὄργανον οἷον τὸ παραγιγνόμενον ἐξ ἐγκεφάλου πνεῦμα. πρὶν φωτισθῆναι δέ, κατὰ τὴν ὑπὸ <τῆς> τοῦ πνεύματος εἰς αὐτὸν ἐκβολῆς ἐναποτελουμένην ἀλλοίωσιν ὁμοιοπαθὲς ὄργανον οὐ γίγνεται. *PHP* 7.7, V.642 K. = 474,5–7 De Lacy (tr. De Lacy).

58 τοῦτο μὲν οὖν αὐτὸ δι' ὅλου λεκτέον ἡμῖν ἐκτετάσθαι τοῦ ἐγκεφάλου, τῇ δέ γε πρὸς αὐτὸ κοινωνίᾳ τὸ κατὰ τὰς ὄψεις [αὐτῶν] πνεῦμα φωτοειδὲς γίγνεσθαι. *PHP* 7.7, V.643–44 K. = 474,27–29 De Lacy (tr. De Lacy). See the summary by De Lacy (1979) 361.

59 Hempel and Oppenheim 1948 (147).

acts in a way which can at least be made capable of explanation on the basis of its constituent parts, even though that explanation may be neither as complete nor as satisfactory as one would wish.[60]

The entire visual process is a pneumatic continuum operating holistically in order to give function to the most important of the senses. It is the supposed hollowness of the optic nerve that allows Galen to think in terms of a continuum between the object of perception and the brain. However, most of the nerves of the body are not hollow, and here Galen uses the notion of a flow of qualitative change, a dynamic pulse flow initiated by *psychic pneuma* to ensure that nervous transmission is 'instantaneous.'[61] However, Galen qualifies this to the extent that it is not possible to state how far *psychic pneuma* travels through the nerves.[62] In any case, *psychic pneuma* remains the indispensable agent of initiation (and implicitly of reception, for it is a two-way process) of nervous action.

4 *Pneuma* and Affected States

Psychic pneuma for its existence depends on the elaborative steps undertaken by and within the blood vasculature and through the agency of the blood vasculature acting as its essential transport system. Any disturbance to the production of blood (and to the quality of the innate heat) will result in changes to *pneuma* at both a quantitative and a qualitative level. Further, anything causing a physical blockage to *psychic pneuma* (in either the ventricles of the brain (as an obstruction within a physical cavity) or in the nerves themselves (where, with the exception of the hollowness of the olfactory and optic nerves, it is more appropriate to speak of an obstruction to pneumatic continuity) will also have its effect on its functional capacity.

In regard to obstruction, Galen, in *On the Affected Parts* (*De Locis Affectis*), remarks that an affection (πάθος) is capable of causing damage to the *encephalon* if a humour (unspecified) physically blocks pneumatic flow:

60 Kupreeva (2014) 177 remarks, in reference to Galen's system, 'the principles of natural design and mixture are sufficient to account for a variety of properties manifest in the organic and inorganic elemental compounds throughout the cosmos ... The elements are legitimate theoretical entities, which are not postulated arbitrarily, but are expected to provide an explanation for the effects we observe in sensible compounds.'

61 'This flow is initiated by action of the brain's *pneuma* on the continuum. This was the case with vision, when the *pneuma* struck the outside air.' De Lacy (1979) 361.

62 *PHP* 7.3, V.612 K. = 448,19–24 De Lacy.

> From all of these [observations] it is reasonable (εὔλογον) that an affection (τὸ πάθος) injures the brain when a humour (τοῦ χυμοῦ) obstructs the passages of the *psychic pneuma* through its channels, since this *pneuma* resides in the ventricles of the *encephalon*. It has been demonstrated in my *On the Doctrines of Hippocrates and Plato* why this agent is called *psychic pneuma* and what is its capacity (δύναμίς). It seems to us reasonable (εὔλογον), since we follow the evidence from dissection (ἐκ τῆς ἀνατομῆς φαινομένοις ἀκολουθοῦσιν), that the soul itself resides in the substance of the brain (ἐν τῷ σώματι τοῦ ἐγκεφάλου) where the thought processes occur and where is deposited the memory of sensory impressions. The first instrument (τὸ πρῶτον ὄργανον) of the soul for all sensory and voluntary activities is the *pneuma* in the cerebral cavities, and especially in the posterior ventricles.[63]

Galen provides clinical evidence, backed by his understanding of ventricular structure and function, as to what happens when there is a physical obstruction to the ventricular system.[64] In trephaning the skull,[65] there is a chance that the operator may cause pressure (either by the instrument itself or by its pressure on the fractured bone) to be applied to the middle ventricle. As a result of this compression, the patient enters a state of torpor (κάρος). This affected condition is ascribed to a change interpreted as a diminution (καταπίπτοντος) in the tension of the psychic *pneuma* (τοῦ κατὰ τὸ ψυχικὸν πνεῦμα τόνου) in this part of the ventricular system.[66] The ascription of a tensional state to *psychic pneuma* is of course unmistakably Stoic.[67]

Health is often tenuous, due to the complex interrelated dynamics of blood and *pneuma* production and distribution, to say nothing of the continuing maintenance of a nominal level of innate heat. There is a delicate balance between humoural physiology and humoural pathology, which is sometimes

63 *Loc. Aff.* 3.9, VIII.174–75 K. (tr. Siegel, slightly modified).

64 An antecedent is found in the Hippocratic text *Sacred Disease*, where, if breath is stopped from moving in a part of the body, then that part becomes paralyzed (ἀκρατές). Blockage of the veins by phlegm (φλέγμα) results in insensibility and loss of speech. *Morb. Sacr.* 10, VI.372 L. = p. 72 Grensemann. See Temkin (1971) 53–54.

65 On trepanation and its effects on the ventricles of the brain, see Rocca (2003) 181–84.

66 *Loc. Aff.* 4.3, VIII.232–33 K. Quite why increased pressure should lead to a diminution of pneumatic tension is not made clear in this passage, unless there is associated damage to ventricular integrity, in which case the increase in pressure from bone fragment or instrument would facilitate the escape of *pneuma* and a consequent overall decrease in pneumatic tension.

67 Alexander *Mixt.* 223,25–36; *SVF* 2.441 = LS 47L. See also the discussion in Trompeter (2016).

overlooked, and which Galen expresses in *On the Natural Faculties* (*De Naturalibus Facultatibus*) as follows:

> Now in reference to the genesis of the humours, I do not know that anyone could add anything wiser than what has been said by Hippocrates, Aristotle, Praxagoras, Philotimus and many others among the Ancients. These men demonstrated (ἀποδέδεικται) that when the nutriment becomes altered in the veins by the innate heat (ὑπὸ τῆς ἐμφύτου θερμασίας), blood is produced when it (sc. the innate heat) is in due proportion (συμμετρίας), and the other humours (οἱ δ' ἄλλοι χυμοὶ) when it is not. And all the observed facts agree with this argument.[68]

Cases of affection to the brain and nerves are ascribed to changed humoural and pneumatic states. For example, the acute onset of apoplexy (ἀποπληξία) is said to be caused by the accumulation of a cold, thick and slippery humour in the more important (κυριωτέρας) of the ventricles of the brain.[69] Attacks of epilepsy (ἐπιληψία) can occur[70] when a 'heavy, atrabilious humour' (παχὺς χυμὸς ὁ μελαγχολικός), in like manner to the accumulation of phlegm (φλέγμα), is retained in the middle or posterior ventricle. The vulnerability of the brain itself is also noted when black bile overflows into its substance, as the following from *On the Affected Parts* attests:

68 *Nat. Fac.* 2.8, II.117 K. (tr. Brock, slightly modified).

69 ἡ δὲ ἀποπληξία διὰ τὴν ἐξαίφνης γένεσιν ἐνδείκνυται ψυχρὸν χυμὸν, ἢ παχὺν, ἢ γλίσχρον ἀθρόως πληροῦντα τὰς κυριωτέρας τῶν κατὰ τὸν ἐγκέφαλον κοιλιῶν). *Loc. Aff.* 3.11, VIII.200 K.

70 However, at *Loc. Aff.* 3.9, VIII.174 K., epilepsy is said to 'always' (ἀεί) be caused by humoural blockage of the channels of the ventricular system. In chapter 11 of *De locis affectis*, Galen also speaks of another form of epilepsy (ἕτερον ἐπιληψίας εἴτε εἶδος), unnamed, and one which 'rarely' (σπανίῳ) occurs, that acts in a retrograde fashion, ascending from the body to the head. Galen states that according to his teacher Pelops, this admits of one of two possibilities: as a quality transmitted (ἤτοι ποιότης ἀναδίδουσθαι) somehow through the contiguous parts of the body which had experienced a change (ἀλλοιουμένων τῶν μορίων κατὰ τὸ συνεχές); or that a *pneuma*-like substance (πνευματική οὐσία) is responsible (3.11, VIII.194–95 K.). In the latter case, it could be that this 'pneumatic substance' is either pathologic in itself or else capable of being affected by a pathological process. Galen then notes that Pelops, held that it was to be expected that a 'humour contrary to Nature' (παρὰ φύσιν χυμόν) would produce an effect similar to that seen in the bite of venomous creatures (3.11, VIII.195 K.). Galen attempts to draw an analogy from the natural world, speculating that in the case of a bite by a spider, stingray and scorpion, there too is passed a 'certain substance, either *pneuma*-like or moist' (τινα οὐσίαν ἤτοι πνευματικὴν ἢ ὑγράν, 3.11, VIII.195 K.). At 421–22 K., Galen notes that the swiftness of action and the severity of the sting of a spider or scorpion, and contact with the torpedo-fish, can be accounted for 'through the capacity of a [transmitted] quality' (κατὰ τὴν ποιότητα δυνάμει). This requires only a minute amount of the noxious substance concerned.

> I am used to calling it melancholic humour or melancholic blood (μελαγχολικὸν χυμὸν ἢ μελαγχολικὸν αἷμα), for I think it is not yet proper to call it black bile. For that humour is generated in some people in large quantity either as a result of their initial mixture or by a habit of eating foods that change into this during the digestion within the vessels. Just like the thick phlegmatic humour, this thick melancholic humour (παχὺς χυμὸς ὁ μελαγχολικός) likewise sometimes causes instances of epilepsy,[71] because it is contained in the places where the cavities of the brain, whether the middle or the posterior cavity, have their exit channels; but when it is present in excess in the very body of the brain, it causes melancholy (μελαγχολίαν ἐργάζεται), just as the other kind of humour of black bile, the one that has arisen as a result of the roasting of yellow bile, results in bestial hallucinations, both without fever and with fever, when it fills the body of the brain excessively (πλεονάζων ἐν τῷ σώματι τοῦ ἐγκεφάλου).[72]

In dizziness or vertigo (σκότωμα), which Galen states arises from the brain, most attacks are caused from rotation of the head resulting in an unequal movement both of humours and of *pneuma* within the *encephalon* (*Loc. Aff.* 3.12, VIII. 201–2 K.). This is not a pathologic change as such. However, Galen also states that the retiform plexus is the reasonable (εὔλογον) source of such afflictions. In these cases, the *psychic pneuma* produced there is referred to as atmospheric and hot (ἀτμώδους καὶ θερμοῦ πνεύματος, *Loc. Aff.* 3.12, VIII.203 K.). This thermal quality does imply an imbalance in the contents of *psychic pneuma*. Galen then remarks that it is possible that within the brain itself, what he terms an 'anomalous dyscrasia' (ἀνώμαλον δυσκρασίαν) arises, which produces this sort of *psychic pneuma*. (3.12, VIII.203 K.). This is presented as evidence of a sort that *psychic pneuma* itself is capable of being affected in the sense of existing in an abnormal state due to change in a part of the body (here the retiform plexus of arteries) charged with its final elaboration.

Syncope (συγκοπή) is defined by Galen in Book 12, chapter 5 of *Method of Medicine* (*De Methodo Medendi*) as follows:

> My predecessors have stated that syncope is an acute collapse of capacity (δυνάμεως). Since, however, the substance of the capacities controlling us lies in the *pneuma* and in the blending of the solid bodies (ἡ οὐσία τῶν

71 At *Loc. Aff.* 3.9, VIII.175 K., where epilepsy can occur in cases of a similar humoural *dyskrasia*, there described as 'thick' (πάχος) and 'slippery' (γλίσχρον).

72 *Loc. Aff.* 3.9, VIII.177–78 K. (tr. Siegel, slightly modified).

> διοικουσῶν ἡμᾶς δυνάμεων ἔν τε τῷ πνεύματι καὶ τῇ τῶν στερεῶν σωμάτων ἐστὶ κράσει), what we must do is to preserve these when they are present and restore them when they are weakened ... Therefore, it is time to add what is lacking. What we must do is preserve the substance of the *pneuma* (τὴν τοῦ πνεύματος οὐσίαν) along with the solid bodies in diseases so that, in terms of both quality and quantity, they are according to Nature (κατὰ φύσιν) as far as possible.[73]

Note here that control of the capacities (δυνάμεις) is a conjoint enterprise, requiring *pneuma* (in its substantive form) together with the blending (κρᾶσις) of the solid bodies. We are given an indication as to what happens when the substance of the *pneuma* is not preserved a little later in the same text (*MM* 12.5, X.840 K.), where Galen admits that a 'collapse of the capacity' occurs after most chronic diseases and in acute colliquative fevers. This is a result of a change in the blending of the solid bodies due to disproportionate changes made by heating, cooling, dryness or moisture. In these instances, a 'change' (ἀλλοίωσις) of the *pneuma* occurs due to the humours being in a 'bad' (κακία) state as well as a bad quality of the outside air from whatever cause. Even the 'noxious capacities or poisons' of venomous creatures may cause a change to *pneuma*.[74] This allows, at the very least, the possibility of *psychic pneuma* being affected by a humoural imbalance in some way, given that blood is an essential ingredient in the processes of pneumatic elaboration.

5 Concluding Comments

Galen's choice of *pneuma* as a psychophysical agent derives principally from Aristotelian and Stoic thought. In Galen's hands it is a holistic construct in the sense that its capacity as first instrument of the rational soul is greater than the sum of its component parts. It functions both as substantial and qualitative agent. The ventricles of the brain are the final destination for *psychic pneuma*. Through the nerves, in a chiefly qualitative continuous flow of capacity, sensation and voluntary motion are made possible. Galen informs us in no little detail of the progressive elaboration of outside air into *psychic pneuma*, but

---

73 *MM* 12.5, X.837–38 K. (tr. Johnston, modified).

74 *MM* 12.5, X.840 K. ἡ δὲ τοῦ πνεύματος ἀλλοίωσις διά τε μοχθηροὺς γίγνεται χυμοὺς καὶ τὴν τοῦ περιέχοντος ἀέρος κακίαν ἄλλοτε ἐξ ἄλλης αἰτίας εἰς τοῦτ' ἀχθέντος, ἔτι τε τὰς δηλητηρίους δυνάμεις ἢ τοὺς τῶν ἰοβόλων ζῴων ἰούς.

does not offer details of precisely how modified elemental air and blood are transformed into *pneuma*. It is telling that *pneuma* is not discussed at all in Galen's great work on elemental blending, *Mixtures*.[75] This may well be because 'Galen has no need to dwell on it, as he is not concerned in this work with the physiology of cognitive and motor processes or with the transportation of blood and nutriment in the body.'[76] Yet this does not get us any closer to an answer. We do encounter *pneuma* as a single reference in a related work to *Mixtures*, *On the Elements According to Hippocrates*, in a passage already discussed.[77] There Galen tasks us to remember first and foremost that in the 'bodies of living beings' (τοῖς τῶν ζῴων σώμασιν), there is nothing 'unmixed' (ἄμικτον).[78] This applies to the 'nature of *pneuma*' (τοῦ πνεύματος φύσις), which is of fire (a reference to the role of vital heat in pneumatic elaboration), but most particularly of air. The passage also states unequivocally that *pneuma* is essential (συστῆναι) to life. While it is clear that *psychic pneuma* is ultimately derived from the elemental components of air and fire mixed and heated in some way, its assigned psycho-physiological role is not to account for the corporeal or structural nature of the sentient organism's existence, but to allow that life form both to exist and to function as a sentient being, as an organized rational totality.

Acknowledgments

I wish to express my gratitude to Chiara Thumiger for the kind invitation to attend this conference and for her exemplary editorial work. I thank the referees for their insightful comments. This paper was funded by the Alexander von Humboldt Foundation through the offices of Professor Philip van der Eijk.

75 *Mixtures* is concerned with how the hot, the cold, the dry and the wet combine and account for 'a large part of the individual nature and peculiarity of a living being.' Singer and Van der Eijk (2019) 3.

76 Singer and Van der Eijk (2019) 14 n. 4.

77 There is of course considerable philosophical overlap between *Mixtures* and *Elements*. In the latter, Galen allows that it is possible for the elements to combine in such as way as to form a 'sentient body' (*Hipp.Elem.* 3, I.432–34 K. = 74,19–76,18 De Lacy).

78 For a discussion of this passage, see Mirrione (2017) 272–75, who notes that in the case of μίξις, 'we perceive the heterogeneous constituents of the body as distinct' (275).

Bibliography

Chiaradonna, R. 'Galen on What is Persuasive (*Pithanon*) and What Approximates Truth.' In *Philosophical Themes in Galen*, ed. P. Adamson, R. Hansberger, J. Wilberding. BICS supplement 114. London: Institute of Classical Studies (2014) 61–88.

De Lacy, P. 'Galen's Concept of Continuity.' *Greek, Roman & Byzantine Studies*, 20 (1979) 355–69.

De Lacy, P. 'The Third Part of the Soul.' In *Le Opere Psicologiche di Galeno: Atti del Terzo Colloquio Galenico Internazionale. Pavia, 1–12 Settembre 1986*, ed. P. Manuli and M. Vegetti. Naples: Bibliopolis (1988).

Durling, R. J. 'The Innate Heat in Galen.' *Medizinhistorisches Journal*, 23.3/4 (1988) 210–12.

Frede, M. 'Galen's "Theology".' In *Galien et la Philosophie*, ed. J. Barnes, J. Jouanna. Vandoevres: Fondation Hardt (2003) 73–126.

Gill, C. 'Psychophysical Holism in Stoicism and Epicureanism.' In *Common to Body and Soul: Philosophical Approaches to Explaining Living Behaviour in Greco-Roman Antiquity*, ed. R. A. H. King. Berlin: De Gruyter (2006) 209–231.

Gill, C. 'Galen and the Stoics: Mortal Enemies or Blood Brothers?' *Phronesis*, 52.1 (2007) 88–120.

Gill, C. *Naturalistic Psychology in Galen and Stoicism*. Oxford: Oxford University Press (2010).

Hahm, D. *The Origins of Stoic Cosmology*. Columbus: Ohio State University Press (1977).

Hankinson, R. J. 'Galen and the Best of All Possible Worlds.' *Classical Quarterly*, NS 39 (1989) 206–27.

Hankinson, R. J. 'Galen's Account of the Soul.' *Phronesis*, 36.2 (1991) 197–233.

Hankinson, R. J. 'Body and Soul in Galen.' In *Common to Body and Soul: Philosophical Approaches to Explaining Living Behaviour in Greco-Roman Antiquity*, ed. R. A. H. King. Berlin: De Gruyter (2006) 232–58.

Hankinson, R. J. 'Teleology and Necessity in Greek Embryology.' In *Teleology in the Ancient World: Philosophical and Medical Approaches*, ed. J. Rocca. Cambridge: Cambridge University Press (2017) 242–71.

Hempel, C. G., and P. O. Oppenheim. 'Studies in the Logic of Explanation.' *Philosophy of Science*, 15.2 (1948) 135–75.

Ierodiakonou, K. 'On Galen's Theory of Vision.' In *Philosophical Themes in Galen*, ed. P. Adamson, R. Hansberger and J. Wilberding. BICS supplement 114. London: Institute of Classical Studies (2014) 235–47.

Kupreeva, I. 'Galen's Theory of Elements.' In *Philosophical Themes in Galen*, ed. P. Adamson, R. Hansberger and J. Wilberding. BICS supplement 114. London: Institute of Classical Studies (2014) 153–96.

Leith, D. 'Elements and Uniform Parts in Early Alexandrian Medicine.' *Phronesis*, 60.4 (2015) 462–97.

Lloyd, G. E. R. *Aristotelian Explorations*. Cambridge: Cambridge University Press (1996).

Lloyd, G. E. R. 'Pneuma between Body and Soul.' *Journal of the Royal Anthropological Institute*, NS 13, supplement 1 (2007) 135–46.

Mirrione, C. *Theory and Terminology of Mixtures in Galen: The Concepts of* Krasis *and* Mixis *in Galen's Thought*. Dissertation Humboldt-Universität zu Berlin (2017).

Pinto, R. 'Air as *Nôesis* and Soul in Diogenes of Apollonia.' *Phronesis*, 63.1 (2018) 1–24.

Rist, J. 'On Greek Biology, Greek Cosmology and some Sources of Theological Pneuma.' In *The Concept of Spirit*, ed. D. W. Dockrill and R. G. Tanner. Prudentia Supplement (1985) 27–47.

Rocca, J. *Galen on the Brain: Anatomical Knowledge and Physiological Speculation in the Second century AD*. Studies in Ancient Medicine 26. Leiden: Brill (2003).

Rocca, J. 'From Doubt to Certainty: Aspects of the Conceptualisation and Interpretation of Galen's Natural Pneuma.' In *Blood, Sweat and Tears: The Changing Concepts of Physiology from Antiquity into Early Modern Europe*, ed. M. Horstmanshoff, H. King and C. Zittel. Leiden: Brill (2012) 629–59.

Rocca, J. 'One Part of a Teleological Whole: Galen's Account of the Lung as an Instrument of Pneumatic Elaboration.' In *The Concept of Pneuma after Aristotle*, ed. S. Coughlin, D. Leith and O. Lewis. Berlin Studies of the Ancient World. Berlin: Edition Topoi (2020) 281–309.

Schiefsky, M. J. 'Galen and the Tripartite Soul.' In *Plato and the Divided Self*, ed. R. Barney, T. Brennan and C. Brittain. Cambridge: Cambridge University Press (2012) 331–49.

Scolnicov, S. 'Atemporal Teleology in Plato.' In *Teleology in the Ancient World: Philosophical and Medical Approaches*, ed. J. Rocca. Cambridge: Cambridge University Press (2017) 45–57.

Sharples, R. W. 'Common to Body and Soul: Peripatetic Approaches After Aristotle.' In *Common to Body and Soul: Philosophical Approaches to Explaining Living Behaviour in Greco-Roman Antiquity*, ed. R. A. H. King. Berlin: De Gruyter (2006) 165–86.

Singer, P. N. 'Galen on Pneuma: between Metaphysical Speculation and Anatomical Theory.' In *The Concept of Pneuma after Aristotle*, ed. S. Coughlin, D. Leith and O. Lewis. Berlin Studies of the Ancient World. Berlin: Edition Topoi (2020) 235–80.

Temkin, O. *The Falling Sickness: A History of Epilepsy from the Greeks to the Beginnings of Modern Neurology*. 2nd edition. Baltimore: Johns Hopkins (1971).

Trompeter, J. 'Die Gespannte Seele: *Tonos* bei Galen.' *Phronesis*, 61.1 (2016) 82–109.

van der Eijk, P. J. 'Galen on the Nature of Human Beings.' In *Philosophical Themes in Galen*, ed. P. Adamson, R. Hansberger and J. Wilberding. BICS supplement 114. London: Institute of Classical Studies (2014) 89–134.

von Staden, H. *Herophilus. The Art of Medicine in Early Alexandria.* Cambridge: Cambridge University Press (1989).

von Staden, H. 'Body, Soul, and Nerves: Epicurus, Herophilus, Erasistratus, the Stoics, and Galen.' In *Psyche and Soma: Physicians and Metaphysicians on the Mind-Body Problem from Antiquity to the Enlightenment*, ed. J. P. Wright and P. Potter, Oxford: Oxford University Press (2000) 79–116.

Primary Texts: Editions and Translations Used

Aristotle, *Generation of Animals* (*GA*). Trans. A. L. Peck. LCL 366. Cambridge MA: Harvard University Press (1942).

[Aristotle] *On Breath* (*De Spiritu*) Ed. and trans. A. Roselli. Pisa: ETS Editrice (1992).

Erasistratus. *Erasistrati Fragmenta: Collegit et Digessit.* Ed. and trans. I. Garofalo. Biblioteca di Studi Antichi, Pisa: Giardini Editori (1988).

Galen, *Method of Medicine* (*MM*). Books 5–9. Ed. and trans. I. Johnston and G. H. R. Horsley. LCL 517. Cambridge MA: Harvard University Press (2011).

Galen, *On Semen* (*Sem.*). Ed. and trans. P. De Lacy. CMG V 3,1. Berlin: Akademie Verlag (1992).

Galen, *On the Affected Parts* (*Loc. Aff.*). Trans. R. E. Siegel. Basel: S. Karger (1976).

Galen, *On the Causes of Symptoms* (*Caus. Symp.*). Trans. I. Johnson. *Galen: On Diseases and Symptoms.* Cambridge: Cambridge University Press (2011).

Galen, *On the Doctrines of Hippocrates and Plato* (*PHP*). Ed. trans. P. De Lacy. CMG V 4,1,2. Berlin: Akademie Verlag (1978, 1980, 1984).

Galen, *On the Elements According to Hippocrates* (*Hipp. Elem.*). Ed. and trans. P. De Lacy. CMG V 1,2. Berlin: Akademie Verlag (1996).

Galen, *On the Natural Faculties* (*Nat. Fac.*). Trans. A. J. Brock. LCL 71. Cambridge MA: Harvard University Press (1916/1979).

Galen, *On the Use of Breathing* (*Ut. Resp.*). In *Galen: On Respiration and the Arteries*. Ed. and trans. D. J. Furley and J. S. Wilkie. Princeton: Princeton University Press (1984) 71–133, 249–57.

Galen, *On the Usefulness of the Parts of the Body* (*UP*). Trans. M. T. May. Ithaca: Cornell University Press (1968).

Galen, *The Art of Medicine* (*Ars Med.*). Ed. and trans. I. Johnston. LCL 523. Cambridge MA: Harvard University Press (2016).

Galen, *Works on Human Nature. Volume I. Mixtures* (*De Temperamentis*). Ed. and trans. P. N. Singer and P. J. van der Eijk, with the assistance of P. Tassinari. Cambridge Galen Translations. Cambridge: Cambridge University Press (2019).

The Hellenistic Philosophers, *The Hellenistic Philosophers*. Volume 1. Translations of the Principal Sources with Philosophical Commentary. Volume 2. Greek and Latin Texts with Notes and Bibliography. Ed. and trans. A. A. Long and D. N. Sedley. Cambridge: Cambridge University Press (1987) = LS.

Hippocratic Corpus, *Die Hippokratische Schrift 'Über Die Heilige Krankheit.'* Ed. H. Grensemann. Berlin: De Gruyter (1968).

Hippocratic Corpus, Hippocrates. Volume II. *Breaths*. Trans. W. H. S. Jones. LCL 148. Cambridge MA: Harvard University Press (1923/1981).

Hippocratic Corpus, Hippocrates. Volume X. *Nature of the Child*. LCL 520. Cambridge MA: Harvard University Press (2012).

The Texts of Early Greek Philosophy (*TEGP*). *The Complete Fragments and Selected Testimonies of the Major Presocratics*. Parts I and II. Ed. and trans. D. W. Graham. Cambridge: Cambridge University Press (2010).

PART 3

Medical Holism beyond the Graeco-Roman World

CHAPTER 12

Humoralism in Āyurvedic Medicine

Francis Zimmermann

Abstract

Sanskrit medical collections offer two alternative approaches to health and disease, which represent two different versions of humoralism in Āyurvedic medicine. A few dissident scholars, who are comparable to the ones denounced by Hippocrates in *On Ancient Medicine*, followed a top-down approach to the patient's body described as an undifferentiated aggregate whose health could only be controlled by acting on its humoral condition. This holistic postulate was best suited for prescribing rejuvenative medications comprised of nourishing and well-balanced foods and drugs to upgrade mental abilities, to sharpen the sensory faculties, to enhance sexual potency, and to maximise life chances. On the other hand, the more authoritative scholars, advocating a bottom-up approach to disease in which clinical investigations came to enhance the holistic concept of disease, started from the observed dispositions of the patient's body to track the distribution of different organic fluids to specific channels, to assess the humoral condition in the different affected parts, and to devise suitable countermeasures. This second version of humoralism, represented by the differentiated integration of channels in the affected parts, was best suited for prescriptions following the principle of opposite treatment. These two modalities of humoralism have been equally constitutive of the Āyurvedic method of treatment.

The following statement opens the Book on Therapeutics (*Cikitsāsthāna*) in the *Carakasaṃhitā* (*Caraka's Collection*): 'Medication is of two kinds, one which promotes vitality in the healthy, and one which dispels diseases in the ailing.' The distinction thus made between two different concepts of therapeutic action in the classical doctrine of Indian medicine is the subject of this chapter. Āyurveda, the name of this medical doctrine, precisely means 'the knowledge for [preserving and prolonging] the lifespan.' The former kind of Āyurvedic medication aims to promote vitality and prolong the lifespan, and the latter aims to preserve the lifespan by dispelling diseases. The rationale is that health and disease are fully determined by the three humours pervading both the world as a whole and the human body which is an epitome of the world. I shall restrict my definition of holism in Indian medicine to the features

 | DOI:10.1163/9789004443143_014

just mentioned: the human body is a microcosm whose physiology is integrally determined by the interplay between the three humours. I shall compare two modalities of the theory of humours and of the nomenclature of bodily constituents, which represent two slightly different forms of holism in Āyurvedic medicine, and I shall underpin the analysis with a few word-by-word translations from Caraka.

The classical doctrine of Āyurveda was laid down in three medical treatises. The oldest one is the *Carakasaṃhitā*, 'Caraka's Collection.' Its author named Caraka cannot have lived much earlier than about 100 BCE nor later than about 200 CE.[1] Most scholars consider that the second one, the *Suśrutasaṃhitā*, 'Suśruta's Collection', was composed slightly later, while the latest of the three core texts, Vāgbhaṭa's *Aṣṭāṅgahṛdayasaṃhitā*, 'The Heart of Medicine', is dated to the seventh century.[2] Cakrapāṇidatta's commentary on Caraka, which is dated to the eleventh century, will be cited at length, in spite of the gap of a millennium between the ancient teacher and his much later disciple. My justification for doing so is that, from the middle of the nineteenth century onwards, authoritative printed editions of the source text have always included Cakrapāṇidatta's commentary,[3] because it alone illuminates a great number of key concepts. Examples will be given of the aphoristic ancient text being explicated by the Medieval commentator.

Sanskrit medical collections offer two alternative approaches to human bodily experiences of well-being and illness, physiological diseases and mental disorders. These are two modalities of humoralism and two complementary methods of treatment. On the one hand, rejuvenative prescriptions addressing healthy patients are comprised of well-balanced and nourishing medications, be they diet foods or regular drugs, meant to upgrade their mental abilities, to sharpen their sensory faculties, to enhance their sexual potency, and to maximise their life chances. On the other hand, specific medicines addressing complaints and disorders, which are nothing else than pharmaceuticals in the modern sense of the word, are prescribed on the basis of clinical investigations to identify material substances and environmental conditions fostering disease outbreaks in particular organs and affected parts of the body. These outbreaks are supposed to result from the humours imbalance, and drugs are selected to make up for this imbalance by following the principle of opposite

1 Meulenbeld (1999) 1A 114.

2 Less well known, Vāgbhaṭa's *Aṣṭāṅgasaṅgraha*, quoted below, was composed broadly at the same time.

3 Meulenbeld (1999) 1B 3.

treatment. Prescriptions which meet healthy people's needs are based on the bookish knowledge of the human body constituents, and they do not require any direct inspection of the individual patient's condition. On the contrary, to prescribe pharmaceuticals directed towards specific medical problems, Āyurvedic practitioners should assess the patient's condition and draw on the empirical knowledge of herbs, minerals and compounded formulas. Being traditionally well-trained pharmacists, they will carefully select and process the appropriate herbs and minerals. The former approach based on the humoral theory and the latter based on pharmaceuticals do not exclude each other. They offer two possible alternatives corresponding to different moments and situations in the physician's action.

1 Humours (*doṣa*) and Diseases (*vyādhi*)

Medical discussions start from lived experiences of health and diseases, whether physiological or mental, as diffuse and dynamic processes, all physicians having in mind an image of the circulation and pervasive distribution of vital fluids through the channels, the aggregate of which constitute the individual body. This humoral and holistic conception of health and diseases is based on the dynamics and interactions of three fundamental imaginary fluids named *dhātu*, 'constituents', or *doṣa*, 'pathogenic forces', which pervade the whole body. By convention called the three humours, they are explicitly disjointed from the identification of specific organs or affected parts. In practice, however, the humoral approach to disease is compounded with the identification of specific organs or affected parts which will be the localised targets of medications.

As a first approximation, humoralism in the classical doctrine of Indian medicine includes the following theses. (1) Mental and physical processes are indissolubly linked, and the human body is an essentially mindful body. (2) Food is the source of all constituents of the living body. Food digestion yields the three humours – wind, bile and phlegm – on the one hand, and the seven organic tissues – chyle, blood, flesh, fat, bone, marrow and semen – on the other hand. (3) Organic tissues are transformed into one another through a series of internal cooking processes, and the fluid ones outweigh the solid ones in the overall framework of metabolisms. (4) Humours and tissues are ubiquitous and circulate through the network of innumerable channels pervading the body. One small note is needed on the first of the seven organic tissues, named *rasa*. Sanskrit *rasa* is a polysemic word, as we shall see later. Here it designates the organic fluid named 'chyle' in sixteenth century European medical texts. This is the fluid separated from food during the first internal cooking process, which in turn will be transformed into blood.

The exact nature of humours, tissues and channels will be explained below, but a fundamental conceptual polarity determines the consistency of the entire medical system, namely, that of 'humours' (*doṣa*) as invisible pathogenic forces which are identified by inference, and 'diseases' (*vyādi*) as visible conditions which are described after the patient's complaints and observation. A choice to be made by the medical practitioner between two methods of treatment is encapsulated in this conceptual polarity which opens Caraka's exposition of the fundamentals of therapeutics:[4]

> Medication is of two kinds (*bheṣajaṃ dvividhaṃ ca tat*): that which promotes vitality (*ūrjaskara*) in the healthy (*svastha*), and that which dispels diseases (*roganud*) in the ailing (*ārta*) ... That which promotes vitality in the healthy is mostly (*prāyas*) included in [the categories of] either virilifics (*vṛṣya*)[5] or rejuvenatives (*rasāyana*), while the second type is mostly (*prāyeṇa*) meant to pacify (*praśama*) diseases (*roga*). The word 'mostly' (*prāyas, prāyeṇa*) denotes the diversity (*viśeṣārtha*) [of uses] because each of the two types of medications produces the two types of effects (*ubhayārthakṛt*).

In drawing the same distinction Suśruta omitted medicines and focussed on patients:[6] 'Āyurveda has two objectives (*prayojana*): freeing from their disease those affected by a disease (*vyādyupasṛṣṭānāṃ vyādhiparimokṣaḥ*), and the preservation of the healthy (*svasthasya rakṣaṇaṃ ca*).' Centred on the patient, Suśruta's phrasing ignores the primary fact that medicines are prescribed. A better interpretation of Caraka's initial statement centred on the prescription should delineate two categories of medicines, those which address the whole person, directly aiming for humoral balance, and those targeted towards specific disorders, which are countermeasures applied to localised body tissues and organs, according to the principle of opposite treatment. In practice, from Caraka down to modern times, humoral medicines based on a global approach to the patient's humoral constitution, and medicines targeted at a specific

4 Caraka, *Cikitsāsthāna* 1, 4; cf. Meulenbeld (1999) 1A 51. The same distinction is repeated verbatim in the *Aṣṭāṅgasaṃgraha, Sūtrasthāna* 12, 5–9 ref. Meulenbeld (1999) 1A 492. All translations are mine. But two other translations listed in the bibliography, one by Ram Karan Sharma and Bhagwan Dash and the other by Priya Vrat Sharma, will be found helpful.

5 Substances which promote virility, sexual performance and male fertility.

6 Suśruta, *Sūtrasthāna* 1, 14.

locus affectus, have coexisted, and they offer two alternative modalities of therapeutic action, complementary to one another.

As expressly stated in the text, quite a few medications which represent a significant minority in each of the two groups, be they basically humoral and secondarily specific, or vice versa, have recourse to one and the same drug having therapeutic indications both to promote vitality and to cure specific diseases. Medicinal substances share this versatility with food substances. They are wholesome or poisonous depending on the situation and conditions of their absorption. Drugs cannot be dissociated from foods in the practice of Āyurvedic medicine. Until recently decoctions and a few other compounded formulas prescribed by the doctor were cooked at home in the kitchen, and conversely, dishes like fermented rice porridge, prepared by the mistress of the house and medicated with garden herbs, were used as family self-medications.[7] Foods and drugs are listed together in the medical texts under the same Sanskrit name *dravya*, 'substances.' They may switch roles and, furthermore, they may either harm or benefit consumers and patients. According to Caraka:[8]

> Substances are of three kinds (*trividhaṃ dravyam*): those which pacify the humours (*doṣapraśamana*), those which corrupt the body constituents (*dhātupradūṣaṇa*), and those which are meant for the maintenance of health (*svasthavṛttau matam*).

The first and third categories present no special difficulty; the first contains medicines and the third includes virilifics and rejuvenatives. The position of *dhātupradūṣaṇa* substances, however, is ambiguous because, besides unhealthy foods, this category may include medicines prescribed as countermeasures to abate every kind of disproportion in the patient's physiology. Thus, in the perspective of therapeutics, *doṣapraśamana* drugs and *dhātupradūṣaṇa* drugs represent two modalities of medication depending on whether the primary objective is to pacify the humours or to devise appropriate countermeasures against the pathological dispositions observed in specific tissues, organs and affected parts of the patient's body. Let me substantiate this analysis which turns on the two facets of the humours, one negative and the other positive. The issue of terminological conventions regarding polysemic words like *doṣa*, *dhātu*, *rasa* and *dravya* will be addressed in greater detail in the third part of

7 The traditional lifestyle in which drugs were processed at home collapsed in the 1980s, due to the rise of pharmaceutical industries.

8 Caraka, *Sūtrasthāna* 1, 67.

this chapter. But for now, suffice it to say that in the above quotation, *doṣa* and *dhātu* designate the humours with opposite connotations.

The three humours of classical Indian medicine, wind, bile and phlegm, when they are in balance in a healthy person, are subsumed under the category of *tridhātu*, 'the three body constituents.' Wind, in short, is a versatile fluid whose essential function is to creep into the finest grooves and gaps, carrying juices and saps, and to drop them off in relevant affected parts of the body. When the humours are corrupted in the physiology of a sick person, they constitute the category of *tridoṣa*, 'the three pathogenic forces.' Depending on the context we must decide whether the humours are *doṣa*, a word which connotes the idea of corruption, or *dhātu*, a word which connotes the idea of constitution. Figures of speech add value to the foregoing quotation. There is a play on words between the verbal form *pradūṣaṇa* and the noun *doṣa*, both from DŪṢ- 'to corrupt', and clearly, *doṣa* (corrupted and corrupting constituents) are to *dhātu* (healthy constituents) what *pradūṣaṇa* (corrupters) are to *praśamana* (pacifiers) – forming a chiasmus, a figure in which concepts are repeated in reverse order. The meaning of this figure of speech is that, following the principle of opposite treatment, you should counteract pathogenic forces with pacifiers, and rebalance the body constituents with countermeasures using corrupters. The essential point is that the three humours, which constitute a self-contained category, are also subsumed under the larger category of bodily constituents which includes both the humours and the tissue elements. Cakrapāṇidatta in his commentary makes explicit first the fact that food and drug substances belonging to the category of 'corrupters of the body constituents' (*dhātupradūṣaṇa*) will attack both humours and tissues, and then the fact that a given substance like *āmalaka*, the celebrated *emblic myrobalan*,[9] in different situations may act either as a panacea, pacifying the three humours, or as a corrupter of humour bile due to its sourness:[10]

> In the foregoing verse, substances (*dravya*) have been divided into three groups according to the kind of power (*prabhāvabhedena*) specific to a given kind of substance (*dravyabhedena*) ... The word *doṣa* here also denotes the tissue dhātus [the seven bodily tissues], chyle, etc. (*rasādayaḥ*), when they are corrupted (*dūṣṭā*). Thus a given substance, like the emblic myrobalan fruit (*āmalaka*) ... on account of its specific power

9 The fruits of Phyllanthus emblica. Extensively used as condiments in South Asian cuisine and highly valued for their invigorating properties, these small plums are pivot ingredients in traditional formulas.

10 Cakrapāṇidatta ad Caraka, *Sūtrasthāna* 1, 67.

(*mahiman*), acts as a pacifier (*śamaka*) of the three humours (*doṣāṇām*) or (*vā*) of the seven tissue dhātus,[11] chyle, etc. (*rasādīnāṃ dhātūnām*), when they are corrupted (*dūṣṭāṇām*). Thus, *āmalaka*, due to its propitiousness (*śivatvāt*), pacifies the three doṣas (*tridoṣahara*). Though (*yadyapi*) Suśruta (*Sūtrasthāna* 46, 144) tries to justify the three-humour pacifying effect (*tridoṣaharatva*) of *āmalaka* on the basis of its perceptible qualities (*guṇa*), saying that 'it pacifies wind due to sourness, bile due sweetness and coldness, and phlegm due to roughness and astringency', however (*tathā'pi*), this panacea effect should better be understood as an outcome of the power (*prabhāva*) specific to *āmalaka*. If it were not for this specific power, its sourness would have vitiated bile.

The disagreement here between Suśruta, who invoked the perceptible qualities of sourness, sweetness and the like, and Cakrapāṇidatta, who favours the concept of *prabhāva*, an invisible power inscribed in the very substance of *āmalaka*, is most relevant to our discussion in this chapter. *Prabhāva* is a holistic concept. It defines the healing power inscribed in the very substance of a given drug as an overall effect, without entering into the details of the drug humoral configuration. When prescribing this drug on the basis of its specific power, physicians will take for granted the complex interplay of perceptible qualities which counterbalance one another to produce a global effect, and they will decide, for example, that in the particular case at hand the risk of *āmalaka*'s sourness being harmful to the patient is negligible. Perceptible qualities are secondary to the material substance itself.

The disagreement between Suśruta and Cakrapāṇidatta should be interpreted from the angle of therapeutics and of practical decisions on the treatment of a given patient. It seems to me that we have here a clear illustration of what I would like to call the two modalities of humoralism in classical Indian medicine. Emblic myrobalans are only one among many substances to which traditional knowledge has ascribed a *prabhāva*, a special healing power on the basis of which they are prescribed when physicians adopt the *doṣapraśamana* modality of treatment, while in other circumstances physicians will avail themselves of an elaborate knowledge of *materia medica* and pharmacology, take into account the minute details of perceptible qualities in the drug and on the patient's body, and use the selected drug as a *dhātupradūṣaṇa*, which amounts to nothing else than applying the principle of opposite treatment. Unhealthy

11 The common practice in Sanskrit studies is to italicise nouns like *dhātu*, *doṣa* and *bhāva* when cited without any suffix, and to keep in standard roman the anglicized plural forms dhātus, doṣas and bhāvas.

foods, as Lord Ātreya will explain later to his pupil Agniveśa,[12] are 'substances (*dravyāṇi*) the nature (*bhūta*) of which is opposite (*pratyanīka*) to the body constituents (*dehadhātupratyanīkabhūtāni*).' Cakrapāṇidatta's commentary elucidates the meaning of this compound phrase:[13] These are substances 'in which their own character (*svarūpa*) is opposite (*pratyanīkasvarūpāṇi*) to the *dehadhātu* of the patient or consumer, namely the bodily tissues, chyle, etc. (*rasādīnāṃ*) and the humours, wind, etc. (*vatādīnāṃ*) which form his *prakṛti* or constitution (*prakṛtisthānām*).' Therefore, in compliance with the principle of opposite treatment, a given substance harmful to such and such body constituents may be used as a medicine against disorders of these constituents in the constitution of a given patient.

In short, these citations and comments have brought to light a dialectic established between humours and diseases. Physicians in devising appropriate treatments alternately make use of the globalising concept of humours, which draw benefits from the prescription of a panacea or of a rejuvenative medication when they are in balance, and of the opposite concept of diseases calling for specific countermeasures.

I would like to extend the analysis of this dialectic and to study how particular dispositions experienced by the patient and retrieved from clinical observation are grafted onto the whole human body structure. The two key concepts are the concept of 'channels' (*srotas*) through the network of which humours and other vital fluids circulate and pervade the patient's whole person, and the concept of 'dispositions' (*bhāva*). In each and every affected part of the patient's body liable to be identified and fleshed out, the clinical evidence collected by the physician points to observable pathogenic dispositions produced locally by some harmful organic fluids brought there through an ubiquitous invisible channel network forming the body at large. The concept of Āyurvedic dispositions, which can partly compare with the concept of *diathesis* in Graeco-Roman medicine,[14] will be described in the next part of this chapter.

---

12 Caraka, *Sūtrasthāna* 26, 81.

13 Cakrapāṇidatta ad Caraka, *Sūtrasthāna* 26, 81.

14 One might like to draw a clear parallel between *bhāva*, explained below, and *diathesis* in Galen's *De Methodo Medendi*, I, 2 passim, which I read in the light of Jacques Boulogne's French translation for the following quotations: 'Any physical condition, whatever it is, is fully contained in a given disposition (*diathesis*)' *MM* I, 2, 3 (X.87 K. = 108 Boulogne), and 'One may call *disease* a damage caused to the body activity, or even the disposition (*diathesis*) which creates the damage' *MM* I, 2, 6 (X.116 K. = 129 Boulogne). This definition applies to *bhāva*.

2 From Transient to Structuring Dispositions (*bhāva*)

A number of drugs, as we have seen, possess a characteristic healing power called *prabhāva*. This word in plain language means 'power', but in medical language a more accurate acception of *prabhāva* is 'predisposition.' The concept of *prabhāva* is akin to the concept of *bhāva*, 'disposition', which is applied to the empirical description of psychological, emotional and physical dispositions. Dispositions and predispositions are key concepts in Āyurveda. The prominent use of the word *bhāva* in the description of the human body cannot be overemphasized. Diseases are the result of 'unfortunate dispositions' (*asukhabhāva*), which phrase designates potential diseases and diatheses leading to various sorts of pathological processes clinically observed. I am speaking of processes because bhāvas are transient phenomena in the sensitive experience as opposed to immutable realities like the soul. The following dialogue opens the Book on Things Relative to the Body (*Śārīrasthāna*) in Caraka's Collection.[15] Agniveśa (the student) asks: 'If the soul is omnipotent, why are we so violently affected by unfortunate dispositions (*asukhaiḥ kasmād bhāvair*)?' Lord Ātreya (the teacher) answers on this particular point fifty verses later:[16] It is because, 'from our disposition (*bhāvāt*) [in the empirical world] or from any [empirical] disposition whatsoever (*na kutaścana bhāvāt*)', we cannot possibly perceive the transcendent soul in us; we are depending on the sensory faculties which perceive only transient dispositions affecting us.

Bhāvas are empirical phenomena and, in the body, *bhāva* denotes emotional states and diatheses that are unstable and constantly changing. Perceptible dispositions are innumerable and cannot be exhaustively taken into account in a clinical examination. The physician must restrict the analysis to the most important ones, a set of dispositions that tend to stabilise and have a structuring effect on the body organs. Now the stability of structuring dispositions is based on material elements found in the environment and shared by the patient's body, following the principle that the body is the world in miniature. Caraka's description of the body as a microcosm, cited at length below, starts from a philosophical statement which reads: 'Man is an epitome of the world.' The Sanskrit word for *man* is *puruṣa*. In medical texts, the word *puruṣa* denotes either 'the patient' or 'the human body.' Most of the time in these pages I am rendering *puruṣa* as 'the human body'; but as an exception, the right translation is 'man' in the following description of the emergence of structuring

15 Caraka, *Śārīrasthāna* 1, 7.

16 Caraka, *Śārīrasthāna* 1, 60–62. Zimmermann (1995) 94, 159.

dispositions in the *puruṣa* who is here defined as comprising the five natural elements – earth, water, fire, air, and ether – plus the soul.[17]

> Lord Punarvasu Ātreya said: 'Man is an epitome of the world (*puruṣo'yaṃ lokasaṃhitaḥ*). For, all the types of dispositions endowed with corporeality (*mūrtimanto bhāvaviśeṣāḥ*)[18] which exist in the world (*loke*) also exist in man (*puruṣe*), and vice versa.' To Lord Ātreya who was making this statement (*vādin*), Agniveśa replied: 'We cannot go deep (*na … avagāhāmahe*) into the meaning of a statement (*vākhyārtham*) expressed (*uktaṃ*) in a sentence (*vākhyena*) of such [a small] extent (*etāvatā*). We want to hear (*śuśrūṣamahe*) a more detailed (*bhūyastaram*) [formulation] than this one (*atas*) which must be explained further (*anuvyākhyāyamāna*) by your enlightened lordship (*bhagavatā buddhyā*).' Lord Ātreya replied: 'Just as innumerable (*aparisaṃkhyeyāḥ*) are the various constituents (*avayavaviśeṣāḥ*) of the world (*loka*), so the various constituents of man are innumerable. Among them (*teṣāṃ*), without detail (*yathāsthūlam*), we want to name (*udāhariṣyāmaḥ*) a few (*katicid*) dispositions (*bhāvān*), taking into account (*abhipretya*) those which are common (*sāmānya*) to the world and man. With the mind concentrated on this particular object (*ekamanā*), Agniveśa, listen (*nibodha*) to them (*tān*); they will be accurately (*samyak*) described (*upavarṇyamānān*). Six dhātus (*ṣaḍdhātavaḥ*) aggregated together (*samuditāḥ*) take the name of 'man' (*puruṣa*). These are: earth (*pṛthivī*), water (*āpas*), fire (*tejas*), air (*vāyu*), ether (*ākāśa*), and the unmanifested brahman (*brahma cāvyaktam*). These very six dhātus aggregated together take the name of 'man' (*puruṣa*). Of this man (*tasya puruṣasya*), earth constitutes the corporeality (*pṛthivī mūrtiḥ*), water the moisture (*āpaḥ kledaḥ*), fire the heat (*tejo' bhisantāpaḥ*), air the breath (*vāyuḥ prāṇaḥ*), ether the cavities (*viyat suṣirāni*), and the brahman the inner soul (*brahma antarātmā*). Similar to the magnificence of the brahman (*brāhmī vibhūti*) in the world (*loke*) is the magnificence of the inner soul (*āntarātmikī vibhūti*) in man (*puruṣe*).

17 Caraka, *Śārīrasthāna* 5, 3–5. However inconvenient it may be, a word-by-word translation with the original Sanskrit phrasing in parentheses is required for the text's grammatical features to make full sense.

18 In all authoritative printed editions, the word *mūrtimant*, 'endowed with corporeality', is placed in parentheses, because it is a modern interpolation added by the nineteenth-century commentator Gaṅgādhara. All scholars agree with him on the exact meaning of Caraka's phrase, which is explained below.

The central contention is that earth (*pṛthivī*) in its material substance is what gives 'corporeality' (*mūrti*) to the patient. A limited number of dispositions 'endowed with corporeality' (*mūrtimant*) exert a structuring effect on both the living body and the world of experience, and for the sake of brevity I shall henceforth render *mūrtimanto bhāvāḥ* as 'structuring dispositions.' Empirical phenomena in the world correspond item by item to the body physiological dispositions. Both the former and the latter are made up of five natural elements plus a transcendent one. The patient's body is a mindful body since it includes the soul (*ātman*) which provides the whole with thought. 'When in death the soul leaves the body, according to Caraka,[19] the body (*śarīra*) remains like an empty house deprived of thought (*śūnyāgāram acetanam*) and it is said to return to the earth and other natural elements.' Cakrapāṇidatta's gloss reads:[20] 'The body made of six constituents (*ṣaḍdhātukaṃ śarīram*), after the sixth one, namely the soul, is gone (*ṣaṣṭhe ātmani gate*), is a body made of only five natural elements (*pañcabhūtamātrakaṃ śarīram*).' Philipp Maas, who will be cited below, has convincingly shown that the treatment of the bodily constituents in Caraka's Collection was quite elusive and that a number of different body concepts which were current at the time of its composition had been integrated into a single comprehensive *dhātu* concept. The three closed lists of the three humours (*tridhātu*), the seven tissues (*saptadhātu*) and the six cosmic constituents (*ṣaḍdhātu*) are equally authoritative. Material elements are at the forefront of clinical investigations. Structuring dispositions (*mūrtimanto bhāvāḥ*), in the physiological constitution of a given patient living on a given soil, derive their stability and their structuring power from the very substance of the soil, to be taken here not as a cosmic constituent but as a material element.

In medical practice, when the physician tries to identify and locate them, the initial distinction made in the classical texts between transient and structuring dispositions must be elaborated further in order to sort out what is visible in the patient's body, under the clinical gaze, from the invisible operation of internal organs that can only be inferred. It takes the form of a distinction between visible dispositions and invisible channels. Ātreya explains that each type of channel in the human body carries a specific structuring disposition:[21]

---

19 Caraka, *Śārīrasthāna* 1, 74.

20 Cakrapāṇidatta ad Caraka, *Śārīrasthāna* 1, 74 (I am adopting the variant *mātraka*, 'only five').

21 Caraka, *Vimānasthāna* 5, 3–4.

> In the human body (*puruṣe*), there are as many (*tāvanta eva*) types (*prakāraviśeṣāḥ*) of channels (*srotasāṃ*) as types of structuring dispositions (*mūrtimanto bhāvaviśeṣāḥ*). For, in the human body, without the channels (*antareṇa srotāṃsi*), either no disposition (*bhāva*) arises, or the body goes to decay. Now (*khalu*), channels, taken in the sense (*arthena*) of running paths (*ayana*), are the conveyors (*abhivāhīni*) of the dhātus undergoing (*āpadyamānānāṃ*) transformation (*pariṇāmam*). However (*api ca*), some scholars (*eke*) hold the view (*icchanti*) that the human body is just (*eva*) an aggregate (*samudayaṃ*) of channels, because of their pervasiveness (*sarvagatatvāt*) and because of the diffusiveness (*sarvasaratvāt*) of [that which they carry] which aggravates or pacifies the humours (*doṣaprakopaṇapraśamanānām*). But it is not so, because that which the channels are made of (*yasya srotāṃsi*), that which they carry, that which they nourish, and that where they are located (*yatra cāvasthitāni*), all that is different from the channels themselves (*sarvaṃ tad anyat tebhyaḥ*).

Stable dispositions inscribed in the body structure are as many customary dispositions carried by specific channels to specific organs and affected parts. Ātreya's position is that, although there are innumerable channels, the types of channels are limited in number and they correspond item by item to the types of dispositions clinically observed. Channels will convey to specific locations in the body the tissues (here named *dhātu*) which undergo a series of internal processes of cooking or coctions transforming chyle into blood, flesh, fat, bone, marrow, and semen; this metabolism here is named *pariṇāma*. At some point in their transformation, tissues may get vitiated and become pathogenic, in which case the corresponding type of channels will convey them to specific locations in the body where the corresponding structuring dispositions may be observed by the physician. The resulting method of treatment is based on the identification of pathogenic dispositions in specific affected parts of the body.

But the foregoing quotation bears the trace of controversies between scholars in ancient times. As many Sanskrit classical texts, the *Carakasaṃhitā* was composed in the form of dialogues between a teacher and his disciples. In the above quotation Ātreya, the teacher, telling his students of the strategy of localisation as a point of departure for diagnosis and therapeutics, reported conflicting views on the matter. Some scholars, otherwise unknown, opposed the very idea of specific channels carrying specific dispositions to specific affected organs. Whereas Ātreya described the human body as a system of differentiated integration, these scholars expressing a dissident view saw the human body as an 'aggregate' (*samudaya*) formed from several elements compacted together and lumped into a whole. Favouring a holism in principle deterring any attempt to visual inspection, they assumed that the fluids flowing through the channels and the fleshy texture of the channels themselves were indistinguishable. They imagined flows of the three humours pervading the whole body without any traceable location. Discussing this approach and eventually rejecting it, Ātreya sets things right. In the classical doctrine, in which pharmaceuticals are devised to aim at localised targets in the patient's body, the humoral qualities of which determine the choice of drugs having appropriate counteractive properties, the primary approach is to identify the type of structuring disposition which accounts for the patient's complaints. The requisites for such a diagnosis, listed above by Ātreya, combine differentiation with localisation in the following way. The physician must look for (1) *what* the channels are made of (bodily tissues transformed from the juice of ingested substances), (2) *what* they carry (the perceptible qualities of ingested substances and of the tissues moving from their previous state to the subsequent), (3) *what* they nourish (organs and tissues), and (4) *where* they are located (affected parts).

To the contrary, the holistic position taken by these unknown scholars advocating the conception according to which the body is an aggregate, led them to a method of treatment quite similar to 'the postulate method' (Jouanna's phrase) denounced in Hippocrates' *On Ancient Medicine*.[22] Introducing arbitrary postulates, some authors, who are to be censured (Hippocrates' phrase), have supposed that there are only one or two causes of disease and death, heat or cold, moisture or dryness, or any other principle they may fancy to postulate. The three humours pervading the whole body conceived of as an aggregate, in the heterodox view evoked above, represented the Indian version of the postulate, since from a metaphysical point of view, the three humours of Āyurveda are said to be the Three Causes of Disease. The comparison may be pursued further. *On Ancient Medicine* makes a distinction between illnesses due to *dunameis*, 'forces', and illnesses due to *schēmata*, 'forms, configurations.'[23] By forces are meant those changes in the constitution of the humours which affect the working of the body. By forms are meant the organs of the body seen from the point of view not of their function but of their configuration. Although the author of *On Ancient Medicine* subscribes to principles such as humoral coction and humoral balance, the interplay of the four fundamental forces of heat and cold, wet and dry, is much less important to the Greek practitioner than the configuration of bodily organs where disease will be located. The same

22 Hippocrates, *On Ancient Medicine* I, 1 (I.570 L. = 118 Jouanna), ref. Jouanna 'la méthode du postulat' in the Notice, ibid. 24.

23 Hippocrates, *On Ancient Medicine* XXII, 1 (I.626 L. = 149 Jouanna). I am following Jouanna's interpretation.

criticism of a philosophical approach, and the very distinction between postulates and the practical knowledge of specific effects, have been at the centre of the classical doctrine of Indian medicine.

In Vedic times, the Great Sages met to decide upon the early origin (*prāg-utpatti*) of the human body. Sage Hiraṇyākṣa propounded the *ṣaḍdhātu* theory that was to become one important tenet of Āyurveda in medicine and Sāṃkhya in philosophy. Caraka recounts the story:[24] 'According to Hiraṇyākṣa, man was born of six constituents, and so were the diseases born of six constituents (*ṣaḍdhātujas tu puruṣo rogāḥ ṣaḍdhātujās tathā*). According to the foremost exponents of the Sāṃkhya school of philosophy (*sāṃkhyair ādyairḥ prakīrtitaḥ*), it was an aggregate of six constituents (*rāśiḥ ṣaḍdhātujaḥ*).' The six constituents were the five natural elements plus the soul, which through the mind controlled the faculties of perception and action. They go by the name of *indriya*, the accurate translation of which is 'faculty, faculties.' Indriyas are usually understood as the sensory and motor organs. But indriyas are not the same as organs, which are the instruments of these faculties. Sensory perception is achieved by the five sensory faculties, each one of which is grafted upon the corresponding material element. Thus, as we shall see now, localisations of disease may be performed through sensory perception within the holistic framework of a dynamic *dhātu* concept of the body. The patient's body on which the physician will endeavour to identify and locate complaints and disorders is not plainly offered to the eyes; it is a dynamic complex made up of faculties producing perceptible manifestations and structuring dispositions produced by the continued use of these faculties.

3 Sensory Faculties (*indriya*) and Material Substances (*dravya*)

In standard operating condition sensory faculties unfold on five levels of reality, named *indriya*, *adhiṣṭhāna*, *artha*, *dravya* and *buddhi*. These five entities may be characterised in the following way: (1) the faculties (*indriya*) as dynamic forces of manifestation; (2) the sites of sensations or sensory organs (*adhiṣṭhāna*) – eyes, ears, nose, tongue, skin – where these faculties are located and which are their instruments; (3) the sense objects (*artha*) which are grasped by the sense organs; (4) the material substances (*dravya*) – ether, air, fire, water and soil – of which the sensory faculties are made; and (5) awareness (*buddhi*) which transforms sensation into perception.[25] Vision is essentially

24 Caraka, *Sūtrasthāna* 25, 15. Quoted in Rosu (1978) 139.

25 I am following Arion Rosu's excellent presentation in Rosu (1978) 197–98.

made of fire in the eyes, hearing made of ether[26] in the ears, smelling made of earth in the nose, tasting made of water on the tongue, and touching made of air on the skin.[27] The materialistic argument that the five sensory faculties have been grafted onto the five natural elements was formulated by Caraka in the Book on Things Relative to the Body:[28]

> The five sensory faculties (*indriyāni*), grafted (*yuktāni*) onto ether, etc., each one of the natural elements being predominant in each one (*ekaikena*) of the sensory faculties, are known by inference (*anumeyāni*) from the action which their respective awareness (*buddhi*) performs.

Each sense organ has a corresponding awareness which transforms sensations into perceptions. For example, fiery sensations in the eyes, when awareness (*buddhi*) brings them to the forefront of our consciousness, are transformed into visual perceptions. Thus, when the eyes exert the action of seeing, from our awareness of fire in the eyes we can infer that vision (the sensory faculty) is grafted onto fire (the natural element). Ten centuries later this verse was elucidated by Cakrapāṇidatta as follows.[29]

> Among the five natural elements beginning with ether (*khādīnāṃ madhye*), the five sensory faculties, the eyes, etc. (*indriyāni pañca cakṣurādīni*), are matched one-to-one (*ekaikena*) with a predominant natural element (*adhikena bhūtena*). The phrase *ekaikādhikayuktāni* [in the verse commented upon] means that each one of the five sensory faculties is electively grafted onto one of the five natural elements (*pañcabhautikāni*). The word *adhika* points for example to the fact that fire is predominant (*param*) in the eyes. The phrase *karmānumeyāni* [predicated upon *indriyāni*] means that the sensory faculties [*indriyāni*, which yield sensations] are known by inference from the subsequent action (*kāryam*) performed by their respective *buddhi* (awareness) [which transforms sensations into perceptions]. The relative pronoun *yāni* in the phrase *yebhyo buddhiḥ pravartate* refers to the five actions by the five *buddhīndriyāni*: visual awareness (*cakṣurbuddhi*) transforms what the eye sees into visual perceptions, etc. And although (*yady api*) in Sāṃkhya sensory faculties

26 *Kha* or *ākāśa* has been alternatively conceived of as ether, space, sky, vacuity. I prefer ether, to connote the idea of a pervading fluid.

27 Rosu (1978) 198.

28 Caraka, *Śārīrasthāna* 1, 24.

29 Cakrapāṇidatta ad Caraka, *Śārīrasthāna* 1, 24.

> (*indriyāṇi*) are said to evolve out of the subject's ego (*āhaṃkārikāṇīndriyāṇi*), as said in *Sāṃkyakārikā*,[30] verse 25: 'The Group of Eleven [i.e., the sensory faculties] evolve out of ego's alterations', nevertheless (*tathā'pi*) due to a difference of opinion (*matabhedāt*) [between Sāṃkhyā philosophers and Āyurvedic physicians], what is taught (*jñeyam*) here is the materiality of the sensory faculties (*bhautikatvam indriyāṇām*). Or if you prefer (*kiṃvā*), this teaching of the materiality of the sensory faculties is metaphorical (*aupacārika*). It says by metaphor (*upacārabīja*) that a feeling which is grasped by a particular sense organ and which is chiefly filled (*bhūyiṣṭha*) with the essential quality (*guṇa*) of a particular element, that feeling is chiefly filled with that element: the eyes grasp fire (*cakṣus tejo gṛṇāti*), therefore they are said to be fiery (*taijasam*).

From the observation of the presence of fire in the eyes, we conclude, by inference, that the eyes are the visible instruments of sight, an invisible but real faculty. Whatever may be the philosophical value of this materialistic argument, we are here tackling medical issues and, even if this argument is merely metaphorical, it has a methodological value. It points to the possibility for physicians to localise the material basis of a complaint and take this localisation as a point of departure for diagnosis and therapeutics. Within a holistic framework, since the six cosmic elements constitute the human body as a self-contained house which the soul inhabits and animates, in practice, diagnosis and therapeutics start from the tracking and tracing of perceptible substances in specific affected locations.

Substances (*dravya*) are of primary importance in this modality of humoralism, and pharmaceutical knowledge plays by far the most essential role in the training of an Āyurvedic practitioner. We already met with the concept of *dravya* in the earlier parts of this chapter. The place granted to material substances in medicine is a very clear criterion for distinguishing between the philosophical modality of humoralism, which downplays the materiality of empirical phenomena in general and of pathogenic dispositions in particular, and another modality of humoralism which prevails in the classical texts and in the mainstream tradition of Āyurveda where material substances (*dravya*) are constitutive of empirical dispositions (*bhāva*). This is not the place to elaborate further on the central position of pharmaceuticals in the actual practice of Indian medicine; entering the field of materia medica would steer us off course; but we have a very simple example at hand. Cakrapāṇidatta's discussion around *āmalaka* (emblic myrobalan), reproduced above, shows that an

30 The earliest text of the Sāṃkhya school of philosophy.

elaborate knowledge of *materia medica* is a requisite for applying a truly informed gaze upon the patient's body. From ancient times down to the early decades of the twentieth century, the training of a student in Āyurvedic medicine began in childhood, and his first concrete observations of living things used to take place in the master's garden. The primary knowledge imparted to these young boys, apart from reading and writing in Sanskrit and learning selected texts by heart, was the ability to recognize the local varieties and perceptible qualities of herbs and fruits like mangoes and myrobalans.[31] The ancient medical collections[32] present a biased view of this practical training because they underscore the interplay of perceptible qualities like sourness, sweetness, coldness, etc., removed from their material basis and from the local context of experience. Remember Suśruta's statement above, saying that *āmalaka* pacifies wind due to sourness, bile due sweetness and coldness, and phlegm due to roughness and astringency. In the classical treatises and formularies that students learnt by heart, *materia medica* was reduced to abstract combinations of humours, tastes and sensory qualities. Expertise in *materia medica*, however, has always been a matter of practice eventually acquired in natural surroundings, that is, in botanical gardens if not in the jungles and forests. Let us try to see things from the physician's garden in traditional India, where young Āyurvedic students used to complete their apprenticeship. Observed in the field, living things and material substances whose names and qualities were taught in the texts will regain their primary position at the centre of the learning experience. In this perspective, there was no real disagreement between Suśruta and Cakrapāṇidatta, in the commentary cited above, about the risks and benefits of prescribing *āmalaka*, but a matter of judgement depending on the particular clinical case. Emblic myrobalans in different situations may act either as a panacea, pacifying the three humours, or as a corrupter of humour bile due to sourness. Building on this primary knowledge of *dravyaprabhāvāḥ*, 'the healing predispositions of substances', and of their sensory qualities which in the end account for these powers, the physician will examine the state of *mūrtimanto bhāvāḥ*, 'the structuring dispositions' in the patient's body. Assuming that the three humours pervading the outside world are also constitutive of the human body, the first step in therapeutics is to match *dravyaprabhāvāḥ* (drug predispositions) discovered in the outside world of experience with *mūrtimanto bhāvāḥ* (structuring dispositions) recognised in the patient's body.

---

31 See Zimmermann (1989) on vestiges of this traditional training observed in Kerala (South India).

32 'Collections' (*saṃhitā*) constitute a literary genre on the model of Caraka's Collection.

Foods and diets make the link between the world and the human body. Philipp Maas highlighted the structural relation between the emergence of the humours as pathogenic forces in the human body and the gradual generation of bodily tissues starting from the intake of food.[33] He cited Caraka's extremely precise description of the process of food digestion separating pure tissues from waste products, which reads as follows.[34]

> From digestion (*tatra*) are produced [1] a juice (*rasa*) called the pure essence of food (*āhāraprasāda*) and [2] waste products called impurities (*mala*). From waste (*kiṭṭāt*) thrive (*puṣyanti*) [1] sweat, urine, feces, wind, bile and phlegm, [2] impure matter oozing from the ears, eyes, nose, mouth, hair follicles and genitals, and [3] body parts (*avayavāḥ*) such as the hair of one's head, beard, the hair of one's body, nails, etc. Thriving from the juice of food (*āhārarasāt*) are [1] chyle (*rasa*), blood, flesh, fat, bone, marrow, semen and *ojas* [an imaginary vital fluid], [2] the five material substances [ether, air, fire, water and soil] of which the sensory faculties are made (*pañcendriyadravyāṇi*), conventionally named (*saṃjñakāni*) the pure essences of the dhātus (*dhātuprasādasaṃjñakāni*), and [3] body parts such as joints, ligaments, mucous membranes, etc.

A number of fixed lists of technical terms have a particular salience in this short extract, as well as a number of figures of speech which will eventually justify the use of polysemic terms like *rasa* and *dhātu*. The underlying theme is one of the tenets of Hinduism: food is the source of life and all living things and phenomena have always been thriving from food. Let us focus on the human body. The very first step in its development is to take food. Then digestion is a refining process yielding the pure essence of food, separated from waste. Apparently, waste is expelled from the body in the form of seeps oozing from all its apertures and in the form of hairs and nails, which in Hindu India daily hygiene routine are taken as impure. But on close reading the three humours, wind, bile and phlegm are included in waste resulting from digestion, and they will not be expelled. Before they become pathogenic forces, the three humours are primarily material waste products of digestion, listed here among other organic fluids. Let us now consider the 'pure essence (*prasāda*) of food (*āhāra*)' yielded by the refining process of digestion. This is *rasa* in the primary sense of this technical term, literally 'the essence' of food, from which through a

---

33 Maas (2008) 136.

34 Caraka, *Sūtrasthāna* 28, 4. I am offering my own translation, which aims to indicate the word-order, collocations and figures of speech.

continuous refinement process the series of seven bodily tissues, chyle, blood, flesh, fat, bone, marrow and semen, will emerge and 'thrive' (*puṣyanti*). The closed list of the seven tissue dhātus is a salient feature here, but this time it is supplemented with an eighth item named *ojas*, the most refined of all dhātus, which represents vitality in the form of a fluid; I shall come back to it in a moment.

There is a play on words in the sentence beginning by *puṣyanti tv āhārarasād rasa-rudhira-māṃsa-*, etc., 'Thriving from the *rasa* [essence] of food [are] *rasa* [chyle], blood, flesh, etc.' In common Sanskrit *rasa* means 'juice'; in Āyurvedic terminology its primary meaning is '[a juice which is] the essence [of food, of life]'; then, following from a figure of speech named *svasaṃjñā*, 'a term used in its conventional meaning', *rasa* comes to mean 'chyle' and denote the first of the seven body tissues. As already mentioned, the chyle, in Āyurvedic as well as in Hippocratic medicine, is the fluid separated from food during the first internal cooking process, which in turn will be transformed into blood. The conceptual distinction here between food essence (which is not yet a body constituent) and chyle (which is the first of bodily tissues) is indisputable. It plays a major role in the assessment of humoralism and holism in Āyurveda, as will be shown below.

Let me explain *svasaṃjñā* and emphasise an interesting feature of medical Sanskrit terminology. Comparable to Galen and his emulators in the West, Āyurvedic scholars of the past were strong logicians and used figures of speech as logical tools in visual inspection and diagnosis.[35] Sanskrit *svasaṃjñā* may be construed as an exact equivalent of English *catachresis* when this figure of speech is used to cross categorical boundaries with words, to give them new specialized meanings, and to incorporate them into a technical terminology. Thus, *rasa*, which denotes juices, comes to mean 'chyle' in medicine. So rich is this excerpt from Caraka that it explicitly mentions another case of *svasaṃjñā*, which is telling in the context of our discussion on the material content of sensory faculties. One set of bodily constituents thriving from the pure essence of food, Caraka says, is the closed list of 'the five dravyas of indriyas conventionally named the pure essences of the dhātus (*pañcendriyadravyāṇi dhātuprasāda-saṃjñakāni*).' In the operation of the sensory faculties, *dravya* denotes the five natural elements all of which are conceived of as fluid or solid materials. As mentioned earlier, the five natural elements supplemented with the soul constitute the closed list of *ṣaḍdhātu*, the six cosmic constituents. Therefore, in the outside world (the macrocosm), the five natural elements named *dravya*

35 Zimmermann (1989) 132–35 gives a detailed description of *svasaṃjñā* and other figures of speech extensively used as logical tools in Āyurvedic medicine.

are five of the cosmic constituents named *dhātu*. But in the human body, our sensory faculties in operation will grasp the material content from the natural elements in the outside world and refine them in order to yield sensations which are the pure essence of material things perceived, just as bodily tissues are the pure essence of food digested. This is why they are 'named by convention' (*saṃjñakāni*) the pure essence of dhātus, a word designating here the natural elements. This is a perfect description of the sensory process in which sensations are given an identifiable and localisable material content.

4 A Final Remark on the Vital Fluid (*ojas*)

To conclude, let us come back to the technical term and concept of *ojas*, the vital fluid par excellence, which is most significant for us in the current discussion. Here is not the place of an elaborate description of its role as a procreative fluid.[36] But clearly, in the present context where *ojas* comes at the end of the series of bodily tissues, the most refined of all, *ojas* represents vitality in the form of a quintessential bodily fluid bound to spread life. Let me recall the distinction from which we started, between two types of medications:[37] 'Medication is of two kinds, that which promotes vitality (*ūrjaskara*) [literally, an *ūrjas*-maker] in the healthy, and that which dispels diseases (*roganud*) in the ailing.' *Ojas*, connected with Latin *augustus*, is a quite frequent term in Āyurveda, whereas *ūrjas*, connected with Latin *urgeo*, does not really belong to the medical domain. Both terms, however, denote 'vigour, vitality', and I would like to suggest that *ūrjas* and *ojas* bear witness to an evolution in the history of Āyurvedic therapeutics. Prior to Caraka, medications for enhancing vitality, virilifics and elixirs of youth did not belong to Āyurveda. They were dealt with in a specialized literature devoted to *rasāyana*, 'rejuvenation.' Philipp Maas in another fine paper has convincingly demonstrated that a process of integration of *rasāyana* into Āyurveda must have occurred, an evolution of which the non-explicit inclusion of *ojas* into the list of bodily tissues bears witness.[38] Another detail in Caraka's Collection which mirrors this process of integration of rejuvenating medications into Āyurveda is the distinction between medications *ūrjaskara*, 'promoting vitality', and medications *roganut*, 'dispelling diseases', which implies a reflection upon holism, humoralism and the causes of disease. On one side rejuvenatives enhancing vitality illustrate a global,

36 Das (2003) 530–35 has exhaustively collected the evidence.
37 Caraka, *Cikitsāsthāna* 1, 4. Quoted above, n. 2.
38 Maas (2017) 76 n. 44.

delocalised approach to lifespan, body integrity and death, and on the other side the physician's choice of drugs for a specific disease takes into account the diversity of empirical dispositions and the localisation of affected parts. In modern and contemporary Āyurveda, practitioners have alternated between the two methods of treatment.

Another significant detail brought to light by Maas in Caraka's definition of rejuvenation is the ambiguous meaning of the first term *rasa* in the compound *rasāyana*. I am following the word-order and indicating the line breaks in translating these two verses:[39]

> A long life, memory, intelligence,
> absence of disease, youthful age, |
> radiance, complexion and voice at their best,
> the greatest strength of the body and sensory faculties (*indriya*), || 7
> successful speech (*vāksiddhi*), authority (*praṇati*), beauty
> [are what] a man obtains through *rasāyana*; |
> because, a means for obtaining better (*śastānāṃ*)
> essence, etc. (*rasādīnāṃ*), [this is] *rasāyana*. || 8

Modern and contemporary practitioners quoting the last hemistich invariably translate it as: '*Rasāyana* is a means for obtaining better chyle, etc., [that is,] better bodily tissues', and in modern and contemporary parlance, this definition of *rasāyana*, taken as a descriptive compound, alludes to the physiological 'circulation and progress' (*ayana*) of a rejuvenating drug intake from *rasa* (chyle) to all the *rasādi* dhātus, that is, from chyle to semen, achieved through successive internal stages of cooking of bodily tissues. Maas, however, has argued that, in the early centuries CE, when a strictly materialistic interpretation of bodily tissues was not yet achieved and fixed in the texts, and in the context of collocations joining youthfulness and radiance to moral and social values like successful speech and authority, it was highly unlikely that *rasa* here meant chyle. The modern explanation of *rasādi* as meaning 'chyle, etc.' might have been a creative innovation for promoting the integration of *rasāyana* into Āyurveda.[40] In the same line, I would suggest that in Caraka's verses above there was a play on the ambiguous meaning of *rasa* – both the essence of food and the essence of life – in accordance with the overall holistic approach inspired from the Hindu concept of food as a source of life.

---

39 Caraka, *Cikitsāsthāna* 1.1, 7–8.
40 Maas (2017) 76.

In the end, once the pursuit of longevity is fully integrated into mainstream Āyurvedic therapeutics, medicine comes to apply a two-pronged approach to health and disease, which both need medication. Health needs to be bolstered using a topdown method, as it were, in the sense that we directly start from the three humours which, taken as an undifferentiated whole, are strengthened by elixirs of long life. The version of holism advocated by the dissident scholars evoked by Ātreya, who described the human body as an 'aggregate', is better suited to this topdown approach resorted to in rejuvenative medications. To the contrary, diseases must be cured using a bottom-up method, in the sense that we start from the observed dispositions of the patient's body from which we can track the distribution of different organic fluids to specific channels, assess the humoral condition in the affected parts, and devise suitable countermeasures. The version of holism represented by the differentiated integration of channels and 'structuring dispositions' described above is better suited to the bottom-up approach in therapeutics following the principle of opposite treatment. But these two modalities of humoralism are equally constitutive of the Āyurvedic method of treatment.

Bibliography

Das, R. P. *The Origin of the Life of a Human Being, Conception and the Female According to Ancient Indian Medical and Sexological Literature*. Delhi: Motilal Banarsidass (2003).

Maas, P. A. 'The Concepts of the Human Body and Disease in Classical Yoga and Āyurveda.' *Wiener Zeitschrift für die Kunde Südasiens = Vienna Journal of South Asian Studies*, 51 (2008) 125–62.

Maas, P. A. 'Rasāyana in Classical Yoga and Āyurveda.' *History of Science in South Asia*, 5.2 (2017) 66–84.

Meulenbeld, G. J. *A History of Indian Medical Literature*. 5 vols. Groningen: E. Forsten (1999–2002).

Rosu, A. *Les conceptions psychologiques dans les textes médicaux indiens*. Publications de l'Institut de Civilisation Indienne. Paris: De Boccard (1978).

Zimmermann, F. *Le discours des remèdes au pays des épices, enquête sur la médecine hindoue*. Paris: Payot (1989).

Zimmermann, F. *Généalogie des médecines douces, De l'Inde à l'Occident*. Paris: Presses Universitaires de France (1995).

Primary Texts: Editions and Translations Used

Carakasaṃhitā, with the *Āyurvedadīpikā* commentary by Cakrapāṇidatta. Ed. Yādavaśarman Trivikrama Ācārya. 3rd ed. Bombay: Nirṇaya Sāgar Press (1941).

Carakasaṃhitā, text with English translation and critical exposition based on Cakrapāṇidatta's *Āyurvedadīpikā*. Ed. Dr Ram Karan Sharma and Vaidya Bhagwan Das., 4 vols. Varanasi: Chowkhamba Sanskrit Series Office (1976–1997).

Carakasaṃhitā, text with English translation and critical notes. Ed. Priya Vrat Sharma, 4 vols. Varanasi and Delhi: Chaukhamba Orientalia (1981–1994).

Galien. *Méthode de traitement*. Ed. and trans. Jacques Boulogne. Paris: Gallimard (2009).

Hippocrate. *L'Ancienne Médecine.* (*On Ancient Medicine*). Ed. J. Jouanna. Paris: Les Belles Lettres (2003).

Suśrutasaṃhitā, text with English translation of text and Ḍalhaṇa's commentary along with critical notes. Ed. Priya Vrat Sharma. 3 vols. Varanasi: Chaukhamba Visvabharati (2001).

CHAPTER 13

A Systemic Etiology of Sicknesses from Ancient Iraq: Organ Systems and the Functional Holism of the Babylonian Body

John Z. Wee

Abstract

From the Late Achaemenid city of Uruk comes a single cuneiform document described here as a *Systemic Etiology*, which attributes to various sicknesses their origins 'from' four ancient organ systems – psychic, alimentary, respiratory, and excretory-reproductive – that bear remarkable resemblance to classifications in modern biology. Features of such a functional holism may already be detected, in varying degrees, elsewhere in the Mesopotamian medical literature. The striking manner in which the *Etiology* re-categorizes certain sicknesses, nonetheless, illustrates how holisms do not organize their constituents in a disinterested fashion, or group them together merely on the basis of previously known characteristics, but can also reframe perspectives in ways that impose new meanings on individual constituents' identities.

Many hundreds of cuneiform medical tablets from ancient Iraq compel us to rethink the ways we write ancient histories of medicine. In contrast to medical manuscripts of papyrus, parchment, or paper that often survive today in relatively late copies, these highly durable clay tablets from Mesopotamia come to us from much closer to their milieus of composition, transmission, and usage, allowing us to envision probable scenarios in which such documents were actually employed in historical contexts. While the cuneiform materials open up new kinds of agenda beyond what have been considered in the study of other ancient medical cultures, there are also issues on which they are particularly intractable – among which is the question of how individual sicknesses and bodily constituents were assigned to separate categories that, when viewed in relation to each other, informed one's understanding of the whole.

Explanatory discourses in Greek or Chinese treatises, for example, have articulated or clearly implied well-defined positions and principles on general topics like nutrition, the environment, medicaments, or categories of sickness.

 | DOI:10.1163/9789004443143_015

By comparison, the medical literature in Mesopotamia consists overwhelmingly of relatively terse statements that simply depict bodily and sickness behaviors in particular scenarios, which are then addressed by diagnoses, prognoses, and therapeutic remedies such as herbal recipes and healing incantations and rituals[1] – with scarce or ambiguous hints in writing on any encompassing medical theory that might provide a comprehensive rationale for sickness or its cure. As a matter of fact, contrary to tendencies in previous generations that took for granted notions and labels such as 'Hippocratic medicine' or 'Daoist medicine,' scholarship today has become increasingly sensitized to the disunities and discontinuities in medical texts, so that we ought to speak more accurately instead of *medicines* in the plural. Against such shifts in methodology, the effort to piece together from diverse cuneiform sources a composite picture of Mesopotamian medical beliefs might well be regarded as regressive – running the risk of smoothing over genuine discrepancies in different texts, in order to promote a coherent narrative. Indeed, it is not without irony that avowals of *ancient* holisms on the basis of inadequate evidence can, in fact, arise out of pressures in *modern* historical scholarship to tell a 'holistic' story of the past.[2]

To avoid the category error of including as collective evidence textual sources that really belong separately, we do well to focus either on a single medical document or on a group of manuscripts tightly defined by their distinctive format or provenance, whose interpretation can be informed largely by its own contents. One such composition, fortunately, comes to us from the ancient city of Uruk in southern Iraq.

1 The *Systemic Etiology* from Uruk

The single cuneiform tablet that is the focus of this essay – whose description as a '*Systemic Etiology*' I will later justify – represents a unique specimen that endeavors to provide a holistic account, apparently, of how sicknesses originate

1 To get a sense of the format and the contents of these statements, see §F, §I, §J, §K, §O, §Q, §R, §S and §T below.

2 Along similar lines, Thumiger (on page 37 of this volume) remarks on how 'many of our historiographic strategies are based on versions of holistic fantasies of exhaustiveness, where the wholes of philological *corpora*, of *opera omnia*, of individual thinkers recomposed from *fragments* to their *whole* are painstakingly pursued with an eye to the ultimate goal of complete reconstruction.'

'from' (*ultu*)[3] one out of four regions in the inner anatomy of the human body. It bears repeated reminding that this document, with no duplicates or closely related texts discovered so far, is a singular item that appears very late in the final centuries of Mesopotamian medicine, whose development up to this point had spanned more than two millennia. So we should not rush to the conclusion that the etiological model here was necessarily normative at other times and localities, or even accepted with consensus in its city of discovery.

The tablet's colophon (§E below) announces its status as a copy from a yet-undiscovered original, and identifies its current owner as Rīmūt-Anu from the prominent magician family of Šangû-Ninurta, which flourished around the fourth century BCE during Late Achaemenid times in the city of Uruk. The family library – containing many manuscripts ascribed to the famous magician Anu-ikṣur (brother of Rīmūt-Anu) – was especially well-stocked in tablets and cuneiform commentaries on medicine, omens, and astrology-astronomy, compositions on magic and ritual, alongside lexical lists, scribal exercises, mathematical texts, and other genres.[4]

The *Systemic Etiology* was excavated in 1969, and its *editio princeps* (labelled *SpTU* I, 43) published in 1976 by H. Hunger, who described it as a 'Liste von Krankheiten, geordnet nach den Körperteilen, aus denen sie kommen,' while observing that the relationships here of sicknesses among themselves and with parts of the human body differed from those in the *List of Medical Terms* associated with the cuneiform lexical tradition.[5] Subsequent publications by Köcher (1978), Geller (2001/2002 and 2014), and Heeßel (2010) adopted minor amendments to points of cuneiform reading, while theories on the *Etiology*'s meaning and significance were additionally proposed at length by Geller (*ibid.*) and Steinert (2016).[6]

Geller correctly noted resemblances here to 'the Hippocratic notion of the 'seat' of a disease being in one of the bodily organs,' but his comparison of the cuneiform *Etiology* to the four *archai* in Galen's *Ars Medica* – i.e., brain,

3 In the *Systemic Etiology*, the Akkadian preposition 'from' (*ultu* or *ištu*) affirms at least the origin of its object – whether understood in spatial, temporal, or more metaphoric ways – without necessarily asserting that this 'origin' is also the 'cause' of the object.

4 Clancier (2009) 81–84, 400–6; Frahm (2011) 290–92.

5 Hunger (1976) 50 (text no. 43). In order to more accurately reflect the contents of the lexical composition, I refer to it as a *List of Medical Terms* instead of the title 'List of Diseases' given by Kilmer (1967) 77–109.

6 Köcher (1978) 22–25; Geller (2001–2002) 60–62 and (2014) 3–8; Heeßel (2010) 30–31, and briefly in (2004) 113–14; Steinert (2016) 230–42.

heart, liver, and testicles – is not entirely persuasive.[7] Steinert offered some helpful insights into the reasons certain sicknesses were attributed to specific organs,[8] but more can be said about the rationales for such associations, as I will explain below. Comparisons to the Greek theory of the four humors or to the Chinese *wuxing* ('Five Processes'),[9] moreover, seem less promising, given how the importance of seasonal changes in these systems is evident to a lesser extent in Mesopotamian medicine, though other calendrical variables could possibly have counterparts in astrological medicine. Looking to developments in the late first millennium BCE, which correlated celestial bodies and zodiacal features with therapeutic ingredients of plant, wood, and stone and with anatomical regions, Geller and also Brown (2018) suggested that hidden in these interconnections is the key to understanding the *Etiology*.[10]

My own work in medical astrology and astronomy during Late Babylonian to Seleucid times, which I will discuss later, is certainly in sympathy with such views that fluidity in professional purviews and efforts at bridging different branches of cuneiform knowledge – particularly involving astrology-astronomy – were characteristic of Babylonian scholarship in the final centuries BCE, partly due to changes in Babylonian institutions resulting from Achaemenid, Seleucid, and even Parthian influences.[11] While it is possible that pathological relationships in the *Systemic Etiology* derived from schemata in astrological and astronomical or other disciplines, I wish to suggest here that motivations indigenous to Mesopotamian medicine already account for the *Etiology* to a high degree of satisfaction. Explanations such as 'the spleen *refers to* Jupiter' and 'the kidney-star is Mars,'[12] in effect, regard these organs in largely atomistic ways, as data points or parameters incidental to the actual physiology of the human body. By contrast, the *Etiology* represents an attempt to map out the Babylonian body holistically – not according to its *physical structure*, as tended to be the practice in Mesopotamian medicine for at least the preceding millennium – but relying instead on categories of basic *functions* essential to the healthy living body.

7 Geller (2014) 23–25.
8 Steinert (2016) 232–39.
9 Steinert (2016) 239–42.
10 Geller (2014) 73–75; Brown (2018) 448–49; cf. Heeßel (2004) 113–14, (2005) 1–22 and (2008) 1–16.
11 Wee (2016) 139–229 and (2017) 236–60.
12 Reiner (1995) 60; Civil (1974) 336; referenced by Geller (2014) 79 and 91.

2 Cuneiform Text of the *Systemic Etiology*

2.1 *Transliteration*[13]

§A1	*ul-tu lib*$_3$*-bi*	GA[Z] ⸢*lib*$_3$⸣*-bi*
§A2	KI.MIN	AN.TA.ŠUB.BA
§A3	KI.MIN	ŠU.⸢DINGIR.RA⸣
§A4	KI.MIN	ŠU.$^{d+}$INNIN.⸢NA⸣
§A5	KI.MIN	*be-e*[*n*]*-nu*
§A6	KI.MIN	^{d}LUG[AL].⸢UR$_3$⸣.[R]A
§B1	*ul-tu* KA ⸢*kar*⸣*-šu*$_2$	*mu-ru-uṣ* SAG.DU *u pi-*[*i*]
§B2	KI.MIN	*pi-i šin-ni b*[*u-u*]ˀ-⸢*ša*$_2$⸣*-nu*
§B3	KI.MIN	MIN ⸢x x x-*mu* (?)⸣
§B4	KI.MIN	MIN ⸢x x x (?)⸣
§B5	KI.MIN	MIN *pa-šit-t*[*u*$_4$] ^{munus}*mar-tu*$_4$
§B6	KI.MIN	⸢*ma-li*⸣ *me-e*
§B7	KI.MIN	Š[U].GIDIM.MA
§B8	KI.MIN	*maš-ka-du*
§B9	KI.MIN	*mi-šit-ti*
§B10	KI.MIN	*a-šu-u*$_2$
§B11	[K]I.MIN	*gi-iṣ-ṣa-tu*$_4$
§B12	[K]I.MIN	*ḫi-miṭ* UD.⸢DA⸣ *nap-ḫar mur-ṣu*
§C1	[*ul-t*]*u ḫa-še-e*	lu.bi
§C2	[KI.MIN]	*ši-i-qu*
§C3	[K]I.MIN	*ša*$_2$*-a-ri*
§C4	KI.MIN	*e-zi-zu*
§C5	KI.MIN	*bu-ša*$_2$*-a-nu*
§C6	KI.MIN	*ṣi-in-na-aḫ-tir*
§D1	*ul-tu* ELLAG$_2$.MEŠ	*ḫi-niq*$_2$*-ti*
§D2	KI.MIN	ŠA$_3$.ZI.GA
§D3	KI.MIN	*du-ur-gig-ga*
§D4	KI.MIN	*sa-gal-lu*$_4$
§D5	KI.MIN	*la a-li-du-ti*

13 Photographs of this cuneiform tablet are available in Geller (2014) 6 fig. 2. Following Assyriological conventions in transliteration, full and half square brackets enclose text restored in varying degrees to damaged portions of the cuneiform manuscript. To facilitate readability, while I mostly retain these brackets in my English translation, I do not allow them to interrupt the spelling of a translated English word.

§D6	KI.MIN	ARḪUŠ *ša*$_2$ *zi-i-ri*
§D7	KI.MIN	*ka-le-e* IM

§E GIM SUMUN-*šu*$_2$ SAR-*ma ba-ri* IM.GI$_3$.DA [m]*Ri-mut*-d*A-nu* DUMU *ša*$_2$ m.d*Ša*$_3$-*maš*$_2$-MU DUMU lu2SANGA-d*Nin-urta* lu2MAŠ.MAŠ *qa-at*$_2$ m*Be-lu-ka-ṣir* DUMU *ša*$_2$ mTIN

2.2 *Translation*

§A1	From the heart	Heart-break
§A2	Ditto (i.e., from the heart)	AN.TA.ŠUB.BA (lit. fallen-from-heaven) epilepsy
§A3	Ditto (i.e., from the heart)	Hand-of-god
§A4	Ditto (i.e., from the heart)	Hand-of-goddess
§A5	Ditto (i.e., from the heart)	*bennu* epilepsy
§A6	Ditto (i.e., from the heart)	dLUGAL.UR$_3$.RA (lit. lord-of-the-roof) epilepsy
§B1	From the mouth (and/of) stomach	Sickness of the head or[14] the mouth
§B2	Ditto (i.e., from the mouth and/of stomach)	Mouth (and) tooth of *bu'šānu* sickness[15]
§B3	Ditto (i.e., from the mouth and/of stomach)	Ditto (i.e., mouth and tooth) of … (?) sickness[16]
§B4	Ditto (i.e., from the mouth and/of stomach)	Ditto (i.e., mouth and tooth) of … (?) sickness[17]
§B5	Ditto (i.e., from the mouth and/of stomach)	Ditto (i.e., mouth and tooth) of *pāšittu* sickness (with) gall[18]
§B6	Ditto (i.e., from the mouth and/of stomach)	Dropsy (lit. full-of-water)
§B7	Ditto (i.e., from the mouth and/of stomach)	Hand-of-ghost

14 Understood as the disjunctive conjunction *ū* ('or'), rather than *u* ('and').

15 My reading tentatively follows Hunger (1976) 50 (text no. 43, obv. 9), contrary to ⸢MUR.DUR$_2$⸣.MEŠ-*šu*$_2$-*nu* ('their toothworms') by Geller (2014) 3.

16 Read as ⸢*gir*$_{11}$⸣-[*gi*]-⸢*iš*⸣-*šum* ('red skin lesions') by Geller (2014) 3.

17 Read as dDIM$_3$.ME ('Lamaštu') by Geller (2014) 3; perhaps intended by the reference '[SpTU 1.43:]12 [sic] (Lamashtu)' in Scurlock (2014) 273.

18 My translation here is influenced by the following statement in a cuneiform commentary on the Diagnostic Handbook Sa-gig: '"*pāšittu* sickness (and) poison" *refers to pāšittu* sickness that contains gall' (*pa-šit-tu*$_2$ *im-tu*$_2$: *pa-šit-tu*$_2$ *ša*$_2$ *mar-tu*$_2$ *u*$_2$-*kal-lu*; *GCBC* 766, obv. 4). Hand copy by Dougherty (1923–1933) vol. II, no. 406; edition and notes by Wee (2019b) 226–27 and 230–31 (Comm. Sa-gig 13+, obv. 4).

§B8	Ditto (i.e., from the mouth and/of stomach)	*maškadu* sickness
§B9	Ditto (i.e., from the mouth and/of stomach)	*mišittu*-stroke
§B10	Ditto (i.e., from the mouth and/of stomach)	*ašû* sickness
§B11	Ditto (i.e., from the mouth and/of stomach)	*giṣṣatu* sickness
§B12	Ditto (i.e., from the mouth and/of stomach)	Burning of *ṣētu*-heat of any sickness[19]
§C1	[From] the lungs	lu.bi (?)[20] sickness
§C2	[Ditto (i.e., from the lungs)]	*šīqu* sickness
§C3	Ditto (i.e., from the lungs)	Wind
§C4	Ditto (i.e., from the lungs)	*ezizzu* sickness[21]
§C5	Ditto (i.e., from the lungs)	*buʾšānu* sickness[22]
§C6	Ditto (i.e., f.rom the lungs)	*ṣinnaḫtiru* sickness
§D1	From the kidneys	Stricture

19 Read as *ḫi-miṭ* UD.⌜DA u_3⌝ *nap-ḫar mur-ṣu* ('"sun-light"-fever and all illnesses') by Köcher (1978) 24; Geller (2001–2002) 61, and (2014) 4. But there does not seem to be enough space for the large sign u_3 ('and') on the tablet.

20 The cuneiform signs lu.bi were read as *dap-pi*$_2$ ('Blutgerinnsel(?)' or 'bloodclot(?)') by Köcher (1978) 24; Geller (2001–2002) 61; Heeßel (2010) 31; and Steinert (2016) 231 n. 106. The meaning 'Blutklumpen(?)' for *dappu* was originally proposed in *AHw*, 162 s.v. *dappu* II on the basis of rather weak lexical evidence, and is unacknowledged in *CAD* Ṭ, 49 s.v. *ṭappu* A. The signs were merely transliterated as LU-*bi*, for possibly *lubu* or *dibbu*, by Hunger (1976) 50–51 (text no. 43, rev. 20). Recently, Geller (2014) 3–8 has suggested the alternative reading *tib-bi* ('throbbing'), though this use is also poorly attested in the dictionaries. I wonder if the signs lu.bi may be a version of or error for BI.LU, which denotes a nasal condition in the diagnostic statement Sa-gig 40: 5: 'If an infant's flesh appears yellowish (but) does not hold heat, his temples are fallen, he rubs his nose a lot but does not have mucus, [BI.LU] sickness seizes him' (DIŠ LU$_2$.TUR UZU.MEŠ-*šu*$_2$ *ur-qa*$_2$ *it-ta-du-u*$_2$ KUM$_2$ *la u*$_2$*-kal* SAG.KI.2-*šu*$_2$ *ma-aq-ta*$_5$ *ap-pi-šu*$_2$ *ma-gal i-si-ir u*$_2$*-pa-ṭi la i-šu* [BI.LU] *ṣab-tu-šu*$_2$). Later, a Babylonian commentator would claim that '"BI.LU" *refers to* (the respiratory sickness) *buʾšānu*' (BI.LU : *bu-ša*$_2$*-nu*) in Comm. Sa-gig 40A, obv. 5 (Wee 2019b, 340, 342 and 344).

21 *ezizzu* is both the name of the lung sickness and the plant used to treat it. Stol (1998) 344; cf. Geller (2001–2002) 62 n. 108; Steinert (2016) 237 n. 129.

22 Steinert (2016) 237 n. 128 drew attention to medical statements like *BAM* 44: 14' // *BAM* 558 i 14: 'If *buʾšānu* sickness seizes a man's lungs and mouth/nose' (DIŠ NA MUR.MEŠ-*ma* ka-*šu*$_2$ *bu-ʾ-ša-nu* DAB-*it*). In addition, I would point out that the logogram (KIR$_4$.ḪAB) for *buʾšānu* is a compound containing the term KIR$_4$ ('nose'). See *CAD* B, 350 s.v. *būšānu*, lexical section.

§D2	Ditto (i.e., from the kidneys)	ŠA$_3$.ZI.GA (lit. aroused-heart) condition[23]
§D3	Ditto (i.e., from the kidneys)	Sick rectum[24]
§D4	Ditto (i.e., from the kidneys)	*sagallu* (lit. large-strands) disorder
§D5	Ditto (i.e., from the kidneys)	Barrenness
§D6	Ditto (i.e., from the kidneys)	Womb (in the case) of hate[25]
§D7	Ditto (i.e., from the kidneys)	Retention of (flatulent) wind

§E Written and inspected, according to (the tablet's) original. Single-column tablet belonging to Rīmūt-Anu, son of Šamaš-iddin, descendant of Šangû-Ninurta the magician. (Written by) the hand of Bēlu-kāṣir, son of Balāṭu.

3 Organ Systems in the *Systemic Etiology*

One of the most useful organizing principles in the discipline of biology today is the hierarchy of complexity that extends from the simplest molecular and cellular levels, to tissues and organs of the body, to organ systems, and to the organism as a whole, its population, community, ecosystem, and beyond. The criteria that define one level are not necessarily of the same kind as those that determine the next. The human heart and its pacemaker cells, for example, may be distinguished in large measure from other organs and tissues by their anatomical or biochemical structures, but constituents of the circulatory system – heart, blood, arteries, capillaries, veins – are grouped together not

23 The expression ŠA$_3$.ZI.GA – literally, 'aroused-heart' – describes sexual virility that is actually functioning properly, rather than impotency resulting from the converse situation. Used as the title for a cuneiform text compilation of incantations for curing sexual impotency (edited in Biggs 1967), this label came to denote also difficulties in achieving arousal and penile erection, despite the positive sense of its literal meaning.

24 The writing *du-ur-gig-ga* stands for *durgigga*, a syllabic representation of the value of the logogram DUR$_2$.GIG meaning 'sick rectum.'

25 Geller (2001–2002) 61 and (2014) 4 and Steinert (2016) 231 interpreted the expression as 'womb which is twisted (*zīri*),' from the root *zâru* ('to twist'; *CAD* Z, 72–73). It is tempting to compare this to the Greek model of the 'wandering womb', which twists and moves about in the female body; cf. Faraone (2011) 1–32. Köcher (1978) 25, on the other hand, assumed partial elision of the expression 'womb which ⟨does not acquire⟩ seed (*zīri*),' apparently with the noun *zēru* ('seed'; *CAD* Z, 89–97). In my tentative understanding, the noun is *zīri* ('hate' or possibly 'hate (magic)'; *CAD* Z, 136–37) and expresses the notion that, contrary to its proper function, the 'womb' (*rēmu*) does not 'love' – the cognate verb *râmu* – i.e., accept and accommodate the unborn child.

primarily on the basis of observable or measurable similarities, but because of their cooperative contributions to the same bodily function.[26]

Although scholars so far have described the *Systemic Etiology* in terms of its four named organs – heart, stomach, lungs, kidneys – their discussions on how a particular sickness relates to an *organ* have tended to lapse into comparisons that belong more properly to *organ systems*. Steinert, for instance, observed the problem of ascribing the sickness *ṣinnaḫtiru* (§C6) to the lungs, since the literal meaning of this expression has to do with the 'evacuation (*ṣinnaḫ*) of the intestines (*tīri*), i.e., diarrhea,' but conceded that actual mentions of this sickness occur 'in connection with respiratory ailments and sicknesses of the mouth and throat region'[27] – a region that is therefore implied to be affiliated with the lungs.

In fact, it is significant that the *Etiology* assigns sicknesses to labels of the inner human anatomy – e.g., 'stomach' (*karšu*, §B) and 'lungs' (*ḫašû*, §C) – even though these labels appear relatively infrequently in descriptions of a patient's medical signs, which represent by far the major source of our anatomical knowledge from the cuneiform medical literature. Furthermore, while the terms *libbu* and *kalâtu* occur with some regularity in such semiotic descriptions, they are usually employed there as signifiers of the 'belly' and 'lateral region' of the human torso,[28] rather than as references to the 'heart' (§A) as a cognitive center and the 'kidney' (§D) as an internal organ, as is the case in the *Etiology*. These disparities result from the divergent aims of medical semiotics and etiology: Whereas medical signs that point to a sickness's identity are those perceptible to the healer's sight, touch, hearing, and smell, the attribution of sicknesses' origins to features of the inner anatomy – removed from sense experience – was aligned with the obscurity surrounding the details of

---

26 This is not to say that physical or chemical similarities could not have developed in response to challenges posed by the same function. The presence of valves both in veins and within the heart, for example, were a common answer to the problem of the backflow of blood, whether resulting from gravity or the pressure exerted by surrounding muscle.

27 'Einen interessanten Fall bildet die Zuordnung der Krankheit *ṣinnahti/uru* zur Lungensektion, da das Wort meist als *ṣinnah tīri* "Durchfall", wörtl. "Entleeren des Darms" analysiert wird. Diese Krankheit wird jedoch in den therapeutischen Texten in Verbindung mit Atemwegsbeschwerden und Erkrankungen des Mund- und Rachenbereichs erwähnt, so dass die genaue Bedeutung von *ṣinnahti/uru* unsicher bleibt.' Steinert (2016) 237.

28 See §G along with these couple more examples from the Diagnostic Handbook: 'If ditto (i.e., he is sick for one day), and he keeps placing his hands on his belly (*libbu*), (and) sucks his fingers, Hand of the great gods, he will die' (DIŠ KI.MIN-*ma ina* ŠA$_3$-*šu*$_2$ ŠU.2-*šu*$_2$ GAR.GAR U.MEŠ-*šu*$_2$ *u*$_2$-*na-ṣab* ŠU DINGIR *rab-bu-ti* GAM; Sa-gig 16: 3) and 'If his left lateral region (*kalītu*, singular of *kalâtu*) is collapsed, his illness will be prolonged' (DIŠ ELLAG$_2$ 150-*šu*$_2$ *muq-qu*$_2$*-ta-at*$_2$ GIG-*su* GID$_2$; Sa-gig 12: 68").

such origins, as well as the notion in Mesopotamian scribal culture that advanced knowledge was secret and hidden.[29]

In my understanding, organs mentioned in the *Systemic Etiology* are emblematic of larger systems defined by function rather than structure, and within which sicknesses were thought to originate. I wish to emphasize that these systems do not precisely map onto organ systems delineated in biology today, so that an exacting reader may for good reason prefer to retain the ancient labels of a 'Heart'-System, 'Stomach'-System, 'Lung'-System, or 'Kidney'-System. There are nonetheless striking similarities to modern counterparts in the *Etiology*'s systems, which possibly hint at universal or converging ways of categorizing bodily processes. In this essay, therefore, I see sufficient value in foregrounding such possibilities by referring to the systems as psychic (§A), alimentary (§B), and respiratory (§C), along with a lower-body system that combines excretory and reproductive functions (§D). I examine all these below, not according to their order of appearance in the text, but in order of decreasing clarity with which they illustrate their respective systems.

3.1 *Psychic System (§A)*

Whereas Hunger's reading of 'jaundice' (^{d}*aḫ̮ḫāzu*) for §A6 was influential for decades,[30] Köcher's proposal early on that the sickness here is actually '^{d}LUGAL.UR$_3$.RA' has gained support in recent times,[31] paving the way for the recognition that epileptic conditions – namely, AN.TA.ŠUB.BA (§A2), *bennu* (§A5), and ^{d}LUGAL.UR$_3$.RA (§A6) – are a particular concern in the first section of the *Systemic Etiology*. That these sicknesses belong together as a group is perhaps no more vividly demonstrated than in Chapter IV (Tablets 26–30) of the Mesopotamian Diagnostic Handbook titled Sa-gig,[32] which includes not only these labels, but also other epileptic states and associated conditions, such as 'Fall' (*miqtu*),[33] Spawn of Šulpaea, and *mišittu*-stroke. The last item will

29 Borger (1957–1971) 188–91; Lenzi (2008); Stevens (2013) 211–53.

30 Written ^{d}DIM$_3$.ME.ḪAB in Hunger (1976) 50 (text no. 43, obv. 6); followed by Geller (2001–2002) 61; Heeßel (2010) 30.

31 Köcher (1978) 35 n. 58; followed by Stol (1993) 16 n. 110; Geller (2014) 3; Steinert (2016) 231.

32 A good English translation and discussion of Chapter IV of the Diagnostic Handbook Sa-gig is provided by Stol (1993) 55–90. For the significance of chapter divisions in the Diagnostic Handbook, see Wee (2019a) 316–53. The modern publication history and differing paginations of the Diagnostic Handbook Sa-gig are too complicated to expound at length in this essay (see Wee, *ibid.* xix–xxv). Here, I refer to quotations from the Handbook using the prefix 'Sa-gig' before the tablet and line numbering in Heeßel (2000) and Scurlock (2014), without necessarily agreeing with the transcribed readings or translations by these authors.

33 The label 'Fall' (*miqtu*, logogram ŠUB) is likely related to 'AN.TA.ŠUB.BA' (lit. fallen-from-heaven).

be of special interest later, since the *Etiology* classifies *mišittu*-stroke (§B9) as originating 'from the mouth (and/of) stomach,' rather than 'from the heart' like the other epileptic sicknesses. In his book on *Epilepsy in Babylonia* (1993), Stol argued that various other afflictions occurred in close proximity to and in the same contexts as epilepsy, among which are the remaining labels at the beginning of the *Etiology* – i.e., Hand-of-god (§A3), Hand-of-goddess (§A4), and Heart-break (§A1), the last of which Stol suggested was a kind of melancholy on the basis of comparative Greek evidence.[34]

On the whole, the epileptic sicknesses in the first section of the *Etiology* are characterized by alterations in mental states and the loss of voluntary control over parts of one's body. Their alleged origin 'from the heart (*libbu*)' attributes these sicknesses to disturbances in one's psyche, rather than identify the person's 'belly' (*libbu*) as the location where they first exhibit their effects. At its most basic root, the Akkadian word *libbu* simply denoted the 'inside,' but the way cuneiform medical works often relied merely on context to distinguish the derived meanings of an abstract 'heart' versus the physical 'belly' could result in confusion – not only for the modern reader, but also in some cases for ancient audiences:

> (§F) [If his cranium] keeps (feeling) crushed all [day/night long], **his heart (*libbu*) keeps rising (*našû*)**, and the bedding keeps turning around about him; Like one who lies down upon a woman, he has arousal of heart (*nīš libbi*), Hand of the *ardat lilî*-demoness.[35]
>
> (§G) '**His *libbu* keeps rising**' *means* his belly (*libbu*) keeps coming up to vomit.[36]

In a description from the Diagnostic Handbook (§F), for example, a patient suffering from the attentions of an *ardat lilî*-demoness – a kind of demon that targets humans of the opposite sex – experiences sexual 'arousal of heart (*libbu*),' so that 'his heart (*libbu*) keeps rising' (in bold print above).[37] A later commentator (§G), however, misunderstood the expression in bold print as a reference to the 'belly' (*libbu*), and imagined that the patient is nauseous, so that his belly keeps heaving upwards in order to vomit. We will shortly revisit

34 Stol (1993) 27–38.

35 [DIŠ UGU-*šu*$_2$] *ka*[*l* U$_4$/GE$_6$ G]AZ.ME ŠA$_3$-*šu*$_2$(!) *i-ta-na-aš*$_2$*-ši-ma* KI.NA$_2$ *it-ta-na-as-ḫar*(!)-*šu* GIM *ša*$_2$ *ana* UGU MUNUS ŠUB-*tu* IL$_2$ ŠA$_3$ TUKU-*ši* ŠU K[I.SIKI]L.LIL$_2$.LA$_2$.EN.NA (Sa-gig 3: 13–14).

36 ŠA$_3$-*šu*$_2$ *i-ta-na-ši*$_2$(si) || Š[A$_3$]-*šu*$_2$ *ana* BURU$_8$ *e-te-ni-la-a* (*STT* 403 obv. 19) in Comm. Sa-gig 1–3, obv. 19 (Wee, *Mesopotamian Commentaries* (2019) 73, 76 and 86–87).

37 The terms translated 'arousal' (*nīš*) and 'rising' (*našû*) are cognates that derive from the same root.

this idea that sexual arousal originates from the heart, when we consider how the *Systemic Etiology* assigns 'ŠA$_3$.ZI.GA (lit. aroused-heart) condition' (§D2) instead to the kidneys.

For our purposes here, it suffices to note that there is no strict necessity to situate the psychic system of a Babylonian body particularly in the anatomical region of the 'belly.' As a matter of fact, in the head-to-foot arrangement of the Diagnostic Handbook Sa-gig (see below), the 'belly' (*libbu*, logogram ŠA$_3$) and a related term 'innards' (*qerbū*, logogram ŠA$_3$.MEŠ) are actually positioned beneath the 'chest' and 'epigastrium' (*rēš libbi*)[38] – so any supposed connection between the psyche and the cardiac organ is not quite explicit, at least in the cuneiform medical literature. On the other hand, the fact that the *Etiology* appears to follow a roughly similar head-to-foot order is tenuous evidence that the psychic system (§A) – mentioned first in the *Etiology* – could have been associated with the brain, since even the cardiac organ may be imagined as situated above the stomach and kidneys, if not also a large part of the lungs. Babylonian ideas about cognition are best considered on their own terms, rather than uncritically through the lens of the well-known dispute in Graeco-Roman antiquity, whether the seat of thought and reasoning resided in the brain or the heart.

The way I have portrayed the 'heart' (§A) in the *Systemic Etiology* as a kind of abstract quality may strike one as incommensurable with concrete organs like the 'stomach' (§B), 'lungs' (§C), and 'kidneys' (§D) subsequently mentioned. As we will shortly learn, however, even the latter were not intended to denote the named organs in isolation from the rest of the human anatomy. Rather, the labels 'stomach,' 'lungs,' and 'kidneys' served as emblems for larger and more intangible alimentary, respiratory, and excretory-reproductive systems – which, like the 'heart,' were defined primarily by function rather than physical features.

3.2 *Lower-Body Excretory and Reproductive System (§D)*

The combination of excretory and reproductive functions into a single system is suggested by the matter-of-fact manner in which the *Systemic Etiology* intersperses sicknesses of the former – Stricture (§D1), Sick rectum (§D3), and Retention of (flatulent) wind (§D7) – among conditions of the latter – ŠA$_3$.ZI.GA (§D2), Barrenness (§D5), and Womb (in the case) of hate (§D6). One obvious similarity between the two functions is the concentration of their organs in the lower half of the human body. Unrecognized was our modern

38 The term translated 'epigastrium' (*rēš libbi*) – literally, 'head / top' (*rēš*) of the 'belly' (*libbi*) – is not unambiguous enough to allow us to distinguish 'the region on top of the belly' from 'the top region of the belly.'

classification of skin and lungs as excretory organs, in that they remove sweat and carbon dioxide as waste products. Moreover, unlike Hippocratic medical schemes for which the regulation of internal humors was crucial for maintaining good health, Mesopotamian medicine did not quite view vomiting as an upper-body behavior symmetrical to bowel evacuations for the purpose of routinely purging the body of its contents.[39]

The perceived affinity between excretory and reproductive functions may also have been encouraged by the issue of their respective emissions from the same genitalia, as well as the cautious regard to which these emissions were subjected. Archaeology and texts on lavatories and sewers affirm the status of excrement as substances marked for disposal,[40] and the lavatory-demon Šulak even had its name pseudo-etymologized to depict its victim as one who failed to observe sanitary practice, so that his 'hand (ŠU) is not (*lā*) clean (KU_3).'[41] While menstrual blood and semen, admittedly, were understood to play vital roles in the reproductive process, they were nonetheless proscribed from certain socio-cultural contexts and even depicted using the language of 'taboo' and 'pollution.'[42] An introduction to a ritual (§H), for instance, labels as 'unclean' a man who appears to have lost control over the emission of his semen, to the extent that its occurrence is decoupled from the usual stimulus of the sexual 'arousal of his heart' (see also §I).

39 For example, the Hippocratic *Aphorisms* recommend that 'in summer purge preferably upwards, in winter downwards' (4.4) and 'pains above the diaphragm signify the need for upward purging, pains below for downward purging' (4.18). Admittedly, though, the Akkadian verb *parû*, which means 'to vomit (from the mouth)' in the large majority of cases, is used a few times in the idiom 'his rectum vomits (*iparru*)' at *BAM* 96 i 16'; 159 iii 13. See also discussion of §M and §N below, where bodily wind may be expelled from the rectum as flatulence or from the mouth as a belch.

40 See, for example, George (2015) 75–106.

41 Hunger (1976) 50 (text no. 47, obv. 2–5); Reiner et al. (1994) 92.

42 van der Toorn (1989) 348–50; Stol (2000) 4–5 and 205–6. Even Frandsen (2007: 81–105), who questioned the conception of a taboo for explaining the avoidance of contact with menstruating women, had to supply a solution rooted in ancient Egyptian culture and belief – namely, that because the Egyptian tomb was 'regarded as a uterus in which the mysterious process of rebirth takes place,' the workmen for the tomb had to separate themselves from influences of a different kind of 'procreation' associated with menstrual blood. To be sure, the sickness 'Spawn/Semen (*riḫûtu*) of Šulpaea' – mentioned above under the section on Psychic System (§A) – or other malevolent roles of 'semen' in medical texts may not depict the vileness of the substance per se, as much as its potential to further propagate agents of harm. So, for example, it is said of the rabid dog whose saliva transmits its sickness: 'it carries its semen in its mouth, where it bit, it left its offspring' (English translation and bibliography in Foster 2005, 190).

(§H) If a man's limbs are drained like a sick man's, … his feet (and) his *piṭru*[43] are limp, he speaks but does not arrive at (a conclusion), he is deprived of the arousal of his heart, his heart keeps becoming angry, he casts forth his semen, whether in his urine or regularly, like one who has had sexual intercourse with a woman – that man is unclean, god and goddess have turned away (?) from him, (so that) his speech is ⟨ not ⟩ acceptable.[44]

(§I) [If] a man's penis stings him, he casts forth semen when he urinates, he is seized [in] his belly/heart and diminished (in his sexual appetite) to go to a woman, (and) pus regularly flows from his penis – that man is sick with *mūṣu*. In order to heal him … (*instructions for preparing and applying medicaments*).[45]

Cuneiform sources do not clearly specify the mechanism by which urine and semen were simultaneously produced (§H and §I), but there was awareness that they derived from different loci in the inner anatomy. Descriptions of urinary problems frequently implicate, not only the penis, but also internal features like the urinary tract and the bladder, often going as far upstream as the kidneys.[46] On the other hand, the testicles were understood to be the source of semen, as implied by the remarkable equation 'testicle = son' in a cuneiform lexical list.[47] Birth anomalies could occur with 'empty' (*rīqu*) testicles, a word that was used also for 'unloaded' donkeys and boats, with the nuance of being 'without work.'[48] Significantly, the practice of castration to create eunuchs for important cultic and palace responsibilities depended on a low enough mortality rate from the procedure, which scholars have argued could have been achieved if – not the male genitalia in their entirety – but only the testicles

43 *CAD* P, 450 s.v. *piṭru* §2 (a part of the body).

44 *šum-ma* LU$_2$ *mi-na-tu-šu*$_2$ GIM *mar-ṣi* D[U]B.MEŠ-*ka* / […]x GIR$_3$.2-*šu*$_2$ *piṭ-ru-šu*$_2$ *ra-mu-u*$_2$ / *i-qab-bi-ma la i-kaš-šad ni-iš* ŠA$_3$-*šu*$_2$ *e-ṭi-ir* / ŠA$_3$-*šu*$_2$ *il-te-nem-men*$_5$(man) *lu-u ina* KAŠ$_3$-*šu*$_2$ *lu-u ka-am-ma ri-ḫu-ut-su* / *ki-ma ša* KI MUNUS *uš-ta-ḫu-u*$_{16}$(um) ŠUB-*su* / LU$_2$.BI *ul e-el* DINGIR *u*$_3$ ^{d}*Iš-tar* [s]*uḫ*-[*ḫ*]*u-ru-šu* (?) / DU$_{11}$.GA.BI ⟨ *ul* ⟩ [*m*]*a-ag-rat* (Ištar and Dumuzi *Hauptritual B*, MS C = *BAM* 319, obv. 1–7) adapted from Farber (1977) 227 and 236–37. The verb *uš-ta-ḫu-u*$_{16}$ derives from the root *šuḫḫû*, 'to have (illicit) sexual intercourse' (*CAD* Š III, 207).

45 [DIŠ N]A GIŠ$_3$-*šu*$_2$ *u*$_2$-*zaq-qa-su* U$_4$-*ma* KAŠ$_3$.MEŠ-*šu*$_2$ *i-ša*$_2$-*ti-nu ri-ḫu-su* ŠUB-*a* / [*ina*] ŠA$_3$-*šu*$_2$ *ṣa-bit-ma ana* MUNUS DU-*ka* LAL LUGUD *gi-na-a ina* GIŠ$_3$-*šu*$_2$ DU-*ak* / [NA.B]I *mu-ṣa* GIG *ana* TI-*šu*$_2$ … (*BAM* 112 i 17–21); cf. *BAM* 112 i 34'–39'; *AMT* 58/6: 2'–5'.

46 Geller (1995) 1811–15.

47 *iš-ku* = *ma-ar* (K 107+4382 rev. 1) in *CT* 18, plate 20.

48 *šumma izbu* XVII 29'–31' in Leichty (1970) 168; De Zorzi (2014) 751. For *rīqu*, see *AHw*, 987–88; *CAD* R, 371–73.

were removed or mutilated, perhaps even allowing high-ranking eunuchs to remain sexually active without the prospect and danger of siring heirs.[49]

It is telling that, as early as in the 2nd millennium BCE, one of the designations for the testicle was 'kidney of the lap' (*kalīt birki*).[50] This very likely alluded to how the testicle resembles the kidney in shape and the fact that each normally belongs to a pair, but it is intriguing to consider also whether the analogous roles of testicle and kidney as sources of penile emissions may have played a part in the naming. As a matter of fact, in contrast to the psychic system represented transpicuously by the abstract notion of the 'heart' (§A), the designation of the 'kidney' – and also the 'stomach' (§B) and the 'lungs' (§C) – as an emblem for its system foregrounded a concrete organ that is, in actuality, seldom explicitly named in the medical signs of sicknesses and conditions attributed to it (§D1–7).

Among these ailments listed in the *Etiology*, stricture (§D1) occurs most closely in association with the kidneys and, even then, appears instead as a descriptor of the urethra and the bladder – along with expressions like 'stricture of a sick rectum' and 'stricture of the loins' that contribute to the obscuration of boundaries between different excretory organs and perhaps also reproductive ones, by assigning all to the same type of sickness.[51] As I suggested earlier, reticent mentions of the kidney in these contexts can be ascribed to the different ends of medical semiotics and etiology. In an effort to represent a system encompassing both excretory and reproductive functions, nonetheless, the choice of kidney as emblem was particularly inspired, given the way it could have been regarded as an analogue of the testicle.

(§J) If a man pours out blood from his penis, **he is struck by a weapon like a woman (variant: wife)**; in order to heal him, you shall crush together legumes, *nuḫurtu*, and horned alkali, ... let (the medicaments) spend the night in the star,[52] (and) in the morning he shall drink (it) on an empty stomach, and he will become healthy.[53]

---

49 Peled (2016) 203–37; Biggs (1969) 100; Adamson (1991) 429.

50 *CAD* K, 74. Though occurring much less commonly than the usual word for 'testicle' (*išku*), the expression 'kidney of the lap' seems to have been sufficiently known to be used also in non-medical contexts and in the cuneiform lexical tradition.

51 Simkó (2013) 48–50 and 56; cf. Geller (2005) 1–2. Instead of the noun 'stricture' (*ḫiniqtu*), a different Akkadian noun was often preferred to indicate the 'constriction' (*kiṣirtu*) of the lungs or the belly.

52 For the celestial irradiation of medicaments and figurines as a means of improving their efficacy for healing, see Reiner (1995) 48–60; Wee (2014) 23–42.

53 DIŠ NA *ina* GIŠ$_3$-*šu*$_2$ MUD$_2$ *u*$_2$*-tab-ba-ka* GIM MUNUS (variant in MS A = *BAM* 396 iv 3: DAM) ^{giš}TUKUL *ma-ḫi-iṣ* / *ana* [T]I-*šu*$_2$ GU$_2$.GAL ^{u2}NU.LUḪ.ḪA NAGA.SI 1-*niš* SUD$_2$ /

(§K) If a man pours out blood from his rectum, **he is struck by a weapon like a woman**; in order to heal him, you shall crush together UGU. SUḪ$_2$.ḪA and seed of *dadānu*-carob, he shall drink (it) in boiled wine on an empty stomach, and he will become healthy.[54]

Most of the cuneiform medical literature employs the male body as shorthand for the human. Of special interest, however, are examples like these (§J and §K) that single out a regular feature of female physiology – i.e., menstruation – and elevate it as the interpretive key for male conditions involving bleeding from the penis or the rectum. Although medical writings make use of the imagery of physical subjugation in depicting the actions of sicknesses, they less commonly address actual physical injuries,[55] and the reference to a 'weapon' here should be understood as a metaphor for a specific kind of blood loss – since the metaphor appears to be restricted, in fact, to the penis and the rectum, and not generally used for bleeding from other orifices like the nose or the ears. Indeed, menstrual blood was clearly recognized as fulfilling vital objectives in the reproductive process – from its role inaugurating a woman's pregnancy[56] to its nourishment of the foetus in the womb[57] – so its comparison to blood loss from the male penis or rectum represented yet one more way that organs functioning in excretion and reproduction could at times be treated without clear distinction from each other.

A final remark needs to be made concerning the sickness *sagallu* (§D4), whose name derives etymologically from the logograms SA ('strands') and GAL ('large'). Because *sagallu* often appears in a group with other muscle disorders (§T), one might easily assume that the 'strands' in its name allude to fibers of muscle. Thus, Labat translated the term as 'dicke Muskeln,' and Geller referred to it simply as 'muscle disease.'[58] Furthermore, in the Standard Babylonian Recension (1st millennium BCE) of the lexical *List of Medical Terms*, a section

[…] *ina* MUL$_4$ *tuš-bat ina še-rim* NU *pa-tan* NAG-*ma* TI (*BAM* 159 i 9–11) = MS XX in Geller (2005) 40–41 (text no. 1, col. iv 3–5).

54 DIŠ NA *ina* DUR$_2$-*šu*$_2$ MUD$_2$ *u*$_2$-*tab-ba-ka* GIM MUNUS ^{giš}TUKUL SIG$_3$-*iṣ* / *ana* TI-*šu*$_2$ UGU.SUḪ$_2$.ḪA NUMUN ^{giš}KIŠI$_{16}$.ḪAB 1-*niš* SUD$_2$ / *ina* GEŠTIN *ba-aš*$_2$-*li* NU *pa-tan* NAG-*ma* TI (*BAM* 152 iii 8–10) = MS AD in Geller (2005) 214–15 (text no. 35, obv. 27–29).

55 Procedures for treating open wounds and fractures were learned mostly manually and mastered by repeated practice, rather than from descriptions in medical texts.

56 Stol (2000) 49.

57 The association of the loss of amniotic fluid and blood with miscarriage in Mesopotamian gynecological texts, for example, suggests 'a pregnant woman's menstrual blood is needed to nourish the foetus'. Steinert (2017) 318 n. 92.

58 Labat (1957–1971) 126–27; Geller (2001–2002) 61, (2010) 123, and (2014) 4. Attia (2000) 53 and Scurlock and Andersen (2005) 729 n. 44 identify *sagallu* with sciatica.

with lines each beginning with the element SA ('strands') includes names of other muscle conditions, such as *maškadu* (§B8 in the *Etiology*) and *šaššaṭu*.[59]

While Kinnier Wilson's proposal to link *sagallu* to filariasis has been unconvincing, he offered a suggestion in the process that should not be overlooked – namely, that the 'large-strands' actually denote, not muscle fibres, but the dilated appearance of varicose veins.[60] These varicose veins occur most commonly in the lower body, causing pain during prolonged standing and walking upright, in agreement with cuneiform descriptions of how '[the strands] of (the patient's) thigh hurt him all at the same time, (so that) he is unable to rise up and walk about' (§T). Pertinent to the *Etiology* is the frequency with which varicose veins develop in the course of pregnancy, with pressures on the lower body exacerbated by weight gain, increased blood volume, and changes to blood flow caused by an enlarging uterus – so that *sagallu* came to be classified in the *Etiology*, not primarily as a muscle disorder, but as an ailment integral to the excretory-reproductive system.

3.3 *Respiratory System (§C)*

The 'lungs' are emblematic of the respiratory system in the *Systemic Etiology*. Certainly, these organs could be vulnerable and affected by conditions of other viscera in the abdominal cavity, so that *su'ālu*-cough, for instance, became known as a medical sign affiliated with stomach sickness.[61] But the specialized role of lungs in breathing and as the production site of phlegm likely explains why they appear here in a separate section on the respiratory system (§C), as opposed to the more broadly defined alimentary system (§B). The metaphor of a musical wind instrument sometimes appears in descriptions of lungs that

59 See statements on *maškadu* (nos. 73–76) and *šaššaṭu* (nos. 79–83) in Kilmer (1967) 93–94.

60 Kinnier Wilson (1962) 61. For the argument that SA ('strands') can refer to blood vessels, see Oppenheim (1962) 27–33.

61 The medical sign of *su'ālu*-cough receives first mention in a therapeutic sub-corpus (VIII) on the STOMACH and therefore becomes prominent as part of its incipit-title: 'If a man is sick with *su'ālu*-cough (and) it turns for him into Constriction of the Belly' (Steinert 2018, 211). Johnson (2017) 112 argued that the *Assur Medical Catalog*, to which this STOMACH sub-corpus belongs, 'involves the conceptualization of the gastrointestinal system in its entirety as a single canal or waterway leading from mouth to anus. The regular movement of food and drink through the alimentary canal is the presupposed norm against which the illnesses found in the STOMACH sub-corpus are defined.' Even if one accepts this model, *su'ālu*-cough may still retain its traditional definition as a condition of the lungs and respiratory system, which are affected by – but not an integral component of – the alimentary canal that Johnson described.

'whistle' and of a trachea that 'whistles its songs like a reed pipe.'[62] Indeed, the logographic depiction of the trachea as the 'long reed' (GI.GID$_2$) of the 'lungs' (MUR.MEŠ) may allude to the same metaphor, while an alternative writing (GU$_2$.MUR) portrays the trachea as simultaneously a feature of the 'neck' (GU$_2$) and the 'lung' (MUR). Both options represent attempts to characterize the trachea in ways that distinguish it from another tube-like passage that runs closely parallel to it – namely, the oesophagus, which constitutes part of the neighboring alimentary canal.

While under the organizing rubric of the 'lungs' in the *Etiology*, medical signs of the sicknesses *bu'šānu* (§C5), *ezizzu* (§C4), and perhaps lu.bi (§C1)[63] tend to focus on observable characteristics of the nasal and oral regions. Furthermore, in many medical descriptions, 'wind' is more commonly portrayed in the context of flatulence. An incantation (§L), for example, depicts both constipation and the 'retention of (flatulent) wind' (§D7) as the result of internal obstruction, which can be clear away by the invocation of divine beings who perform roles analogous to workmen on a blocked canal – so it is understandable that the *Etiology* assigns the problem of flatulence to the lower body excretory and reproductive system.

(§L) Of what are your insides full? [Of what] are your insides [full]? ... your insides ... Whom shall I send to the canal inspector inside you, so that they may take up spades of silver (and) shovels of gold, open the rivers (and) open the canals? May his excrement escape and come out! May the whirlwind inside him come out and see the sun! ...[64]

(§M) ... He has been blown into by the wind of the steppe, he keeps pouring out a libation for it. His eyes fill the steppe, his lips [keep] becoming dry. He keeps flopping about like a fish, he keeps bloating up like a snake. Gula, who provides human health, saw the young man and brought him to the temple of Asalluhi. Merciful Ea looked upon him (and said): 'Belch and get well, young man!' If it is wind, may it go out through the rectum! If it is a belch, may one make it go out through the throat![65]

62 'His lungs whistle' (*ḫa-šu-šu i-ḫal-lu-la*; Sa-gig 22: 71–72); '(My) trachea ... let whistle its songs like a reed pipe' (*ur-u$_2$-du* ... *i-ra-tu-ša$_2$ ma-li-liš uḫ-ta*[*l-lil*(?)]; Lambert (1960) 52–54; cf. *CAD* U/W, 268 s.v. *ur'udu* §1a.1').

63 For interpretations on this sickness, see footnote 20 on lu.bi (§C1) in my translation of the *Systemic Etiology* above.

64 Composite edition titled 'Belly 9' in Collins (1999) 134–36.

65 Edition of *BAM* 574 ii 21–27 (titled 'Belly 25') in Collins (1999) 166–67.

(§N) The chest is his fermenting vat, wind is his fermenting mixture. This incantation, which Marduk brought to existence in the land, [is for] his belly and [his] head ...[66]

Other incantations, however, suggest an alternative passage for the escape of bodily wind, namely, 'through the throat' (§M). It must be emphasized that the identity or the quality of wind was not a determining factor in the way it had to be expelled – rather, that healing occurred via the removal of the offending wind from any opening accessible, whether through the mouth or the anus.[67] This is illustrated by the imagery in §N, which compares the body to an ancient fermenting vessel, with outlets at the top and at the bottom for the release of gases produced in fermentation.[68] The double mention of 'wind' in the *Etiology* as an issue both of the excretory-reproductive system (§D7) and, here, of the respiratory system (§C3) should be understood in this light.

(§O) If the breathing of a man's nose is difficult, (he is sick with) *ṣinnaḫtiru* (and) the burning of *ṣētu*-heat ... (*instructions for preparing and applying medicaments*).[69]

The problem with the etymology of *ṣinnaḫtiru* (§C6) – literally, 'evacuation (*ṣinnaḫ*) of the intestines (*tīri*)' – has already been noted, and the best solution may be to assume that perceptions of the sickness expanded or altered over time. In the medical statement above (§O), which in fact comes from a therapeutic tablet from the same Šangû-Ninurta library as the *Etiology* itself,[70] breathing difficulties are listed as a stand-alone sign that can point to *ṣinnaḫtiru*. This statement is illuminating, also, because of the way 'burning of *ṣētu*-heat' (§B12) is included in the diagnosis, which has implications for its discussion later. Finally, *šīqu* (§C2) is listed in close proximity with *su'ālu*-cough in a vademecum of therapeutic plants,[71] and descriptions of *šīqu* 'in (the

66 Edition of PBS 7 87 (CBS 1690) rev. (titled 'Belly 6') in Collins (1999) 129–30.

67 The different terms 'wind' (*šāru*) and 'belch' (*gišâtu*) in §M were used for poetic variation – as is common in such incantation narratives – and should not be misunderstood as references to different types of gaseous substances.

68 Collins (1999) 81.

69 DIŠ NA *na-piš* KIR_4-$šu_2$ DUGUD *ṣi-in-[na-aḫ]-ti-ru ḫi-miṭ* UD.[DA ...]. Hunger (1976) 51 (text no. 44, line 1).

70 This detail on provenance is correctly emphasized also in Steinert (2016) 237 n. 132.

71 *BAM* 1 ii 27–33 and 37–40.

patient's) belly' or appearing at the 'lips' may be suggestive of sputum of some kind.[72]

3.4 *Alimentary System (§B)*

In terms of interpretation, this is the most difficult section in the *Systemic Etiology*. At stake are four issues: (1.) The identity of the bodily organ(s) at §B1 emblematizing the system, (2.) the anaphoric referents of the extra 'ditto' notations in §B3–§B5 and their meaning, (3.) the rationale for gathering under this system a miscellany of sicknesses that belong elsewhere in diverse categories, and (4.) the meaning of the expression 'any/all sickness' (§B12), which appears to contradict the practice of listing only a specific name or type of sickness per line.

The internal organ (§B1) that represents this section has been understood by scholars as 'stomach'[73] or 'mouth (KA) of stomach,'[74] with the latter interpreted as the throat or oesophagus. I lean towards this latter opinion, while also allowing for the possibility of asyndeton, i.e., 'mouth (and) stomach,' so that the organizing principle in any case is the alimentary system.[75]

Furthermore, most were of the view that 'mouth (*pi-i*)' in a line below (§B2)[76] belongs to the *left* column, and that this term 'mouth' is the referent of the extra 'ditto' notations (§B3–§B5). The resulting explanations have been unsatisfactory. Those who thought the *Etiology* introduces the 'stomach' at §B1 had to believe that it almost immediately switches focus to the 'mouth (allegedly, of the stomach)' (§B2–§B5), before returning again to the topic of the 'stomach' proper (§B6–§B12) – and, indeed, that the ancient scribe supposed

---

72 *ina* ŠA$_3$-*šu*$_2$ *ši-qu* (Sa-gig 13: 92); NUNDUN.MEŠ-*šu*$_2$ *ši-qa*$_2$ ŠUB-*a* (Sa-gig 13: 89). Suggested as 'colored sputum' by Scurlock and Andersen (2005) 42 and 688 n. 84; 'bronchitis' by Fincke (2000) 148.

73 '*ul-tu ka-*⌈*ar*⌉*-šu*$_2$ … Aus dem Magen' in Köcher (1978) 24; '*ul-tu ka-ar-šu*$_2$ … from the belly' in Geller (2001–2002) 61; 'Aus dem Magen' in Heeßel (2010) 30; cf. '*ul-tu* KA.KA?.ŠU$_2$' in Hunger (1976) 50 (text no. 43, obv. 7).

74 '*ul-tu* KA *kar-šu*$_2$ … from the throat' in Geller (2014) 3–8; 'Aus dem Magen-Mund (*pī karši*)' and 'Der "Magen-Mund des Mundes" bezeichnet offensichtlich die obere, zur Speiseröhre hinführende Öffnung des Magens' in Steinert (2016) 231 and n. 103.

75 But note also the contrary opinion that, 'as several of the diseases originating in this organ are diseases of the head, "the head" (or a part of it) seems to be more likely' and 'this would require at least one emendation, like SAG instead of KA, unless we may read *ka-li-šu*$_2$: *kallu* is "the crown of the human skull" …' in Stol (1993) 26–27 and n. 31.

76 The word 'mouth' is written as the logogram KA in §B1, but as the syllable signs *pi-i* in §B2, even though it would have been very natural and easy for the same orthography to have been adopted in both cases. One wonders if this distinction in writing served to emphasize the fact that different referents were intended – the 'mouth' (KA) of stomach (i.e., throat/oesophagus) versus the oral cavity (*pi-i*).

he could convey the relatively rare expression 'mouth of stomach' lucidly enough and without confusion by using only the term 'mouth' (§B2–§B5).[77] Those who preferred the reading 'mouth of stomach' from the very start (§B1) were obligated to explain why the term 'mouth' needed to be explicitly written out as *pi-i* (§B2) and not simply implied by KI.MIN ('ditto') as is the practice in all the other sections (§A, §C, and §D), as well as why the double 'ditto, ditto' (§B3–§B5) later reverts back to a single 'ditto' (§B6–§B12). Geller argued that the entire phrase '(from the throat and) mouth and tooth' (§B2) – referring to the actual oral cavity, not the stomach – was meant by the extra 'ditto' notations (§B3–§B5).[78] Steinert suggested that these notations in fact designate the ordinal number 'second,' so that the resulting phrase 'second stomach-mouth' denoted 'the lower exit of the stomach leading to the duodenum,' and that the single 'ditto's thereafter (§B6–§B12) referred particularly to the duodenal region.[79]

In my understanding, the phrase 'mouth and tooth' (§B2) belongs instead to the *right* column and is replicated by the extra 'ditto' notations (§B3–§B5).[80] The names of sicknesses in §B3 and §B4 are unfortunately too damaged to read on the manuscript. The labels 'mouth (and) tooth of *bu'šānu* sickness' (§B2) and '(mouth and tooth) of *pāšittu* sickness (with) gall' (§B5), on the other hand, depict the diseased condition of the oral cavity in the event of these sicknesses, which the *Etiology* classifies as problems of the alimentary system. This interpretation finds support in a second mention of *bu'šānu* (§C5) as trouble for the respiratory system – presumably referring to features of the sickness like cramped innards, feverish chest and back, and copious and bloody phlegm, which were regarded as separate from 'mouth (and) tooth' conditions such as oral *bubu'tu*-vesicles and difficulty using one's mouth.[81]

77 Köcher (1978) 24; Heeßel (2010) 30 nn. 37–38.

78 Or, more precisely, 'mouth and teeth (plural)' (§B2) in Geller (2014) 7. He did not clearly say what the 'ditto' notations in §B6–§B12 exactly mean.

79 Steinert (2016) 231 nn. 104–5.

80 Admittedly, the phrase 'mouth and tooth' (§B2) is written farther left than the left margin of the right column, but a transgression of column boundaries was not uncommon, particularly since the scribe here must have known in advance that the signs he intended to write could not all fit into the right column on a single line, and that the format of this tablet assigned to each line preferably a new sickness or condition. Steinert (2016) 231 n. 103 objected that '*pi-i* [§B2] nicht zu den rechts davon aufgezählten Krankheiten gehören kann, welche im Nominativ stehen.' But case endings are not reliably reflected in the orthography of late texts like the *Systemic Etiology*, as evident also from the supposedly nominative terms *mi-šit-ti* (§B9), *ša*$_2$*-a-ri* (§C3), *ḫi-niq*$_2$*-ti* (§D1), and *la a-li-du-ti* (§D5) that look like genitive forms.

81 '[If his mouth] is full of [*bubu'tu*-vesicles], and his saliva flows, *bu'šānu* is [its] name. [If an infant's saliva] holds blood, *bu'šānu* is [its] name. [If an infant's innards] are cramped, and his mouth is difficult, *bu'šānu* is [its] name. [If an infant's cranium, his chest], and his

(§P) Gall, gall, gall (from) *pāšittu* sickness! Gall keeps walking about like a yellow heron.[82] It keeps standing on the reed enclosure of the wall. It looks upon those eating bread, (and) it looks upon those drinking beer, (and says): 'When you eat bread (and) when you drink beer, I will fall upon you, and you will belch like an ox!'[83]

The short narrative in the incantation above (§P) illustrates the *Etiology*'s categorization of *pāšittu* (§B5) as an ailment arising from the consumption of food and drink through the alimentary system, along with its manifestation by means of gall. Similarly, in a curse for the violation of a treaty, the god Ea is asked to give the offender 'deadly water to drink,' and to 'fill (him) with dropsy (§B6).'[84] Other sicknesses in this section may not be as unambiguously connected to nutrition or to the digestive organs. As we already learned, *maškadu* (§B8) was considered a muscle disorder (§T), and *mišittu*-stroke (§B9) associated with epileptic conditions otherwise assigned to the psychic system (§A). Meanwhile, both *ašû* (§B10) and *giṣṣatu* (§B11) appear as sicknesses that affect the skin. It is not difficult to speculate about possible reasons these were classified as alimentary conditions, especially when the category is defined so broadly as to include any 'sickness of the head or the mouth' (§B1) – so that an eye that is pressed down and fixed in place due to *mišittu*-stroke,[85] or the inflammation of the face and diminished eyesight owing to *ašû*,[86] could all have been grounds for ascribing the sickness to an alimentary complex that

---

back keep becoming hot, *buʾšānu* is [its] name.' ([DIŠ KA-*šu*$_2$ *bu-bu-ʾ*]-*ta* SA$_5$ *u il-la-tu-šu il-*⸢*la*⸣-*ka bu-ʾ-ša*$_2$*-nu* MU.[NI] / [DIŠ LU$_2$.TUR *il-la-tu-š*]*u*$_2$ MUD$_2$ *u*$_2$*-kal-la bu-ʾ-ša*$_2$*-nu* MU.[NI] / [DIŠ LU$_2$.TUR ŠA$_3$.MEŠ-*šu*$_2$] *eb-ṭu*$_2$ ⸢*u*⸣ KA-*šu*$_2$ *k*[*a-b*]*it bu-ʾ-ša*$_2$*-nu* MU.[NI] / [DIŠ LU$_2$.TUR UGU-*šu*$_2$ GABA-*s*]*u u ša*$_2$*-šal-la-šu*$_2$ KUM$_2$.MEŠ *bu-ʾ-ša*$_2$*-nu* MU.[NI]) in Sa-gig 33: 87–90. 'If an infant's cry is stifled, but he does not have mucus, BI.LU sickness seizes him' (DIŠ LU$_2$.TUR *ik-kil-la-šu*$_2$ *e-sir*$_2$ *u*$_2$*-pa-ṭi* NU *i-šu* BI.LU *ṣab-tu-šu*$_2$) in Sa-gig 40: 114. The label BI.LU is defined as (a kind of) *buʾšānu* in Comm. Sa-gig 1–3, obv. 19 (Wee, *Mesopotamian Commentaries* (2019) 73, 76, and 86–87).

82 I wonder if the reference here is to the yellow eyes of several heron species, which resemble the jaundiced appearance of the whites of the eyes in cases of patients who suffer from high levels of bilirubin – i.e., a contributor to the yellow color of gall.

83 Edition of *BAM* 578 ii 39–44 (titled '*martu* 1') in Collins (1999) 230–31.

84 Esarhaddon's Succession Treaty, §60 (lines 521–22) in Parpola and Watanabe (1988) 51.

85 'If a man has *mišittu*-stroke of the face, his eye is pressed down (and) constantly fixed day and night, (so that) he cannot sleep, (and) he cannot stop rubbing his face incessantly with honey and ghee …' (DIŠ NA *mi-šit-ti pa-ni i-šu* IGI-*šu*$_2$ *i-*⸢*ṣap-par*⸣ [*u*]*r-ra u* GE$_6$ *ur-ta-na-at-t*[*i*] / *la it-ta-na-a-a-al ina* LAL$_3$ I$_3$.NU[N.N]A IGI.MEŠ-*šu*$_2$ *ka-a-a-nam-ma muš-š*[*u-da*] / *la i-kal-la* …) in *AMT* 76/5: 11'–13'.

86 '[If] his face keeps becoming inflamed, his eyesight is diminished, his body is full of *birdu*-marks, and his belly seizes him – *ašû* is its name.' ([DIŠ *pa*]-*nu-šu*$_2$ MU$_2$.MEŠ-*ḫu di-gil*$_2$*-šu*$_2$ *ma-ṭi* SU-*šu*$_2$ *bir-di ma-lu u* ŠA$_3$-*šu*$_2$ [D]AB-*su a-šu-u*$_2$ MU.NI) in Sa-gig 33: 5.

influenced the head and that extended downwards into the inner parts of the human anatomy.

Indeed, in the head-to-foot organization of the Diagnostic Handbook Sa-gig (discussed below), it is remarkable that about two-thirds of medical statements[87] begin with a sign from the head and the neck, illustrating the disproportional attention given to manifestations of sicknesses in the facial, nasal, and oral regions – not to mention the effects of maladies felt in the area of the stomach or abdomen. To be sure, the mouth appears positioned at the junction between alimentary and respiratory systems, being implicated in activities of eating, drinking, and vomiting, along with those of breathing, coughing, and the expectoration of phlegm. In the *Systemic Etiology*, however, one gets the impression that respiratory conditions and ailments were the more rigidly defined, and that the alimentary system seems to display the character somewhat of a catch-all category.

The phrase 'any/all sickness' (§B12) sticks out in an *Etiology* that otherwise appears interested to identify specific ailments or to narrowly describe certain types of illnesses. One solution is to view it as an extension of the nature of *ṣētu*-heat (§B12), referring therefore to 'all sickness (of this kind),' i.e., all kinds of fevers.[88] Another proposal links the phrase to the logographic expression TU.RA KILIB$_3$.BA – meaning 'all sickness' – that appears as the title of *one among other* cuneiform text series on medicine,[89] and as *one among other* analogous statements in a Late Babylonian composition on medical astrology,[90] thereby placing TU.RA KILIB$_3$.BA on parity with other specifically named sicknesses despite the literal meaning of 'all sickness.'

> (§Q) If a man's innards keep becoming inflamed, his bowels keep making much noise like (the call) of an *iš qippu*-bird ... that man is sick with bloating of wind and *ṣētu*-heat. Should its effects prolong, Hand-of-ghost ... (*instructions for preparing and applying medicaments*).[91]

87 In the head-to-foot arrangement of the Diagnostic Handbook Chapter II (Tablets 3–14), the contents of Tablets 3–10 focus on the head and neck region.

88 'Brennen der Hitze(-Fieber) (*ḫimiṭ ṣēti*) und alle Krankheiten (dieser Art?)' in Steinert (2016) 231.

89 Composite edition of the *Exorcist Manual*, line 9 in Jean (2006) 65.

90 *LBAT* 1597, obv. 5' in Geller (2014) 80.

91 DIŠ NA ŠA$_3$.MEŠ-*šu*$_2$ MU$_2$.MEŠ-*ḫu ir-ru-šu*$_2$ GIM *ša*$_2$ MAR.GAL *ma-gal* GU$_3$.G[U$_3$-*u* ...] / NA.BI *ni-kim-tu*$_2$ IM UD.DA GIG KIN-*šu*$_2$ *i-la-bir-ma* ŠU.GI[DIM.MA ...] (*BAM* 51, lines 66–67).

(§R) If a man (has) burning of *ṣētu*-heat, blast of wind, *šimmatu*, *rimûtu*, *šaššaṭu*, Hand-of-ghost, Hand-of-oath-curse, sick rectum, (or) **any sickness** – in order to heal him, (*instructions for preparing and applying medicaments*).[92]

(§S) If a man *ditto* (i.e., is overcome with *ṣētu*-heat), (or) **any (type of) burning of *ṣētu*-heat**; [You shall dry] *aprušu*-plant (and) *elkullu*-plant from the well, mix (them) with oil of *kukru*-plant, keep salving him, and he will become healthy.[93]

In translating 'Burning of *ṣētu*-heat of any sickness' (§B12), I have taken the phrase to mean that *ṣētu*-heat can occur in connection with other kinds of sicknesses – even those belonging to other organ systems – and that the *ṣētu*-heat component of such situations is nevertheless to be attributed to the alimentary system. Elsewhere, for example, we find that *ṣētu*-heat can arise together with the respiratory ailment *ṣinnaḫtiru* (§O) or the muscle disorder *kiṣṣatu* (§T), and it is paired above with 'bloating of wind' (§Q) that could be a sickness of the respiratory or the excretory-reproductive system. In other instances, the phrase 'any sickness' is used to ensure that no sickness relevant to the purpose at hand is inadvertently forgotten (§R) – occurring at the end of a list of sicknesses that can appear somewhat unrelated to each other, but that in fact are relieved by the same remedial prescription. Finally, the reference to 'any (type of) burning of *ṣētu*-heat' (§S) comes closest to the sense expressed in the *Etiology*. In fact, this medical statement (§S) comes from a tablet devoted to *ṣētu*-heat that belongs to a therapeutic text sub-corpus on the stomach region,[94] shedding light on the *Etiology*'s rationale for treating *ṣētu*-heat as an alimentary condition.

3.5 *Unrepresented Modern Organ Systems*

It is worth briefly musing on possible reasons for the absence of Mesopotamian analogues to other modern organ systems. Muscular, skeletal, and integumentary systems were not separately categorized, because the ancient authors probably considered their constituents of muscle, bone, skin, and hair, among other features, to be part of the general architecture of the human body, which operated in the background of each of the systems discussed above. Revealingly,

92 DIŠ NA TAB UD.DA *ši-biṭ* IM *šim-ma-tu*$_2$ *ri-mu-tu*$_2$ *ša*$_2$*-aš*$_2$*-ša*$_2$*-ṭu* / ŠU.GIDIM.MA ŠU.NAM.ERIM$_2$ DUR$_2$.GIG DU$_3$ GIG *ana* TI-*šu*$_2$ (*BAM* 168 obv. 18–19).

93 DIŠ NA EŠ$_5$ TAB-*iṭ* UD.DA DU$_3$.A.BI-*ma* ^{u2}*ap-ru*$_3$*-ša*$_2$ ^{u2}*il*$_3$-⸢*kul*$_2$*-la*⸣ *ša*$_2$ TUL$_2$ *tu*(!)-[*bal*] / *ina* I$_3$ ^{šim}GUR$_2$.GUR$_2$ ḪE.ḪE ŠEŠ$_2$.MEŠ-⸢*su*⸣-*ma* T[I] (*BAM* 66 rev. 14'–15').

94 *BAM* 66 rev. 14'–15' = MS C of Tablet 4 of the therapeutic text sub-corpus titled SUALU (or, elsewhere, STOMACH). See Johnson (2014) 30–31 (line 11 in composite edition).

therapeutic descriptions of patients whose sickness 'appears in her flesh and in her strands,' or concerning whom 'the flesh (and) strands of his feet are stiff,' suggest that 'flesh' and 'strands' were thought to compose the soft substance of the human body that clothed the bare skeleton.[95] Much remains unclear of ancient Mesopotamian conceptions of brain material, or the extent to which nerves were recognized as a different kind of 'strand' from blood vessel and muscle fiber, so the failure to articulate a nervous system is unsurprising.

Mesopotamian myths require the incorporation of some element of divine origin in the process of creating humankind. In the *Babylonian Creation Myth* (*Enūma eliš*), the spilled blood of the enemy god Qingu becomes the material from which humans are formed, who accordingly inherit the penalty of servitude towards the gods.[96] In the Babylonian Flood Story (also known today by the title *Atra-ḫasīs*), the god *Wê-ila* hatches a 'scheme' (*ṭēmu*) to rebel against the great god Enlil, but is eventually slaughtered and his flesh and blood used to create the 'human' (*awīlu*) with his 'ghost' (*eṭemmu*), whose heartbeats are described as a drum that would resound for the rest of time.[97] It is likely, therefore, that Babylonian healers viewed blood as a substance infused with the vitality of human life itself, similar to what we find as well in other ancient cultures.[98] But it is less certain that the ancients appreciated the role of blood as a medium conveying nourishment throughout the body – much less as a carrier of oxygen and carbon dioxide, hormones, and immunological elements – so we cannot expect much progress on the formulation of circulatory, endocrine, and lymphatic systems.

4 Holisms of Form and Function

Already in the first half of the second millennium BCE, an Old Babylonian cuneiform lexical list titled Ugu-mu ('My Cranium')[99] inventoried parts of the human body, beginning at the cranium on top of the head and moving down

95 *ina* UZU.MEŠ-*ša*$_2$ *u* SA.MEŠ-*ša*$_2$ ⸢GAL$_2$-*ši*⸣ (*BAM* 240 obv. 59'); UZU SA GIR$_3$.2-*šu*$_2$ ⸢*ša*$_2$-*gu-ma*⸣ (*AMT* 68/1 rev. 5); cf. the ambiguity of whether to read UZU SA ('flesh (and) strands') or ^{uzu}SA ('strands,' with *flesh* as a determinative or noun-classifier) in *AMT* 44/4: 1.

96 *Enūma eliš* VI, 29–36 in Lambert (2013) 110–13.

97 *Atra-ḫasīs* (Old Babylonian Version) I, 208–30 in Lambert and Millard (1999) 58–59.

98 Keyser (2017) 168–203.

99 Cuneiform compositions conventionally derive their title from their incipit – i.e., the first words or line of the composition – which, in the case of this head-to-foot list, consists of the words 'my cranium.'

towards the foot. Owing to a preference for acrophonic and orthographic criteria[100] in the cuneiform lexical tradition, however, Ugu-mu seems to have been phased out over time, though its principle of enumerating the body *a capite ad calcem* would manifest itself repeatedly in narratives of literary, religious, and magic genres, and came to shape how later medical works were organized.[101]

According to a remarkable paragraph ascribed to the venerated Babylonian scholar Esagil-kīn-apli from the eleventh century BCE,[102] he is said to have 'deliberated within himself, and (descriptions of the human body in) the Mesopotamian Diagnostic Handbook Sa-gig from the cranium to the feet became held together 'as a new weave' and ratified as knowledge.' The metaphor envisioned older diagnostic textual traditions as threads that were unraveled and rewoven together to create a new edition, a prominent feature of which was the arrangement of medical statements in Chapter II of the Handbook (Tablets 3–14) in head-to-foot order of their first medical sign. Therapeutic works such as the *Assur Medical Catalog* likewise favored this anatomical organization, applying it not to signs but to the sicknesses themselves.[103]

As part of developments in medical astrology during the final centuries BCE, the pairing of zodiacal signs with regions of the human body from head to foot gave rise to the Zodiac Man – a figure that would appear centuries later in Medieval Latin manuscripts as *Homo signorum* (see, for example, Figure 13.1), whose images adorn calendars, devotional Books of Hours, and academic treatises of the time. Already when describing the Zodiac Man discovered in a cuneiform tablet, moreover, I made these observations:

> 'The stereotypical Zodiac Man seems to be the product of purely metrical considerations that dissected the human frame into sections of roughly equal height, so that only one zodiacal sign (Aries) deals with the head, while an extraordinary total of four zodiacal signs (Sagittarius–Pisces) concern themselves with the legs,' and 'symmetry between cosmos and body in the Zodiac Man was achieved by projecting the spatial and

100 Acrophonic lists group together lexical terms that each begin with the same sound or syllable, while orthographic lists group together terms that each begin with the same written cuneiform sign or signs.

101 Couto-Ferreira (2017) 43–68.

102 I refer to this paragraph as *Esagil-kīn-apli's Manifesto* in Wee (2019a) 29–35; earlier edited in Finkel (1988) 148–50.

103 For an edition of the *Assur Medical Catalog*, see Steinert (2018) 209–19.

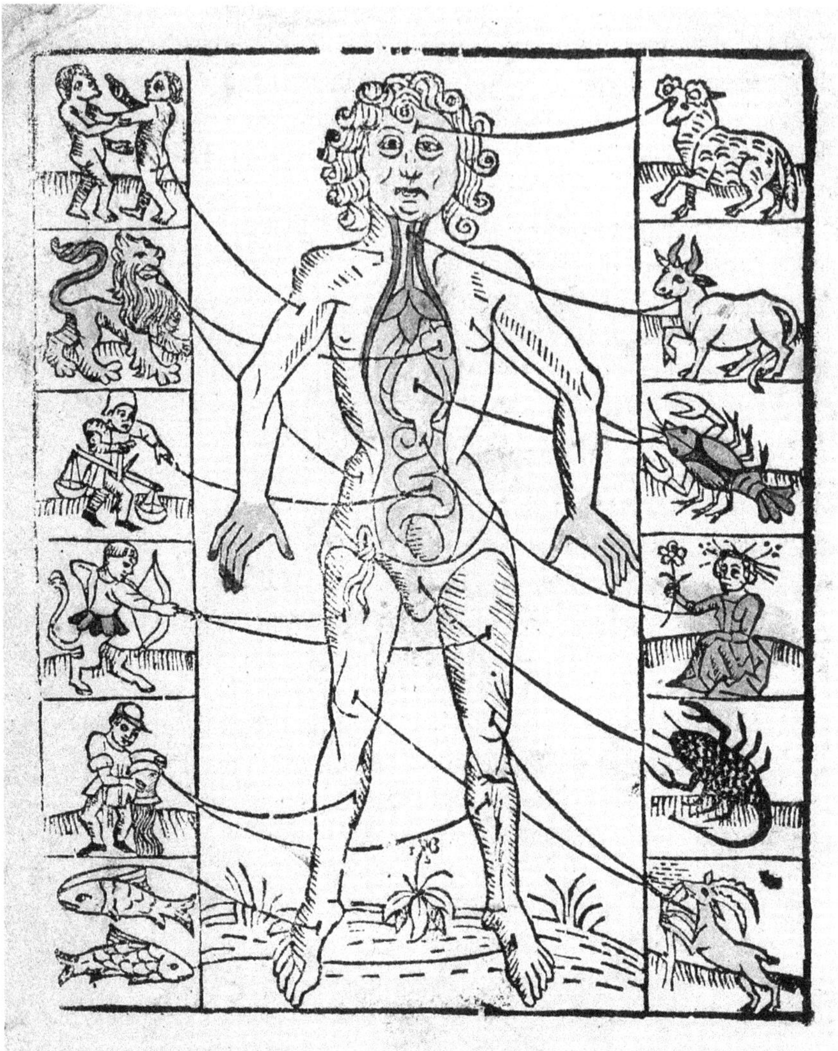

FIGURE 13.1 Zodiac Man. Showing the parts of the body controlled by the signs of the Zodiac. The zodiacal signs down the right column are Aries (I), Taurus (II), Cancer (IV), Virgo (VI), Scorpio (VIII), and Capricorn (X), while those down the left column are Gemini (III), Leo (V), Libra (VII), Sagittarius (IX), Aquarius (XI), and Pisces (XII). Der 'Teutsch Kalender.' 'Meister Almansor spricht.'

temporal dimensions of the zodiac onto the merely external human form, with apparently little regard for the biological functions of its parts.'[104]

It takes only a cursory glance at Figure 13.1 to recognize a typical adult human figure. Certainly, we may speak of an abstract kind of holism in the Zodiac Man, which views the human stature as a comprehensive summation of the heavens, as symbolized by all twelve zodiacal signs constituting the zodiac circle. Among the possible ways that these signs could have been linked to different body parts, however, it is difficult to suggest a criterion more prominent than the body's physical structure and proportions.

For the Zodiac Man described in cuneiform, for instance, it is remarkable how little this description seems to have relied on erudite scholarly hermeneutics, of a kind that otherwise characterized Mesopotamian commentaries and esoteric compositions around the same centuries BCE and earlier. True to the final position of Pisces in the zodiac, for example, the Fishes find themselves at the Zodiac Man's feet (see Figure 13.1) – while their Babylonian name 'The Tails' (KUN.MEŠ) was not invoked to connect the sign instead to the human 'coccyx / tail-bone' (GIŠ.KUN or UR_2.KUN).[105] Similarly, whereas a Babylonian medical commentary linked Sagittarius (Pa-bil-sag) to the feverishness of a 'hot head' (bil + SAG),[106] this logic played no part in determining Sagittarius's position within the cuneiform Zodiac Man. The proportions of the stereotypical Zodiac Man, therefore, may be said to represent one end of a spectrum that privileges physical form and structure over function and meaning in the partitioning of the human body.

Towards the opposite end of this spectrum, on the other hand, may be situated modern illustrations of Sensory and Motor Homunculi, as popularly depicted by the neuroscientist Wilder Penfield and his collaborators (Figure 13.2).[107] In these depictions, images of human body parts are mapped onto the brain's hemispheres, in proportion to the sizes of cerebral regions that determine the sensory and motor functions of these body parts. The results are distorted forms that scarcely resemble the appearances of human bodies observed in real life, but which more accurately reflect the brain's disproportional investment in certain body parts, such as the face, the organs of vocalization, the hands, and the feet/legs.

104 Wee (2015) 219 and 232.

105 Wee (2015) 231–32.

106 Wee (2019a) 171–72. To be precise, the root 'to become hot' (*emēmu*) typically used in medical descriptions is expressed by the logogram KUM_2, which happens to be one among several values of the cuneiform sign bil.

107 Penfield and Boldrey (1937) 432 (fig. 28); Penfield and Rasmussen (1950) 25 (fig. 10), 44 (fig. 17), 57 (fig. 22), and 214–15 (figs. 114–15). Actual three-dimensional models of these homunculi have been constructed and exhibited in museums or as display pieces.

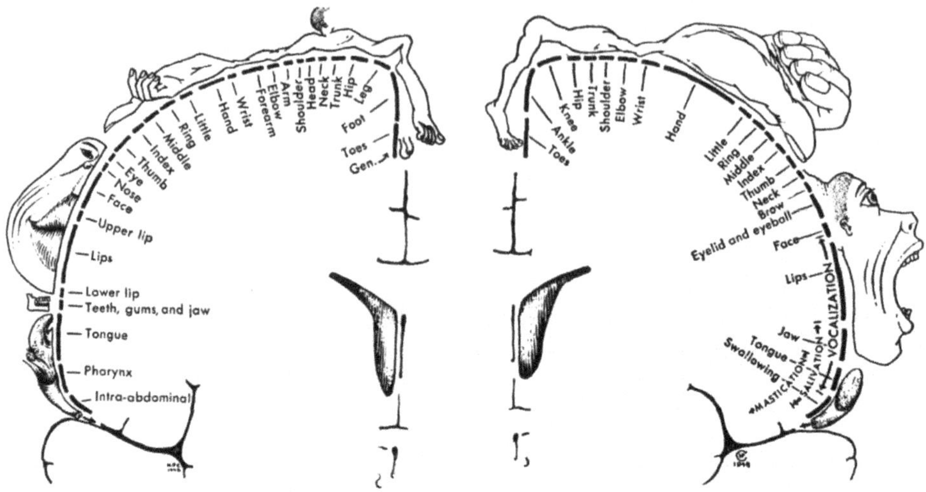

FIGURE 13.2 Sensory Homunculus (left) and Motor Homunculus (right). The right side of each human body part is laid upon a cross section of the hemisphere of the human brain, drawn somewhat in proportion to the extent of the sensory or motor cortex devoted to it. Original by Penfield and Rasmussen (1950) Figs. 17 and 22

A similar analysis can be applied to the head-to-foot organization in Chapter II (Tablets 3–14) of the Diagnostic Handbook, in order to sketch a mental image – not of the brain's relationship to the body (i.e., Figure 13.2) – but of the significance of each bodily region for medical diagnosis. In these diagnostic tablets, an overwhelming two-thirds of the contents give priority to the head and neck (Tablets 3–10), while only one-twelfth focus on the upper limbs (Tablets 10–11), one-sixth on the torso (Tablets 12–13), and one-twelfth on the lower body and genitalia (Tablet 14). While both the Diagnostic Handbook and the Zodiac Man enumerate the body *a capite ad calcem*, therefore, a different image emerges because of the Handbook's concern not merely for the body's physical proportions, but also for the behaviors of individual body parts in response to sickness.

Indeed, when organizing the Diagnostic Handbook, the scholar Esagil-kīn-apli recognized the fact that certain bodily features and behaviors were not comfortably assigned to a single locus in the head-to-foot scheme of Chapter II – so that passages addressing *bubu'tu*-vesicles (Tablet 18),[108] 'strands'

108 Sa-gig Tablet 18, lines 21–23 constitute a distinct section, with statements each beginning with 'If from his head to his feet, he is full of *bubu'tu*-vesicles {of some color} …' In addition, this section is awkwardly incorporated into the head-to-foot sequence of the

(Tablet 21)[109] throughout the entire body, and the vomiting of gall (Tablet 23) were instead relegated to *later* chapters,[110] as were discussions on less tangible entities like mood, mentality, and love sicknesses (Tablet 22), as well as the epileptic states and conditions (Chapter IV) that would later characterize the psychic system (§A) in our *Systemic Etiology*. A similar solution was adopted in the *Assur Medical Catalog*, which begins by arranging its therapeutic tablets from the (I) cranium, (II) eyes, (III) ears, (IV) neck, etc., down to the (X) kidney, (XI) anus, and (XII) hamstring, before launching into themes unbound by head-to-foot considerations, such as (XIII) the skin, (XVIII) mental illness, (XX) sex, and even (XXIII) the veterinary.[111]

In other words, therefore, the manner in which one defines the whole – whether by prioritizing the human body's physical stature, its pathological responses, or its healthy normal functions – determines what qualifies as its constituents. The fact that both diagnostic and therapeutic text corpora were not restricted to head-to-foot schemes, as I observed, was an acknowledgement that such schemes could not adequately address the variety of scenarios involving the body and sickness that were encompassed by medicine as a discipline, and that both anatomical structure and physiological processes had important roles to play in the construction of holisms. If the Zodiac Man represents one extreme in the valuation of bodily form over biological function, the *Systemic Etiology* may be said to exemplify a move in the opposite direction, towards a functional holism of the Babylonian body.

5 Re-categorizing Sickness

Typical of laconic cuneiform compositions, however, the *Etiology* does not articulate its views on organ systems in straightforward fashion, framing its presuppositions instead in negative terms by listing sicknesses and conditions that *hinder* the proper function of these systems. It is instructive, then, to consider precisely what is meant when we speak of a sickness's origin or derivation 'from' (*ultu*) a named organ like the 'lungs' (§C) or 'kidneys' (§D). Without

---

Diagnostic Handbook Chapter II (Tablets 3–14), appearing in the 'head' section (i.e., at Sa-gig Tablet 3: 100–4) on rather contrived grounds that the phrase 'from his **head** to his feet' starts out by mentioning the 'head'!

109 Cf. Fincke (2011) 473–74.

110 The chapter divisions of the Diagnostic Handbook Sa-gig go as follows: Chapter I = Tablets 1–2; Chapter II = Tablets 3–14 (head-to-foot); Chapter III = Tablets 15–25; Chapter IV = Tablets 26–30; Chapter V = Tablets 31–35; Chapter VI = Tablets 36–40.

111 Steinert (2018) 209–19.

precluding the possibility that ailments like *mišittu*-stroke (§B9) or Stricture (§D1) were imagined as having some substantive basis, sicknesses involving actual concrete components appear to acquire them from sources other than those identified in the *Etiology* – with gall (§B5) coming from the gall bladder as Babylonian healers would have known, and wind (§C3 and §D7) being 'blown into' the human body from the outside (§M).[112] Furthermore, while a word's etymology is not always a firm indication of its perceived meaning, there are at least suggestive dissonances in the way AN.TA.ŠUB.BA (lit. fallen-from-heaven, §A2) and ^{d}LUGAL.UR$_{3}$.RA (lit. lord-of-the-roof, §A6) are 'from the heart,' while ŠA$_{3}$.ZI.GA (lit. aroused-heart, §D2) is instead 'from the kidney,' not to mention hints of external agency in the labels Hand-of-god (§A3), Hand-of-goddess (§A4), and Hand-of-ghost (§B7).

The language of origins (i.e., 'from') and the composition's self-presentation as an etiology, nevertheless, should be taken seriously. Short of positing a radical break with earlier medical ideas, one can still acknowledge that, say, wind and AN.TA.ŠUB.BA have links to the exterior and the celestial, while at the same time affirm with the *Systemic Etiology* that they *become* sicknesses 'from' the lungs, kidneys, or heart. The model of origination in the *Etiology*, in other words, is less concerned with the sources of materials or agencies, than with the derivation of pathological identities. Indeed, as we have observed repeatedly, the actual organs of stomach, lungs, and kidneys are often not directly named elsewhere in roles involving sicknesses ascribed to them here, and make more sense as emblems of larger systems to which they belong. Ironically, then, one might even view the *Etiology* as driven by a kind of teleology, in that it identifies as the *origin* of a sickness the organ system that the sickness impedes from fulfilling its intended *purpose*.

The formulation of a functional holism in the *Systemic Etiology* was not a project embarked upon from scratch, but absorbed and recategorized elements that had long been defined in earlier holisms, which were often constructed on the basis of other considerations. Earlier, for instance, we noted how Chapter IV (Tablets 26–30) of the Diagnostic Handbook addresses epileptic sicknesses like AN.TA.ŠUB.BA (Tablets 26–29), *bennu* (Tablets 26, 29),[113] and ^{d}LUGAL.UR$_{3}$.RA (Tablets 28–29) – alongside a section on *mišittu*-stroke (Tablet 27),[114] presumably because of how commonly victims of a stroke also

112 Echoing this idea that wind derives from the outside (§M), another incantation (titled 'Belly 3' in Collins (1999) 126) addresses wind inside the human body with the question: 'Pure Wind that dwells on the mountain, who brought you here?'

113 Sa-gig 26: 4' and Sa-gig 29: 21, 83'–84'.

114 Sa-gig 27: 1–10.

experience epileptic seizures. In the *Etiology*, however, *mišittu*-stroke (§B9) is separated from these epileptic conditions originating in the psychic system (§A), and is instead assigned to the alimentary system (§B), possibly owing to the highly conspicuous and permanent disfigurement of the face by partial paralyses, which can also interfere with the sufferer's ability to feed himself or to consume food. The realignment of sickness categories is also illustrated by the excerpt below, which is typically viewed as a discourse on muscle disorders.

(§T) [If his head], his cervix, and his inguinal region hurt him all at the same time – *šaššaṭu* is [its name].
[If his neck], his waist, his hands, and his feet are stiff – *šaššaṭu* is [its name].
[If] he twists [his neck], and his eye is jittery, (and) he shudders *ditto* jitters now and then – *šaššaṭu* is [its name].
[If] his strands are tense [from] his neck [strands] to his heel, his eyebrows are knitted, and his [jaw] feels covered up – [*šaššaṭu* is its name].
[If the strands] of his thigh hurt him all at the same time, (so that) he is unable to rise up and walk about – *sagallu* is [its name].
[If] his thigh hurts him from his hips to his ankles, (but) he rises up and walks about – *maškadu* is [its name].
[If] his strands hurt him [from] his coccyx to his toes – *maškadu* is [its name].
[If] they hurt him [from] his hip to the *piṭru* of his ankles, (but) he acquires no harm – *kiṣṣatu* is [its name].
If his strands keep becoming sluggish from his hip to his toes – *kiṣṣatu* of *ṣētu*-heat is [its name].[115]

This excerpt comes from Tablet 33 of the Diagnostic Handbook and defines the different muscle ailments, in part, based on the extent of their effects on the

115 [DIŠ SAG.DU-*su t*]*i-ik-ka-šu*$_2$ *u ša-pu-la-šu*$_2$ 1-*niš* GU$_7$.MEŠ-[*š*]*u*$_2$ *ša*$_2$*-aš-*[*ša*$_2$*-ṭu* MU.NI] / [DIŠ GU$_2$-*su* MUR]UB$_4$-*šu*$_2$ ŠU.2-*šu*$_2$ *u* GIR$_3$.2-*šu*$_2$ *aš-ṭa ša*$_2$*-aš-*[*ša*$_2$*-ṭu* MU.NI] / [DIŠ GU$_2$-*su i*]*-zu-ur-ma* IGI.2-*šu*$_2$ *gal-ta-at pi-qa la pi-qa i-par-ru-ud* KI.MIN *i-gal*(!)-⸢*lu-ut ša*$_2$⸣*-a*[*š-ša*$_2$*-ṭu* MU.NI] / [DIŠ TA SA.G]U$_2$-*ni-šu*$_2$ EN *eq-bi-šu*$_2$ SA.MEŠ-*šu*$_2$ *šag-gu*$_5$ *šu-*ʾ*-ra-šu*$_2$ *kaṣ-ra u i*[*s-sa-š*]*u*$_2$ *ḫe-sa-a* [*ša*$_2$*-aš-ša*$_2$*-ṭu* MU.NI] / [DIŠ SA.M]EŠ ^{uzu}UR$_2$-*šu*$_2$ 1-*niš* GU$_7$.MEŠ-*šu*$_2$ ZI-*a u* DU.MEŠ-*ka la i-le-*ʾ*-e* SA.GAL [MU.NI] / [DIŠ ^{uzu}]UR$_2$-*šu*$_2$ TA *giš-ši-šu*$_2$ EN *ki-ṣal-li-šu*$_2$ GU$_7$-*šu*$_2$ ZI-*bi u* DU-[*a*]*k maš-ka-d*[*u*$_3$ MU.NI] / [DIŠ TA] ^{uzu}GIŠ.KUN-*šu*$_2$ EN ŠU.SI.MEŠ GIR$_3$.2-*šu*$_2$ SA.MEŠ-*šu*$_2$ GU$_7$.MEŠ-*šu*$_2$ *maš-ka-d*[*u*$_3$ MU.NI] / [DIŠ TA *giš*]*-ši-šu*$_2$ EN *pi-ṭir ki-ṣil-li-šu*$_2$ GU$_7$.MEŠ-*šu*$_2$ *ḫi-ṭam*$_2$ NU TUKU *ki-iṣ-ṣa-t*[*um* MU.NI] / ⸢DIŠ⸣ TA *giš-ši-šu*$_2$ EN ŠU.SI.⸢MEŠ GIR$_3$.2-*šu*$_2$ SA⸣.MEŠ-*šu*$_2$ *it-te-nen-ṣi-l*[*a-šu*$_2$ *k*]*i-*⸢*iṣ-ṣat*⸣ UD.D[A MU.NI] (Sa-gig 33: 94–102).

human body, as considered from the familiar perspective beginning at the head and moving downwards to the toes. In contrast to manifestations of *šaššaṭu* that affect the upper as well as lower body, both *sagallu* and *maškadu* appear to be restricted to the latter. Because of how anatomy is subsumed under the functional holism of the *Systemic Etiology*, however, *maškadu* (§B8) could not be identified primarily as a lower body condition – since it is not easily implicated in the excretory and reproductive functions that characterize this bodily region – and instead ends up in the catch-all category of the alimentary system. On the other hand, because pregnancy is frequently accompanied by the swelling of varicose veins, the sickness *sagallu* (lit. large-strands)[116] (§D4) could be acknowledged as a feature of reproductive functions belonging to the lower body system.

In other cases, a single sickness under earlier schemata is apportioned among the organ systems of the *Etiology*. Wind trapped within the human body is compared elsewhere to fermentation gases that leak out of any available opening in their container, whether 'through the rectum' or 'through the throat' (§M and §N). In the *Etiology*, however, organ systems are defined in such a way that they serve non-overlapping purposes, each making a non-dispensable contribution to the organism's survival. The surfeit of wind (§C3) in the respiratory system, which interrupts the regularity of breathing through burps, hiccups, or a sensation of bloating in the chest, therefore represents a separate category of problem from wind (§D7) and feces that are retained in the bowels due to impediments in lower body excretory functions (§L).

An interesting thought experiment can be contemplated in the case of *bu'šānu* sickness, whose effects on alimentary (§B2) and respiratory (§C5) systems are separately noted. Certainly, the perception of bodily wind as a single problem was made easy by the involvement of a common substance (i.e., wind) and situation (i.e., entrapment within the body), regardless of whether its escape occurred via the mouth or anus. By contrast, respiratory aspects of *bu'šānu* involving blood in the phlegm and fevers in the chest and back can be distinguished – perhaps more easily – from alimentary features such as

116 The fact that the excerpt (§T) from the Diagnostic Handbook – devoted to muscle disorders – does not always mention 'strands' as part of medical signs may be an argument that these 'strands' do not exclusively refer to muscle fibers. While 'large (GAL) strands (SA)' are explicit in the etymology of *sagallu*, this does not exclude the possibility that swollen veins could also have occurred in the muscle problems *šaššaṭu* and *maškadu*, even if not associated with pregnancy in the *Systemic Etiology*. Note, for instance, the following equations involving the element sa ('strands') – sa-ad-gal = *maš-ka-du* (no. 75), sa-me-el-gal = *ša-aš*$_2$*-ša*$_2$*-ṭu* (no. 80), and sa-ad-gal = *ša-aš*$_2$*-ša*$_2$*-ṭu* (no. 81) in Kilmer (1967) 94.

the proliferation of *bubu'tu*-vesicles in the mouth, as well as pain or discomfort in oral movements. Most likely, definitions of *bu'šānu* encompassing all these medical signs arose out of practical observations that they tended to occur together, around the same time or experienced by the same patients. Nonetheless, it is worth considering – if ideas about the sickness had been, from the very beginning, shaped by the functional holism of the *Systemic Etiology* – whether *bu'šānu* would necessarily have been defined in such a way that straddled two organ systems, or whether it could have been perceived instead as two related sicknesses each belonging to a separate system, perhaps analogous to the manner in which the alimentary sickness *ṣētu*-heat occurs in connection with the respiratory illness *ṣinnaḫtiru* (§O).

Holisms therefore possess the power and potential to reshape perspectives and to provide alternative interpretations of objects and events. The construction of a holism is not merely a disinterested gathering of its constituents in one place, or even the structuring of their relationships on the basis of known affinities – rather, holisms dictate the very terms by which their constituents' identities are construed, sometimes even bestowing new meanings or emphases on old names like 'wind' and *sagallu*. Indeed, while alleging to be comprehensive in their treatment of entities as a coherent *whole*, holisms involve *a priori* suppositions of what entities are correctly assigned to the group, while excluding other entities as category errors to be removed from consideration. So, for example, while body parts enumerated in the head-to-foot (I–XII) schema of the *Assur Medical Catalog* must have been imagined with their usual covering of skin, the topic of (XIII) skin itself could be discussed only as a separate category outside this constructed schema.

• • •

It behooves us to do a final, critical check on the extent to which our interpretation of the *Systemic Etiology* so far may have been influenced by modern impulses to treat ancient data – however fortuitously made available to us – as components of a 'holistic' account. Suspicions may be warranted, particularly since the proposal of psychic (§A), alimentary (§B), respiratory (§C), and excretory-reproductive (§D) systems appears to resonate so profoundly with biological constructs of the human body acknowledged in the present.

With the *Systemic Etiology*, nonetheless, we are dealing with the following: (1.) A single, sufficiently well-preserved ancient document and text object, rather than separate sources whose affiliation as a group may be questioned. (2.) Sections that group together entities in ways explicitly replicated elsewhere – e.g., the sicknesses of the psychic system (§A) in Chapter IV of the

Diagnostic Handbook – or are implied to do so, as in the occasional blurring of boundaries between the excretory and the reproductive. (3.) An effort to minimize repetitions of entities across separate sections, and to clarify entities that may be affiliated with more than one section – so that 'mouth (and) tooth of *bu'šānu* sickness' (§B2) is differentiated from respiratory aspects of *bu'šānu* sickness (§C5), and the burning of *ṣētu*-heat is affirmed to be a feature of the alimentary system even when occurring alongside 'any (other) sickness' (§B12). Each section is therefore deemed to make a non-dispensable contribution to the whole, as is often characteristic of constituents in a holism.

All evidence considered, the *Systemic Etiology* may indeed be regarded as an *ancient* endeavor to map out the human body in holistic ways, by looking beyond structures and forms so often operative in Mesopotamian medicine, towards the idea of an organism comprised of functional systems.

Bibliography

Adamson, P. B. 'Surgery in Ancient Mesopotamia.' *Medical History*, 35 (1991) 428–35.

Attia, A. 'A propos de la signification de šer'ânu dans les textes médicaux mésopotamiens: une question d'anatomie.' *Histoire des Sciences Médicales*, 34 (2000) 47–56.

Biggs, R. D. 'Medicine in Ancient Mesopotamia.' *History of Science*, 8 (1969) 94–105.

Borger, R. 'Geheimwissen.' In *Reallexikon der Assyriologie und Vorderasiatischen Archäologie*, vol. 3, ed. E. Ebeling, B. Meissner, E. Weidner and W. von Soden. Berlin: De Gruyter (1957–1971) 188–91.

Brown, D. 'Astral Magic and Medicine.' in *The Interactions of Ancient Astral Science*, ed. D. Brown. Bremen: Hempen Verlag (2018) 443–49.

Civil, M. 'Medical Commentaries from Nippur.' *Journal of Near Eastern Studies*, 33.3 (1974) 329–38.

Clancier, P. *Les bibliothèques en Babylonie dans la deuxième moitié du* Ier *millénaire av.* J.-C. Alter Orient und Altes Testament 363. Münster: Ugarit-Verlag (2009).

Couto-Ferreira, M. E. 'From Head to Toe: Listing the Body in Cuneiform Texts.' In *The Comparable Body: Analogy and Metaphor in Ancient Mesopotamian, Egyptian, and Greco-Roman Medicine*, ed. J. Z. Wee. Studies in Ancient Medicine 49. Leiden: Brill (2017) 43–71.

Faraone, C. A. 'Magical and Medical Approaches to the Wandering Womb in the Ancient Greek World.' *Classical Antiquity*, 30.1 (2011) 1–32.

Fincke, J. C. *Augenleiden nach keilschriftlichen Quellen. Untersuchungen zur altorientalischen Medizin.* Würzburger medizinhistorische Forschungen Band 70. Würzburg: Verlag Königshausen & Neumann GmbH (2000).

Fincke, J. C. 'Neue Erkenntnisse zur 21. Tafel der diagnostischen Omenserie SA.GIG und zur Überlieferung diagnostischer Omentexte in Hattuša.' *Bibliotheca Orientalis*, 68 (2011) 472–76.

Finkel, I. L. 'Adad-apla-iddina, Esagil-kīn-apli, and the Series SA.GIG.' In *A Scientific Humanist: Studies in Memory of Abraham Sachs*, ed. E. Leichty, M. de J. Ellis and P. Gerardi. Occasional Publications of the Samuel Noah Kramer Fund 9. Philadelphia (1988) 143–59.

Frahm, E. *Babylonian and Assyrian Text Commentaries: Origins of Interpretation*. Guides to the Mesopotamian Text Record 5. Münster: Ugarit-Verlag (2011).

Frandsen, P. J. 'The Menstrual 'Taboo' in Ancient Egypt.' *Journal of Near Eastern Studies*, 66.2 (2007) 81–105.

Geller, M. J. *Ancient Babylonian Medicine: Theory and Practice*. Chicester: Wiley-Blackwell (2010).

Geller, M. J. 'Kidney and Urinary Tract Disease in Ancient Babylonia, with Translations of the Cuneiform Sources.' *Kidney International*, 47 (1995) 1811–15.

George, A. R. 'On Babylonian Lavatories and Sewers.' *Iraq*, 77.1 (2015) 75–106.

Heeßel, N. P. 'Astrological Medicine in Babylonia.' In *Astro-Medicine: Astrology and Medicine, East and West*, ed. A. Akasoy, C. Burnett, and R. Yoeli-Tlalim. Florence: Edizioni del Galluzzo (2008) 1–16.

Heeßel, N. P. 'Diagnosis, Divination and Disease: Towards an Understanding of the Rationale Behind the Babylonian Diagnostic Handbook.' In *Magic and Rationality in Ancient Near Eastern and Greco-Roman Medicine*, ed. H. F. J. Horstmanshoff and M. Stol. Studies in Ancient Medicine 27. Leiden: Brill (2004) 97–116.

Heeßel, N. P. 'Stein, Pflanze und Holz: Ein neuer Text zur 'medizinischen Astrologie.' *Orientalia Nova Series*, 74.1 (2005) 1–22.

Johnson, J. C. 'The Stuff of Causation: Etiological Metaphor and Pathogenic Channeling in Babylonian Medicine.' In *The Comparable Body: Analogy and Metaphor in Ancient Mesopotamian, Egyptian, and Greco-Roman Medicine*, ed. J. Z. Wee. Studies in Ancient Medicine 49. Leiden: Brill (2017) 72–121.

Keyser, P. T. 'The Lineage of 'Bloodlines': Synecdoche, Metonymy, Medicine, and More.' In *The Comparable Body: Analogy and Metaphor in Ancient Mesopotamian, Egyptian, and Greco-Roman Medicine*, ed. J. Z. Wee. Studies in Ancient Medicine 49. Leiden: Brill (2017) 168–203.

Labat, R. 'Fußkrankheiten.' In *Reallexikon der Assyriologie und Vorderasiatischen Archäologie* vol. 3, ed. E. Ebeling, B. Meissner, E. Weidner and W. von Soden. Berlin: De Gruyter (1957–1971) 126–27.

Lenzi, A. *Secrecy and the Gods: Secret Knowledge in Ancient Mesopotamia and Biblical Israel*. State Archives of Assyria Studies 19. Helsinki: The Neo-Assyrian Text Corpus Project (2008).

Oppenheim, A. L. 'On the Observation of the Pulse in Mesopotamian Medicine.' *Orientalia Nova Series*, 31 (1962) 27–33.

Peled, I. *Masculinities and Third Gender: The Origins and Nature of an Institutionalized Gender Otherness in the Ancient Near East*. Alter Orient und Altes Testament 435. Münster: Ugarit-Verlag (2016).

Penfield, W., and E. Boldrey. 'Somatic Motor and Sensory Representation in the Cerebral Cortex of Man as Studied by Electrical Stimulation.' *Brain*, 60 (1937) 389–443.

Penfield, W., and T. Rasmussen. *The Cerebral Cortex of Man: A Clinical Study of Localization of Function*. New York: Macmillan Company (1950).

Reiner, E. *Astral Magic in Babylonia. Transactions of the American Philosophical Society*, New Series 85.4. Philadelphia: The American Philosophical Society (1995).

Reiner, E., J. H. Johnson and M. Civil. 'Linguistics in the Ancient Near East.' In *History of Linguistics*, Volume 1, The Eastern Traditions of Linguistics, ed. G. Lepschy. Longman Linguistics Library 1. London: Longman (1994) 61–96.

Simkó, K. 'The Abrasive Stone in Assyrian and Babylonian Medicine.' *Le Journal des Médecines Cunéiformes*, 22 (2013) 24–60.

Steinert, U. 'Concepts of the Female Body in Mesopotamian Gynecological Texts.' In *The Comparable Body: Analogy and Metaphor in Ancient Mesopotamian, Egyptian, and Greco-Roman Medicine*, ed. J. Z. Wee. Studies in Ancient Medicine 49. Leiden: Brill (2017) 275–357.

Stevens, K. 'Secrets in the Library: Protected Knowledge and Professional Identity in Late Babylonian Uruk.' *Iraq*, 75 (2013) 211–53.

Stol, M. *Birth in Babylonia and the Bible: Its Mediterranean Setting*. Cuneiform Monographs 14. Groningen: Styx (2000).

Stol, M. 'Einige kurze Wortstudien.' In *Festschrift für Rykle Borger zu seinem 65. Geburtstag am 24. Mai 1994: tikip santakki mala bašmu …*, ed. S. M. Maul. Cuneiform Monographs 10. Groningen: Styx (1998) 343–52.

Stol, M. *Epilepsy in Babylonia*. Cuneiform Monographs 2. Groningen: Styx (1993).

van der Toorn, K. 'La pureté rituelle au Proche-Orient ancien.' *Revue de l'histoire des religions*, 206.4 (1989) 339–56.

Wee, J. Z. 'Lugalbanda Under the Night Sky: Scenes of Celestial Healing in Ancient Mesopotamia.' *Journal of Near Eastern Studies*, 73.1 (2014) 23–42.

Wee, J. Z. 'Discovery of the Zodiac Man in Cuneiform.' *Journal of Cuneiform Studies*, 67 (2015) 217–33.

Wee, J. Z. 'Virtual Moons Over Babylonia: The Calendar Text System, Its Micro-Zodiac of 13, and the Making of Medical Zodiology.' In *The Circulation of Astronomical Knowledge in the Ancient World*, ed. J. M. Steele. Time, Astronomy, and Calendars 6. Leiden: Brill (2016) 139–229.

Wee, J. Z. 'Pan-astronomical Hermeneutics and the Arts of the Lamentation Priest.' *Zeitschrift für Assyriologie und Vorderasiatische Archäologie*, 107.2 (2017) 236–60.

Wee, J. Z. *Knowledge and Rhetoric in Medical Commentary: Ancient Mesopotamian Commentaries on a Handbook of Medical Diagnosis (Sa-gig)*. Cuneiform Monographs 49.1. Leiden: Brill (2019a).

Primary Texts: Editions and Translations Used

Biggs, R. D. *ŠÀ.ZI.GA: Ancient Mesopotamian Potency Incantations*. Texts from Cuneiform Sources 2. New York: J. J. Augustin (1967).

Campbell Thompson, R. *Assyrian Medical Texts from the Originals in the British Museum*. London: Milford (1923).

Collins, T. J. 'Natural Illness in Babylonian Medical Incantations.' PhD diss., University of Chicago (1999).

De Zorzi, N. *La serie teratomantica šumma izbu: testo, tradizione, orizzonti culturali*, 2 vols. History of the Ancient Near East, Monographs 15. Padua: S.A.R.G.O.N. Editrice e Libreria (2014).

Dougherty, R. P. *Goucher College Cuneiform Inscriptions*. New Haven: Yale University Press (1923–1933).

Farber, W. *Beschwörungsrituale an Ištar und Dumuzi: attī Ištar ša ḫarmaša Dumuzi*. Wiesbaden: Franz Steiner Verlag (1977).

Foster, B. R. *Before the Muses: An Anthology of Akkadian Literature*, 3rd ed. Bethesda: CDL Press (2005).

Geller, M. J. *Melothesia in Babylonia*. Science, Technology, and Medicine in Ancient Cultures 2. Berlin: De Gruyter (2014).

Geller, M. J. *Renal and Rectal Disease Texts*. Die babylonisch-assyrische Medizin in Texten und Untersuchungen 7. Berlin: De Gruyter (2005).

Geller, M. J. 'West Meets East: Early Greek and Babylonian Diagnosis.' *Archiv für Orientforschung*, 48–49 (2001–2002) 50–75.

Gurney, O. R., and J. J. Finkelstein. *The Sultantepe Tablets*, vol. 1. Occasional Publications of the British Institute of Archaeology at Ankara 3. London: Lund Humphries London and Bradford (1957).

Gurney, O. R., and P. Hulin. *The Sultantepe Tablets*, vol. 2. Occasional Publications of the British Institute of Archaeology at Ankara 7. London: Percy Lund, Humphries and Co. Ltd. (1964).

Heeßel, N. P. *Babylonisch-assyrische Diagnostik*. Alter Orient und Altes Testament 43. Münster: Ugarit-Verlag (2000).

Heeßel, N. P. 'Diagnostische Texte.' In *Texte zur Heilkunde*, ed. B. Janowski and D. Schwemer. Texte aus der Umwelt des Alten Testaments, Neue Folge 5. Gütersloh: Verlagsgruppe Random House GmbH (2010) 8–31.

Hunger, H. *Spätbabylonische Texte aus Uruk I.* Ausgrabungen der Deutschen Forschungsgemeinschaft in Uruk-Warka 9. Berlin: Mann Verlag (1976).

Jean, C. *La magie néo-assyrienne en contexte.* State Archives of Assyria Studies 17. Helsinki: Vammalan Kirjapaino Oy (2006).

Johnson, J. C. 'Towards a Reconstruction of SUALU IV: Can we localize K 2386+ in the therapeutic corpus?' *Le Journal des Médecines Cunéiformes*, 24 (2014) 11–38.

Kilmer, A. D. 'List of Diseases.' In *The Series ḪAR-ra* = ḫubullu *Tablet XV and Related Texts*, ed. B. Landsberger and M. Civil. Materialien zum sumerischen Lexikon 9. Rome: Pontificium Institutum Biblicum (1967).

Kinnier Wilson, J. V. 'The Nimrud Catalogue of Medical and Physiognomical Omina.' *Iraq*, 24.1 (1962) 52–62.

Köcher, F. *Die babylonisch-assyrische Medizin in Texten und Untersuchungen*, vols. 1–6. Berlin: De Gruyter (1963–1980).

Köcher, F. 'Spätbabylonische medizinsche Texte aus Uruk.' In *Medizinische Diagnostik in Geschichte und Gegenwart: Festschrift für Heinz Goerke zum Sechzigsten Geburtstag*, ed. C. Habrich, F. Marguth, and J. H. Wolf. Munich: Werner Fritsch (1978) 17–39.

Lambert, W. G. *Babylonian Creation Myths.* Mesopotamian Civilizations 16. Winona Lake IN: Eisenbrauns (2013).

Lambert, W. G. *Babylonian Wisdom Literature.* Oxford: Oxford University Press (1960).

Lambert, W. G., and A. R. Millard. *Atra-ḫasīs: The Babylonian Story of the Flood.* Winona Lake IN: Eisenbrauns (1999).

Leichty, E. *The Omen Series šumma izbu.* New York: J. J. Augustin (1970).

Parpola, S., and K. Watanabe. *Neo-Assyrian Treaties and Loyalty Oaths.* State Archives of Assyria 2. Helsinki: Helsinki University Press (1988).

Pinches, T. G., and J. N. Strassmaier. *Late Babylonian Astronomical and Related Texts.* Providence: Brown University Press (1955).

Scurlock, J. *Sourcebook for Ancient Mesopotamian Medicine.* Writings from the Ancient World 36. Atlanta: Society of Biblical Literature Press (2014).

Scurlock, J., and B. R. Andersen. *Diagnoses in Assyrian and Babylonian Medicine.* Urbana and Chicago: University of Illinois Press (2005).

Steinert, U. 'Körperwissen, Tradition und Innovation in der babylonischen Medizin.' In *Körperwissen: Transfer und Innovation*, ed. A.-B. Renger and C. Wulf. Paragrana: Internationale Zeitschrift für historische Anthropologie, 25.1 (2016) 195–254.

Steinert, U. 'The Assur Medical Catalogue (AMC).' in *Assyrian and Babylonian Scholarly Text Catalogues*, ed. U. Steinert. Die babylonisch-assyrische Medizin in Texten und Untersuchungen 9. Berlin: De Gruyter (2018) 203–91.

Wee, J. Z. *Mesopotamian Commentaries on the Diagnostic Handbook Sa-gig: Edition and Notes on Medical Lexicography.* Cuneiform Monographs 49.2. Leiden: Brill (2019b).

CHAPTER 14

Epidemic Disease in a Humoral Environment: From *Airs, Waters and Places* to the Renaissance

Vivian Nutton

Abstract

Studies of humoralism have rightly concentrated on the balance or imbalance of humours in individuals, but ancient medical texts, including the *Epidemics* and *Airs, Waters and Places*, also discussed diseases within the wider community. The so-called *Constitutions* in the *Epidemics* are a remarkable record of collaboration, as well as of the collection and analysis of information over a long period of time. This paper looks at some of the attempts made by humoralist physicians in the Middle Ages and Renaissance to investigate the diseases of groups or of regions, raising the question why little trace remains of similar studies in Antiquity. It argues that the complexity of record-keeping and the absence of any civic organisation hampered such efforts. Although commentators on *Airs, Waters and Places* offered advice on town-planning and a healthy environment, this remained largely at the level of theory.

Holism, whether singular or plural, has become relevant today in ways that would have been thought unlikely half a century ago when modern biomedical science seemed on the brink of providing a universal explanation and a potential universal cure for illness. Those who doubted this reductionism were dismissed to the very fringes of medicine, and investigators into the history of one of the longest-lived theories of holism, humoralism, were accused of antiquarianism and of supporting ideas that had delayed for centuries the practice of effective medicine.[1] Yet humoralism, whether in its classical form that focused on health and disease as dependent on a balance of basic fluids, humours, or, more broadly, on a constitution of the body that involved both physical and psychological components in relation to the wider environment and life-style, is a long time a-dying. It is not only that, in its Arabised form as Yunani medicine, it remains a living medical tradition in the Islamic world, promoted by governments in several countries, but also that modern

1 Wooton (2006).

 | DOI:10.1163/9789004443143_016

genomics and gene therapy has allowed new insights into individual receptivity as a cause of illness. Galen's belief that many harmful changes were the result of mutations at the deepest level of the body that could be conceived is confirmed, at least at an intellectual level. Recent DNA analysis of the plague bacillus has resulted in new ideas and new understanding of the factors influencing its behaviour that would have been entirely acceptable to a doctor in the sixteenth, the fourteenth, or even the second century. This is not to claim any direct influence from humoralism, but merely to state that medical ways of understanding health and illness are returning to problems of individuality and its relationship to a wider whole that exercised Galen and his Hippocratic predecessors long ago.

This paper looks at the relationship between humoralism and epidemic disease, or rather, since the word epidemic has a very specific connotation, simply 'common' or 'widespread' states of ill health, whether we are talking of the Thucydidean plague, localised (or endemic) conditions, or the remarkable *Constitutions* in the *Epidemics*. There are few discussions of such diseases in ancient medical texts, and medical historians have had to work perforce on the basis of scattered reports by historians or theologians. It might be argued that this absence of information simply reflects the absence of widespread diseases in Antiquity, but, leaving aside the great pandemics, such as the Antonine Plague in the time of Galen, the plague of St Cyprian in the next century, and the Justinianic plague – and one might include in this also the Thucydidean plague – there is abundant evidence for more localised outbreaks from Egypt and Syria through Italy to the yellow plague, *y fad felen*, of remote Wales in the sixth century. Such reticence is all the more surprising since the environment, and specifically air, became one of the famous six non-naturals of late Antiquity, and in Medieval and Renaissance Europe was a standard element in medical advice literature, both for individuals and for groups.[2] This later literature not only shows the influence of classical texts, but also contrasts with ancient Hippocratic Galenic humoralism.

The name of the Augsburg physician Ulrich Ellenbog may well be unknown today, but in the days when medical history was often a search for ancestors, he enjoyed a certain reputation as the first printed author to write on industrial diseases. Ellenbog has been relegated to at best a footnote, an unfortunate demotion since both he and his books are well worth studying for what they reveal about early German humanism and medicine in the years before the arrival of Greek texts in the late 15th century. Born in 1435, he travelled to universities in Germany and Italy before setting up practice in Memmingen and

2 Mikkeli (1999) 41–68; Nicoud (2007).

marrying a wealthy wife. In 1472 he was appointed the first professor of medicine at the new university of Ingolstadt. He then became doctor to the Bishop and Chapter of Augsburg, before returning to Memmingen as Stadtarzt. He next moved on to similar posts at Ravensburg and Biberach before ending his life in 1499 as the personal physician to Archduke Sigismund of Austria. This was a typical career of a wealthy university-trained doctor.[3]

In 1473, he wrote a *consilium* for the goldsmiths of Augsburg entitled *On the Poisonous Evil Vapours and Fumes of Metals such as Silver, Quicksilver, and Lead*, a short text that was printed in 1524 also in Augsburg.[4] It falls into two sections. The first deals with the effect of smoke from furnaces, for which Ellenbog's advice is always to work in the open air, or, at least, in a well-ventilated forge, to avoid damp coal, if possible, and sprinkle incense on the fire when it is started up. In the second part he distinguishes this coal smoke from the far more poisonous fumes given off by various metals being smelted. He appreciates the difference between diseases of those who work with gold and silver, and those who work with lead, rightly attributing it to the differences between the nature of the metals, and he offers slightly different prescriptions for their conditions.

His advice as printed is typical of the late Middle Ages in form and structure and is a useful guide to the strengths and weaknesses of humoralism in general. Humoralism depended on close observation to determine the individuality of the patient's bodily mixture of humours, both innate and in its response to change, and its Galenic version it required attention to an almost infinite range of possibilities that became multiplied over time. The plan in Schöner's *Viererschema*, still the most valuable study of the notion of the four humours, shows neatly how further complications were introduced over the centuries, some, we might think, much more relevant than others.[5] But how were humoral practitioners taught to observe? We know Galen's ideas on the best way of taking the pulse, and his Medieval and Renaissance successors only added detail to his advice; we know about uroscopy, and urine charts; and from the late Western Middle Ages we have handbooks on medical astrology, as well as the handy tables, largely from British sources, that tell us about the information carried round on his belt by a physician when visiting a patient.[6] For the sixteenth century, we have the notes taken by students of consultations at the bedside in Padua, where Giambattista da Monte and his colleagues discussed

3 Assion (1980).
4 Ellenbog (1524); English translation by Barnard (1932).
5 Schöner (1964). See also Arika (2007).
6 O'Boyle (2005).

for the benefit of students the cases they could see in front of them.[7] Such riches are on the whole missing for Antiquity. We have also a fair number of references in the Hippocratic Corpus and still more in Galen on how the physician should observe, what he should see, and what he should prioritise. And no one can afford to neglect the short text by Rufus, *Medical Questioning*, which offers explicit advice on how the doctor may gain valuable information about the patient.[8] But, as with so much in practical matters, how to observe will have been something learned almost by osmosis from contact with a superior, from seeing, from listening, from being shown, something that is experienced rather than being written down, and hence hard for a historian dependent on written material to pick up. We need a study of medical observation comparable to recent work on gesture.

Ellenbog's little tract is interesting for many reasons. It is unusual in being a *consilium*, for a group, rather than an individual. This is one of the reasons why his prescriptions are made in general terms, although still in the standard humoral categories. The fumes of lead, silver and antimony are cold, hence require a heating remedy, drinking wormwood to provoke sweating; those of aqua fortis, verdigris and nitre are hot, but also can be treated similarly to the others by using theriac. That is because Ellenbog classifies all these substances as poisons, and poisons act by their total substance, largely independently of the humoral balance of those who have been poisoned. Recent work on poisons has also emphasised how much, still within a humoral context, the late Middle Ages and Renaissance developed new ideas on pharmacology, and particularly poisons, that went beyond what they had learned from their predecessors.[9]

Specific discussions about the diseases of specific groups are not found in Antiquity – I make this assertion somewhat hesitantly, since one might include under this heading works such as the Hippocratic work *On Young Girls* and even Soranus' *Gynaecology*. But compared with the humoralist doctors of the sixteenth and seventeenth century, Girolamo Mercuriale and Bernardino Ramazzini chief among them, there is relatively little. Mercuriale (1530–1606) produced several volumes largely based on classical sources in which he considered the diseases of different groups such as children, and in at least part of his most famous book, *De Arte Gymnastica*, those of athletes and fitness fanatics.[10] Ramazzini, a later successor to Mercuriale in Padua in the next century, wrote a large book *De Morbis Artificum*, covering a whole series of occupations from

7 Giambattista Da Monte, *Discursus et consilia*, London, Wellcome Library, WMS 567.
8 Rufus of Ephesus, *Quaestiones medicinales*; Letts (2015).
9 Pastore (2008).
10 Arcangeli and Nutton (2008).

gondoliers and blacksmiths to nuns, always prey to housemaid's knee because of their constant praying.[11] We have no ancient text that can compare with these that deals with localised or group diseases, which is somewhat surprising considering the range of individual observations and the familiar presence within the Hippocratic Corpus of two works that encouraged doctors to think in terms of groups, the *catastaseis* (*Constitutions*) within *Epidemics* I and 3, and *Airs, Waters and Places*. This is not to deny that, like Mercuriale and Ramazzini, one could draw up a nice list of ancient observations on the diseases of groups. The pallor of miners is a commonplace, and the healthiness of hilltop towns is contrasted with the deadliness of the city.[12] Galen's diatribe against athletes derives in part from his own experiences in the gym, and in part from, in his view, the theoretical impossibility of attaining and maintaining a perfectly balanced health.[13] But none of them is developed into a specific treatise or into any wider correlation.

In this context the achievement of the writer of *Epidemics* I and 3, deserves further attention even after the magisterial edition by Jacques Jouanna.[14] Alongside *Aphorisms* and *Prognostic*, the *Epidemics*, and particularly its books 1 and 3, are the most influential of all medical tracts in the Hippocratic Corpus. They consist of two distinct types of document. One is a series of brief case-descriptions, describing important features of an individual illness over several days, and indeed over months. The second is the *catastaseis*, 'constitutions', broader surveys of diseases in one place, Thasos, over a year.[15] First and foremost they attempt to link notes on individual cases together and to relate them to the weather conditions under which they occurred, which, in the author's view, can in some way be thought of as a cause. I am being deliberately vague in my formulation here. Bringing this information together in one place thus will serve as a guide to predicting what sort of diseases are likely to occur at any particular time in the future, should a similar climatic condition reoccur. To create this wider picture is a remarkable intellectual achievement, and the writer has deservedly been praised over the centuries. But he may not have been the first to do so, or, at any rate, he had himself already prepared a similar summary, since he mentions something 'from the earlier *Constitution*', and he was not the last, to judge from the fragmentary *catastaseis* in *Epidemics* 5 and 7.[16] What he did was much more complicated than the simple process of

11 Ramazzini (1713); English translation by Cave Wright (1940).
12 Nutton (2013) 27–28.
13 König (2005) 254–300.
14 Jouanna (2016).
15 Jouanna (2016) XXXIII–XLIII.
16 Hippocrates, *Epid.* I,5 = p. 2 Jouanna.

selection that he carried out when he abbreviated and perhaps organised his original notes to form the case histories. He had to amalgamate material drawn from both his, and, since there is some evidence that other healers were also involved, from others' notes, and then categorise and arrange it to provide a clear account of climate and disease over a long period of time. One should not underestimate the difficulties involved in such a procedure at both an intellectual and an organisational level. We appear to be dealing with a group of doctors, sharing information in the form of written material within a permanent building of some sort, for texts of this kind cannot have been easily transported on visits even in a village, let alone around the countryside. We are not dealing with *Wanderärzte*, but with an *iatreion* somewhere on Thasos.[17] This is more than a problem of literacy; these are written records composed in a sophisticated manner, and preserved in a way that will allow consultation, and consultation by others. What was written down was arguably more complex than the material so far found on the lead tablets of merchants but whatever material form was chosen, it required to be conserved in some way. How this was done is unclear, except that it can only have been carried out in a specific work-place as a record of cases seen over a long period.[18] This would fit with Elizabeth Craik's suggestion that the word *Epidemiai* refers to something broader than just as simple visit, but may be a record of a doctor's journey or series of journeys around a variety of communities before returning to base, a practice we can document from later times.[19] But neither *Constitutions* nor the stylistically far less elaborate individual case notes can be easily regarded as a finished article; they are both work in progress. This may well help to understand why there is so little trace of similar productions in Antiquity; these are private notes requiring a specific occupational and physical context that is not always easy to reproduce, and, as private notes, they are much less likely to survive that something than is finished and available to be copied. But one should not criticise too much the doctors of Antiquity for failing to develop some of the ideas found in the *Constitutions*, for such detailed attention to the relationship between weather and disease is not found again until Guillaume De Baillou in his *Ephemerides* in the early seventeenth century, although the general point that is at issue had long been commonplace.[20] Air, at least since late antiquity, had been one of the six non-naturals that every humoral physician

17 Diller (1934).
18 For some suggestions, see Perilli (2012–2013).
19 Craik (2015) 64.
20 De Baillou (1640), but written in the last decades of the sixteenth century.

was expected to consider in advising a patient, and one can see how easily Ellenbog's discussion of fumes and dampness fitted into this pattern.

Air, of course, is the first component in another famous text, *Airs, Waters and Places*, perhaps written between 450 and 420.[21] Like *Epidemics* I and III, it can be divided into two related sections. The first, 1–11, explains the necessity for a doctor to consider the effects of changing seasons, winds and waters, which are then described in order of the importance of a town's orientation, the various types of water, and finally the seasons. The second and most original part is a description of the differences between different people, which are then explained in environmental and anthropological terms. A long section deals with the Scythians, explaining their physique and the behaviour in terms of their mode of life in their region, and, famously, suggesting that some of their physical peculiarities can be the result of changes originally brought about by their customs but later transmitted genetically. The work originally contained a similar excursus on the Libyans of N. Africa, but this seems to have been lost at an early stage.[22]

The two parts are neatly linked together by an elegant transition, and share the same aim, that of providing a doctor whether visiting or resident, with a way of understanding the conditions he is likely to meet. The first part explains the sort of medical condition that is likely to arise in a particular area, the second the generalities, the *phuseis* and *ideai* of the population in a particular area, that can be used as a base from which to consider everything else relating to the individual patient. Both parts thus serve the same purpose, providing the physician with some of the essential data upon which to base a diagnosis, information that is not otherwise available from a physical examination of the patient. It confirms and supplements rather than opposes a humoral explanation for individual illness.

All this is well known; less so is the later reception of its ideas, and here we meet a paradox. Clarence L. Glacken's *Traces on the Rhodian Shore: Nature and Culture in Western Thought from Ancient Times to the 18th Century*, first published in 1967, is a justly celebrated exposition of ideas on the relation of mankind and the environment.[23] His judgment on *Airs, Waters and Places* is double-edged. On the one hand, he praises the influence of this text on subsequent theorists in history, ethnology and geography, while criticising it for suggesting that if environmental influences on the physical and mental qualities of

21 Cf. also the programmatic statement in *The Nature of Man* 9, distinguishing individual diseases from 'common' ones, the latter caused by the air we breathe.

22 Jouanna (1996) is the best modern edition.

23 Glacken (1967).

individuals can be shown, they can by extension be applied to whole peoples. Glacken argues that it is the nature of the legacy of this tract that is of most interest. He then goes on to talk about the quotations and allusions to it in some of the later sections of the Aristotelian *Problems*. But if one turns to the index to Glacken's large volume, this Hippocratic legacy becomes slight, indeed, a couple of references to Bodin and Burton, and, somewhat more detailed discussions of eighteenth-century writers such as Arbuthnot, Montesquieu and Herder. From then on in academic discussions, it is Hippocrates the ethnographer rather than Hippocrates the doctor that takes precedence, a representative of Greece's encounter with the barbarian in what Rosalind Thomas calls the ethnography of health.[24]

But, leaving Galen aside for the moment, until the sixteenth century, any interest in the second half of the tract is extremely limited. True, Rufus of Ephesus, the most underrated of all ancient medical writers, knew his *Airs, Waters and Places*, and recommended to the physician the need to enquire of the inhabitants of each locality what diseases were endemic there – his example is the guinea worm in Egypt and Arabia – and how they were treated by the locals. But he excuses himself from going further by saying that the possibilities are infinite, and need to be described on the basis of local information.[25] This is not, he argues, contrary to what Hippocrates says in the prologue to *Airs, Waters and Places*, where the author promises a method of discovering what conditions are likely to present themselves, sound in itself, says Rufus, but in need of supplementation.

Such reluctance to deal with widespread diseases, both endemic and epidemic, seems to have been shared with other doctors in Antiquity. Indeed, it is, I think, not until we reach the Islamic period that we find such an interest, although in the absence of most medical writing from Antiquity such comments must be provisional at best. This is a book entitled *On the Prevention of Bodily Ills in Egypt*, written around 1020 by the Egyptian Galenist physicians, Ibn Riḍwān. It was written as a riposte to a work by Ibn al Jazzār, who died around 980, that dealt with the causes, prevention and treatment of epidemic diseases.[26] Ibn Riḍwān accused al-Jazzār, a Tunisian, of writing about Egypt despite never having set foot in it – a reproach that might also be levelled at Ibn Riḍwān, who seems never to have left his native Cairo. Ibn Riḍwān shared the view of Ibn al-Jazzār that bad air was the cause of epidemic disease, but argued that the Egyptian air was bad in a very different way from what Ibn

24 Thomas (2000) 42–74.
25 Rufus, *Quaestiones* 12,64–13,72.
26 Dols (1984).

al-Jazzār had suggested, and hence that it produced a range of different endemic diseases. His explanation is fully in the Galenic tradition. He begins with a description of Egypt, and of the temperament of the land along the lines of *Airs, Waters and Places* – its wind, its situation, its seasons, and its water supply, mainly the Nile, often turbid like sludge, and filled with rotten substances, but elsewhere, as in the Fayyum, in swamps. He then proceeds to deal with the local diseases in accordance with the Galenic six non-naturals. Some of his observations ring very true: in time of famine, prices rise, and starvation and disease increases; others are less so – mass panic is likely to result in sleeplessness, and hence greater susceptibility to disease. He is also aware that, save for the swampy Fayyum, the urban environment of Cairo is far unhealthier than towns elsewhere in Egypt, such as Alexandria or Memphis, and that crowded, low-lying parts of town, such as Fustat, are worst of all. Nonetheless, says this proud Egyptian, Egypt is on the whole healthier than many other regions and its diseases, thanks to long experience, are easier to cure. His book shows how an intelligent author could write up the diseases of his own locality within a Hippocratic-Galenic framework, but he seems to have had few followers – or even readers, for Dols lists a mere seven manuscripts.

His example seems not to have been followed again until the sixteenth century, when there are a variety of studies of local, and often epidemic, disease – the English Sweat, the *lues Morava*, the *plica polonica*, or syphilis, almost all of them written within the Galenist tradition, as well as an enormous number of plague tracts. A Paduan professor for example, can contrast almost in passing, the arrival of a plague there with local endemic diseases of neighbouring towns, the diseases of liver and spleen in Forli, the leg tumours of Ferrara, and the goitres of Brescia.[27] Why we have this lack of information in earlier periods has long been a puzzle, not least because all these later writers, from Ibn Ridwan to Girolamo Fracastoro, Julien le Paulmier and Guillaume de Baillou in the sixteenth century, are writing within the Hippocratic tradition.[28]

One reason may be that the perspective of surviving ancient medical writers remains very much within the geographical boundaries of the Hippocratic Corpus. Galen is a wonderful observer, not least of food and drink, and our understanding of life in the ancient countryside of Greece, Asia Minor and around Rome owes much to him, but one would be hard pressed to find much within his writings about diseases within Rome and Latium, let alone beyond the Alps. Rufus mentions almost in passing an outbreak of buboes in Libya,

27 Trincavella (1586) 19r–20r.
28 Fracastoro (1546); Le Paulmier (1578); De Baillou (1640).

Egypt and Syria, and he refers also to Arabia, but we know little about anything further East, where travellers, doctors possibly among them, had visited.[29]

Rufus' references to water are from the first part of *Airs, Waters and Places*. He is not unique in this. With two exceptions, authors who cite or paraphrase it overwhelmingly cite the first part.[30] The exceptions are the glossators and Galen himself in *The Soul's Habits follow the Body's Temperaments*, the one tract above all in which he deals with generalised characteristics.[31] The parallel with physiognomics is obvious – and a passage al-Masudi, writing around 940 in his *The Meadow of Gold*, claims, rightly or wrongly as coming from Galen has similar links with physiognomy. Galen mentions ten particular properties of the negros: curly hair, thin eyebrows, splayed nostrils, thick lips, sharp teeth, smelly skin, black colour, long feet and hands, large genitals, and excessive petulance (explainable by the imperfect organisation of their brain, hence their feeble wits) – Galen has a lot to answer for, if he is al-Masudi's source.[32]

Rufus' uses the section in *Airs, Waters and Places* on water twice, once in *Medical Questions*, the other, at much greater length, excerpted by Oribasius under the heading *On Waters*.[33] Whether this is the title of a book or merely of a section in a longer work on foodstuffs or his medical encyclopedia, *For the Layman*, is impossible to tell. The latter seems more plausible especially as, following *Airs, Waters and Places*, Rufus indicates the varied qualities of water that are likely to be encountered by a travelling doctor. In this he does not deviate from the Hippocratic classification, an indication that this, like so much else, may well as become standard in Alexandrian Hippocratic education, and is repeated by Galen in his commentary on the treatise and elsewhere.

But, on the whole, water receives little attention in the humoral tradition. We have interesting snippets of information from travellers on how water can be kept cool or be purified, or the difference in quality between the water in the Tiber in its upper reaches and once it reaches the city of Rome. Galen, the great observer, notes the polluting stench of a river that carries away the scourings from toilets, restaurants and baths, as well as the filthy water in which

29 Rufus, p. 304 ed. Daremberg-Ruelle = Oribasius, *Collectiones* 44,14: CMG VII,2,1, 131–2; *Quaestiones* 12,67–69. But in the long fragment on water quoted by Oribasius, *Collectiones* V 3,3: CMG VI 1,1,117–19, he mentions Thrace, a lake among the Sauromatae and another in Persia, as well as a spring near Susa, which causes the teeth of anyone who drinks from it to fall out.

30 Anastassiou and Irmer (2006) 23–39; (1997) 25–53; (2001) 30–36.

31 Rufus, *Quaestiones* 13,72.

32 Barbier de Meynard and P. De Courtelle (1871) I, 163–64.

33 Rufus, p. 298, 341–48 ed. Daremberg-Ruelle = Oribasius, *Collectiones* V 3,3: CMG VI 1,1,117–19. For the problem of authenticity, see Anastassiou and Irmer (1997) I, 33, where there appears to be a divergence of opinion expressed in the *apparatus criticus* and the footnote.

clothes and blankets have been washed. It is the same with water near an army camp, or one that has had rotting animals, fruit and vegetables dumped in it but there is little, in the Galenic texts so far published, that goes beyond the message *of Airs, Waters and Places*, or medical warnings against marshes, fens and stagnant pools that would not have been echoed by writers of all persuasions from Plato and Aristotle down to Cato, Columella and beyond.[34]

Anne Liewert in her 2015 study of meteorological medicine in the Hippocratic Corpus has argued that, while the environment provides the background against which to place the health of the individual patient, there is a crucial difference between the attention given to water and places, on the one hand, and climate and weather on the other. The latter is constantly changing, and it is these changes that are seen as crucial in the causation of illness. Hence, she suggests, the relatively little attention paid to other environmental factors in the Corpus, and well beyond.[35] Since, on the whole, one could not change one's environment, the most that one could be done was in the way of prediction and prophylaxis: knowing what was likely to happen allowed the doctor to take precautions, and for that one needed to be aware of the environment.

This does not mean that some ancient doctors did not offer wider prescriptive advice. Fragments of writers from the century or more before Galen, preserved in the 4th century writer Oribasius, and now shortly to be supplemented from Galen's own commentary on *Airs, Waters and Places*, reveal a remarkable series of observations and discussions about the health of cities. One can talk of a Hippocratic tradition, if not a specifically Alexandrian tradition, going back three or four generations before Galen, and including Rufus of Ephesus as well as some of his teachers and his teachers' teachers.[36] Sabinus, for instance, compared the clean air of a city at dawn with that later in the day when it has become altered by the smoke, smells, dust and the other effusions, *apophorai*, and odours of the town. Athenaeus of Attaleia, the earliest of Oribasius' doctors, explains how the movement of air is blocked by buildings. In a crowded centre, it becomes thick, befouled by exhalations and increasingly unhealthy. Allowing the air to move leads to better digestion, better appetite, and greater sensitivity.[37] Sabinus goes further in offering medical advice about town planning. A city should have straight roads, orientated east, west, north and-south, and with straight roads leading in from the suburbs to allow gentle winds to sweep away the smoke and fumes; the sun can reach every house. By contrast,

34 Borca (2000).
35 Liewert (2015).
36 Nutton (2000) 69–70.
37 Cf. also Rufus, p. 517 ed. Daremberg-Ruelle.

with narrow winding streets, the winds cause turbulence as they meet obstructions in a veritable battle of the winds. Sunlight never penetrates in some areas, and the exhalation, *anathumiasis*, cannot be dispersed. The air becomes thick and hard to breathe. This relates to a city on the plain: one on a hill top is better off with winding streets, which block the foul air rising up from the plain.

It will be interesting to compare Sabinus' account with Galen's commentary on *Airs, Waters and Places*, when it is published, but for the moment two points are worth stressing. This is a confident extension of ideas that had long been familiar; how far back such discussions among medics went back is unclear, but certainly for some time. Secondly, Sabinus is writing within an academic situation, and using the academic form of a commentary. That it was possible to range widely within such a commentary is well known, and what is so far known of Galen's confirms that he too used the Hippocratic text as a basis for observations and discussions that are remarkable in both depth and quality. Sabinus and Galen were not alone in choosing to comment on *Airs, Waters and Places*, evidence that by the late 1st century, if not much earlier, this text had already become in some way authoritative within the Hippocratic humoral tradition. But are these medical discussions likely to have travelled far outside the classroom or the library? We have the example of Vitruvius to show that at least one architect was interested in building a healthy city, but he too is a theorist as much as a practitioner. No one, as far as I know, believes that any of Sabinus' prescriptions or advice were taken: we are not in the world of planned cities such as Karlsruhe or Washington DC. Neither one should imagine that it had no link with the real world, with the massive rebuilding of cities and towns all over the Greek world in the first and second centuries, a building programme in which Galen's father participated. Colonnaded streets, splendid public buildings, *exedrae*, fountains and aqueducts were being built afresh almost everywhere, streets that had formerly been mud tracks were paved with stone. One only has to compare the descriptions of cities in Pausanias with those of Strabo a century earlier to feel the change, and a wander around any ancient site will only confirm the enormous amount of building that took place in this period; villages became towns, towns cities, and suburban living was not confined to Rome or Athens. At the very least, all this activity provides a background against which to view Sabinus' comments.

This paper began with an example of a Renaissance physician, Ulrich Ellenbog, writing a *consilium* for a group, as a way of approaching a wider problem in humoral medicine, the lack of attention in our surviving medical sources given to epidemic disease, or of anything that might come under the heading of *loimos*, plague. Galen, as always, is well versed in theory, and his distinction between epidemic and endemic diseases goes back to *Airs, Waters and Places*. Although both affect large numbers of individuals, the former are sporadic and universal, the latter confined to one area or region and always present. The latter may have the origin in the local environment, but epidemics are widespread, *pankoinos*, and indiscriminate. It is precisely for that reason that epidemics seem to challenge humoral beliefs in the importance of the individual.

They seem to present a challenge, because the notion that air was in some way responsible is accepted by almost everyone in Antiquity, and, effectively, down to the nineteenth century, whether doctors or not. The historian Herodian is a typical representative of ancient views, twice describing outbreaks of mass disease. In 188 CE, during an outbreak of *loimos*, plague, in Rome, doctors advised Commodus to leave Rome for Laurentum, a town in Latium, where the redolent fragrance of the surrounding laurel trees purified the noxious air.[38] Those left behind in the steamy city followed medical advice to make constant use of perfumes, incense and aromatic herbs, whose sweet odours, once in their nostrils, prevented the foul air from entering the body. Later in his history, describing how many soldiers died in an outbreak of disease in a camp in North Syria, Herodian explained that this was the result of troops being recently moved there from Illyria, where they had enjoyed moist cooler air as well as better rations. Bad air and diet were thus responsible for this outbreak, which was ended when the troops retreated to Antioch, with its less stifling air and an abundance of good water.[39]

Herodian's comments are a typical example of ancient ideas on epidemics, not least because, as already stated, we have a singular lack of information from medical sources. That outbreaks of epidemic disease were common in Antiquity is abundantly clear from a variety of sources, and especially historians, from Thucydides, via Livy and Lucian, to Procopius and Joshua the Syriac chronicler of events in Edessa.[40] This contrasts with what we find in our medical sources. Galen, of course, provides us with many snippets of information on a variety of epidemic diseases in Rome and in Asia Minor, but his comments can be criticised in exactly the same way as he himself criticised Thucydides; they are partial, and do not always easy to fit together. The same goes for Rufus, particularly if one interprets the heading in Oribasius and Aetius, 'Rufus on plague', to refer to a section taken from another larger work.[41] Other writers

38 Herodian, *Hist*. 1.12.2.
39 Herodian, *Hist*. 6.6.2.
40 Nutton (2013) 24–27.
41 Rufus, pp. 309, 351, 440 ed. Daremberg-Ruelle; the section on the health of towns, p. 517 ed. Daremberg-Ruelle, is ascribed to a book on regimen.

are strangely silent: nothing in Aretaeus, for example, despite his interest in disease and diseases. Caelius Aurelianus, is at first sight more promising, for he refers to a work, now lost, by Asclepiades that dealt with plague or epidemic disease under a title that Caelius gives in Latin as *De lue*, a word he also uses to characterise epilepsy as the sacred *lues*. Others, like Celsus in a single short paragraph in *De medicina* I, 10 on the writers on theriac, prescribe remedies or prophylaxis.[42] We can also dimly hear ancient debates about the causes of the epidemic among doctors, veterinarians like Vegetius, philosophers like Plutarch, and theologians, but we have to rely on brief comments rather than extended explanations. Besides, whether one believed in a judgment of God, a disturbed balance of the natural order, pestilent exhalations, plague-bearing seeds transported by winds or clouds, changes in the climate or putrefaction, the acknowledgment of the principal involvement of the air was universal.[43]

What, under such circumstances, could a humoral physician do? Or, to put it another way, what could be done to reduce the effect of epidemic disease? It is worth reverting for examples to Ulrich Ellenbog and the doctors of the sixteenth century, the great age of epidemics. By then Western doctors had already had over two hundred years of experience with bubonic plague, to say nothing of other diseases. They had long established protocols for treating illness based on the six non-naturals, and, compared with their predecessors in the fourteenth century, they had two new weapons at their disposal: the civic organisation of plague control, and the printing press, which allowed for the easy dissemination of advice and information. For example, Ellenbog's own little tract on plague, *Instruktion wider die Pestilentz*, was among the first medical books printed in German, in 1484, and was republished ten years later.[44] A brief survey of Renaissance plague literature shows both the influence of the classical physicians and the ways in which those trained in the classical tradition developed those ideas.[45]

These plague tracts were written for a general public, and their advice is applicable to all. They accept religious remote causes in some version of divine anger and of God punishing his people, but while religious and civic authorities might demand a religious remedy involving prayer, processions and public fasting, most medical writers take the view that they alone to can take effective action to reduce the effects of the disease. They accept all or most of

42 Véronique Boudon-Millot provides a good survey of the ancient literature on theriac in her edition of the pseudo-Galenic *De theriaca ad Pisonem*, Galen (2016) VIII–XLI.

43 Conrad and Wujastyk (2000).

44 Ellenbog (1524).

45 Cohn (2010).

the explanations in classical authors, planetary conjunctions, changes in the weather, or something such as an earthquake that would change air.[46] This adds a certain authority to their explanations, but does not help with any treatment or contribute much to the ongoing debate. Where there is debate, it is over precisely what it is that makes the air so deadly. It is a debate about classification, for the classification in turn determines treatment.

The standard view, which goes back to Galen and beyond, is that the air has become in some way foul: it has become hot and sticky and causes the body to become putrid.[47] (There is a subsidiary debate as to whether the air itself is already putrid or simply incites the body to become so.) Putrefaction, the result of heat and moisture, thus fits perfectly into the standard humoral model: it can be treated by drugs that will dry and cool the body, and it can be predicted atmospherically, by noting changes in the stars and season, and physically, by specifying those individuals who are most likely to be at risk. Others, again following Galenic precedent, argued that even if plague might be the result of exhalations from the earth, the population needed to be reassured and avoid becoming fearful, for fear, *timor*, lessened resistance to the infection.

Others, like Ellenbog himself, had a slightly different explanation. In his *consilium* for the Augsburg goldsmiths, he concluded that the air had become poisonous, and thus had to be treated as one would a poison, with heating, evacuants, and particularly with antidotes such as theriac, that operated on all bodies alike. Similar writers who think in terms of poison tend not to spend much time in prophylaxis or in specifying who is most at risk but concentrate on therapy. Simone Simoni, for instance, who became professor at Leipzig and elsewhere, is scathing in 1576 about his fellow doctors who spend time on identifying the best humoral characteristics for withstanding plague.[48] This is useless, in his view, for plague attacks people of all humoral types indiscriminately, and spending time on this rather than in successfully treating sufferers once they have fallen ill is just a waste of time.

Others took a middle view: it was not the air itself that was the causative agent, but what it contained. Girolamo Fracastoro in 1546 put forward a view, ultimately deriving in part from Lucretius and from the Aristotelian *Problems*, that in contagious diseases the air carried with it seeds of disease, that differed according to the particular disease, plague, measles, smallpox, but also rabies, scabies and the evil eye.[49] Some were spread by touch, others by seeds

46 Beroaldo (1505) sigg. B. iii.r., A viii.v, citing Seneca with approval.
47 Cohn (2010) 161–207, gives a good survey of these theoretical debates.
48 Simoni (1576); Nutton, (2006).
49 Fracastoro (1546); Pellegrini (1950); Nutton (1990); Pennuto (2008).

left in clothing and the like, others by air-borne seeds. Such a view, however, revolutionary it might have seemed to later historians in an age familiar with bacilli and germs, could be, and was, easily adopted by anyone who believed in a theory that bad air caused epidemic disease, and who recommended that one should take in less of the bad air. Hence the recourse to pomanders and perfumes, exactly as earlier Romans did in 188 AD, to drive away smells and bad air, or the bonfires in the streets that Hippocrates was said to have organised in his cure of the plague of Athens.[50]

But Fracastoro's theories, and his belief in contagious diseases, also gave support to the advocates of civic action. Here is the major difference between Antiquity and the Middle Ages and Renaissance By 1400, all around Europe, royal and local authorities had imposed regulations for cleaning the streets to prevent infection. Ineffective, these might usually have been, and one hears the same complaints noted earlier about the blockage of drains and water-courses and the foetid mass of rubbish that poured into rivers. Modern locks on the river at Padua in 1541, said the College of Physicians, were to blame for a deadly fever, because they did not allow the filthy waste of tanneries and other rubbish to be carried swiftly away, and instead created a stinking, putrefying mass that attracted an unprecedented number of insects and visibly turned the air bad.[51] A slightly earlier outbreak in Oxford was ascribed to a similar problem with its locks, blocked among other things by a dead horse. Stronger civic action, at least in theory, was needed.[52]

A second development, beginning also in the fourteenth century but two hundred years later still largely confined to the bigger and better organised cities of Italy, was the publication of plague regulations, banning potential carriers of infection from outside and removing from society those who developed signs of the disease, and usually, those associated with them. Some were removed to a special hospital, a lazaretto, others were shut up in their own houses. As with street cleaning, rules might be broken and disregarded, and authorities reluctant to declare a plague for fear of the expense of setting up hospitals and the resentment of citizens thrown out of work as the town closed down.[53] But procedures there were, and could be implemented, possibly successfully. Such action had been indeed considered in Antiquity, but then the only effective remedy, it was argued, was segregation, the fumigation

50 Rubin Pinault (1992) 35–60.
51 Da Monte (1583) 1106–20.
52 Mitchell (1977–1978) 71–94.
53 Bamji (2016); Cohn (2010).

of infected buildings and the slaughter. But these prescriptions were for sick animals, not humans, and no ancient town ever developed the health structures that are found in-the Renaissance.

This hurried survey of later ideas on plague show that it was possible to combine an individualist humoral approach with a concern for 'common' diseases, whether of groups like the goldsmiths or of whole communities, and the question must at least be posed of the reasons why ancient medical writers say so little about them. In a tradition that took back a discussion of health and illness to Plato's ascription to the historical Hippocrates of the need to consider the individual against the 'whole', however one might choose to interpret this version of holism, it is *prima facie* surprising to find so little on wider diseases. One must, of course, admit that what survives of ancient medicine is but a tiny fraction of what was written, and that a Latin or Greek Fracastoro could have discussed at length contagious diseases such as the Thucydidean plague in a treatise that is now lost to us. After all, both the *Epidemics* and *Airs, Waters and Places* emphasise environmental causes, principally the weather and the seasons, and, at least in the Roman period, there was a tradition of doctors in the Hippocratic tradition writing about urban pollution and the healthy city. By late Antiquity also students in Alexandria were taught to consider the relationship of the individual to everything around as one of the so-called six non-naturals that influenced the body for good or ill, a holistic precept that became standard in both Arabic and late-Medieval Western medicine. Two factors are certainly at play, one intellectual, the other organisational. For Galen and others like him, the nature of any locality, its climate, situation and water supply, was to be used as a basis for judging the nature of its inhabitants. But to go beyond these Hippocratic generalities is difficult in two ways. Rufus of Ephesus noted the problem: the sheer range of possibilities that could not easily be set down in a single text. But collecting and evaluating the material, despite the precedent of the Hippocratic *Constitutions*, presented its own problems, and may explain why we have no examples later than the early fourth century BCE. Writing up a single case history was an easier task than tracking the diseases of a community over a long period of time in the absence of archival documentation. The second, and perhaps more significant factor, was the absence of an effective civic organisation that would allow any official reaction to the arrival of an epidemic beyond the dispatch of a religious embassy to a shrine or the introduction of a non-local healer. The earliest 'quarantine' was created by a city state, Ragusa/Dubrovnik, in the fourteenth century, but it had already been preceded by regulations on street cleaning and, in Ragusa and gradually elsewhere, it was followed by the creation of health boards with strong powers of control as well as with a relatively long tradition of effective civic administration by members of the local elite.[54] This administrative gap may in part explain why similar practices were not put in place in Antiquity, with the possible exception of Christian charitable assistance in times of plague, and why, despite the reputation of *Airs, Waters and Places*, so well chronicled by Glacken, its direct influence on humoral physicians and on ideas about 'common' diseases among in Antiquity was limited, and that of the Hippocratic *Constitutions* even less. However much one might subscribe to a humoral and holistic theory of health and disease that went beyond the individual, practical considerations imposed constraints that were extremely hard to overcome.

Bibliography

Anastassiou, A., and D. Irmer, D. *Testimonien zum Corpus Hippocraticum, Teil I.* Göttingen: Vandenhoeck & Ruprecht (2006). *Teil* II,1 (1997). *Teil* II,2 (2001).

Arika, N. *Passions and Tempers. A History of the Humours.* New York: Ecco (2007).

Assion, P. 'Ulrich Ellenbog.' In *Die deutsche Literatur des Mittelalters.* Verfasserlexikon, ed. 2, ed. G. Keil and K. Ruh. Berlin and New York: De Gruyter (1980) II, 495–501.

Bamji, A. 'Medical Care in Early Modern Venice.' *Journal of Social History*, 49.3 (2016) 483–509.

Barbier de Meynard, C., and P. De Courtelle. *Al-Masudi, Les prairies d'or*, vol. I. Paris: Imprimerie nationale (1871).

Barnard, C. 'Ulrich Ellenbog.' *The Lancet*, 219, issue 5657 (January 30, 1932) 270–71.

Beroaldo, F. *De terraemotu et pestilentia.* Bologna: J. de Herbona, (1505).

Blazina Tomic, Z., and V. Blazina. *Expelling the Plague. The Health Office and the Implementation of Quarantine in Dubrovnik, 1377–1533.* Montreal, Kingston, Ithaca and London: McGill-Queen's University Press (2007).

Borca, F. 'Towns and Marshes in the Ancient World.' In *Death and Disease in the Ancient City*, ed. V. M. Hope and E. Marshall. London and New York: Routledge (2000) 74–84.

Cohn, S. K., Jr. *Cultures of Plague. Medical Thinking at the End of the Renaissance.* Oxford: Oxford University Press (2010).

Conrad L. I., and D. Wujastyk (eds.) *Contagion. Perspectives from Pre-Modern Societies.* Aldershot, Burlington, Singapore and Sydney: Ashgate (2000).

Craik, E. M. *The 'Hippocratic' Corpus. Content and Context.* London and New York: Routledge (2015).

Da Monte, G. B. *Consultationes Medicae.* Basel: n.p. (1583).

54 Blazina Tomic and Blazina (2015).

Daremberg, C., Ruelle, C-É. (eds.) *Œuvres de Rufus d'Éphèse*. Paris: Imprimerie Nationale (1879).

De Baillou, G. *Epidemiorum et ephemeridum libri*. Paris: J. Quenel (1640).

Diller, H. *Wanderarzt und Aitiologe*. Philologus Suppl. 26. Leipzig: Dieterich'sche Verlagsbuchhandlung (1934).

Dols, M. W. *Medieval Islamic Medicine. Ibn Riḍwān's Treatise 'On the Prevention of Bodily Ills in Egypt.'* Berkeley, Los Angeles and London: University of California Press (1984).

Ellenbog, U. *Von den gifftigen Besen Temmpffen un[d] Reüchen, der Metal, als Silber, Quecksilber, Bley und anders So die edlen Handtwerck des Goltschmidens, und ander Arbaiter in des Feür sich gebrauchen müssen.* Augsburg: M. Ramminger (1524).

Fracastoro, G. *De Sympathia et Antipathia Rerum. De Contagione, et Contagiosis Morbis et Curatione Libri III*. Venice: Heirs of L. A. Giunta (1546).

Galen, *Theriac for Pison* (*Ther.Pis.*). Ed. V. Boudon-Millot. Paris: Les Belles Lettres (2016).

Glacken, C. L. *Traces on the Rhodian Shore: Nature and Culture in Western Thought from Ancient Times to the 18th Century*. Princeton: Princeton University Press (1967).

Jouanna, J. (ed.) *Hippocrates, Airs, Waters and Places* (*AWP*). Paris: Les Belles Lettres (1996).

Jouanna, J. (ed.) *Epidemics I, III* (*Epid.*) Paris: Les Belles Lettres (2016).

König, J. *Athletics and Literature in the Roman Empire*. Cambridge: Cambridge University Press (2005).

Le Paulmier, J. *De Morbis Contagiosis*. Paris: D. Duval (1578).

Letts, M. *Questioning the Patient, Questioning Hippocrates: Rufus of Ephesus and the Limits of Medical Authority*. Dissertation Oxford University (2015).

Liewert, A. *Die meteorologische Medizin des Corpus Hippocraticum*. Berlin: De Gruyter (2015).

Mikkeli, H. *Hygiene in the Early Modern Medical Tradition*. Helsinki: The Finnish Academy of Science and Letters (1999).

Mitchell, W. T. (ed.) *Epistolae Academicae 1508–1596*. Oxford: Clarendon Press (1977–78).

Nicoud, M. *Les Régimes de Santé au Moyen Âge. Naissance et Diffusion d'une Écriture médicale (XIII*e*–XV*e *siècle)*. Rome: École française de Rome (2007).

Nutton, V. 'The Reception of Fracastoro's Theory of Contagion: the Seed that fell among Thorns.' *Osiris, ser.* 2.6 (1990) 196–234.

Nutton, V. 'Medical Thoughts on Urban Pollution.' In *Death and Disease in the Ancient City*, ed. V. M. Hope and E. Marshall. London and New York: Routledge (2000) 65–73.

Nutton, V. 'With Benefit of Hindsight: Girolamo Mercuriale and Simone Simoni on Plague.' *Medicina & Storia*, 6 (2006) 5–20.

Nutton, V. *Ancient Medicine*. 2nd ed. London and New York: Routledge (2013).

O'Boyle, C. 'Astrology and Medicine in Later Medieval England. The Calendars of John Somer and Nicholas of Lynn.' *Sudhoffs Archiv*, 89 (2005) 1–22.

Pastore, A. 'Il trattato *De venenis* e la tradizione tossicologica del suo tempo.' In *Girolamo Mercuriale. Medicina e Cultura nell'Europa del Cinquecento*, ed. A. Arcangeli and V. Nutton. Florence: Leo S. Olschki (2008) 233–46.

Pellegrini, F. *La Dottrina Fracastoriana del* Contagium Vivum. *Origini e Primi Sviluppi da Autografi Inediti Conservati nella Biblioteca Capitolare di Verona*. Verona: Tipografia Valdonega (1950).

Pennuto, C. *Simpatia, Fantasia e Contagio. Il Pensiero Medico e il Pensiero Filosofico di Girolamo Fracastoro*. Rome: Edizioni di storia e letteratura (2008).

Perilli, L. 'Writing, Preserving, and Disseminating Scientific Knowledge: Some Remarks on Manuscripts and Other Writing Supports in Ancient Greece.' *Manuscript Cultures*, 5 (2012–2013) 20–32.

Ramazzini, B. *De Morbis Artificum Diatriba*. 2nd ed. Padua: G. B. Conzetti (1713).

Ramazzini, B. *Diseases of Workers*. Trans. W. Cave Wright. Chicago: The University of Illinois Press (1940).

Rubin Pinault, J. *Hippocratic Lives and Legends*. Leiden and New York: Brill (1992).

Rufus of Ephesus, *Medical Questions* (*Quaestiones Medicinales*). Ed. H. Gärtner. Corpus medicorum graecorum IV. Berlin: Akademie-Verlag (1962).

Schöner, E. *Das Viererschema in der antiken Humoralpathologie*. Wiesbaden: Steiner Verlag (1964).

Simoni, S. *Artificiosa Curandae Pestis Methodus*. Leipzig: J. Steinman (1576).

Thomas, R. *Herodotus in Context. Ethnography. Science and the Art of Persuasion*. Cambridge: Cambridge University Press (2000).

Trincavella, V. *Opera omnia*. Lyons: Giunta and Guittius (1586).

Wooton, D. *Bad Medicine. Doctors doing Harm since Hippocrates*. Oxford: Oxford University Press (2006).

CHAPTER 15

Mind-Body Interaction: The Influence of Ancient Ideas in Twelfth-Century England

Claire Trenery

Abstract

The twelfth century witnessed the wide dissemination of Latin texts and translated Greek and Arabic medical works through western Christendom, which brought with them a wealth of new ideas. The materialistic fundamentals of ancient Graeco-Roman medicine were introduced to a Christian philosophical tradition that distinguished between the material body and the immaterial soul. This chapter focuses on one of the most significant phenomena that emerged within this new cultural and intellectual environment: the proliferation of hagiographical writing that recorded, often in large collections, acts of wonder that were performed by the saints. Through the records made in English miracle texts, I explore representations of the physical, mental and spiritual suffering of pilgrims, which are indicative of the close interaction between religion and medicine. This chapter analyses the reception of ancient 'holistic' medical ideas in the central Middle Ages and the impact of Christianity on representations of physical, mental and spiritual illness and healing.

> There was a sick person in whose case the remorseless critical phase terminated his acute fever in madness. The dementia doubled his strength, and it took eight sane men all their time to restrain the single madman from desiring and having the strength to devour his children and wife. He was rolled before the feet of the bishop, so that Saint Hugh might pour holy water over him; and the demon, conjured with stern words, left him. The patient lay there, imaging the sleep of death. Colour and warmth left his face, sight was lost, his senses gone and his pulse sunk to stillness. The bishop hastened to call back the latent senses to the outer world and drenched him more profusely with the holy water. The spirit, as it raged about in the tepid blood, felt the cold. Each thing rebounds at the sensation of its opposite, and, in this case, the contrary cold stirred up substantial heat. Thus, simultaneously, the sickness collapsed and the patient rose up, his mind no longer agitated by madness nor his blood

 | DOI:10.1163/9789004443143_017

> by the acute fever. On this account, he gave thanks to God and to Saint Hugh, he who had been in control of neither mind nor body but now was in control of both.[1]

This remarkable cure was recorded in the *Metrical Life of Saint Hugh of Lincoln*, which was composed in Latin in around 1220 to celebrate the late Bishop of Lincoln's canonisation. Hugh had died in 1200, and it is likely that his encounter with this fevered madman occurred sometime in the 1190s. The poet's description of the madman is striking and reveals his belief in a connection between physical, mental and spiritual health and sickness. It seems that the source of the man's madness (*rabies*[2]) was initially physical; excessive heat from his fever (*febris*) had caused his mind (*mens*) to become agitated by insanity (*dementia*). Madness, in this case, was both a corporeal and a mental condition since the agitation of the mind (*mens*) was dependent on the fevered body (*corpus*). This man's madness was also a spiritual condition, and his cure required the expulsion of a demon using holy water. When the demon departed, the madman was left in a death-like state, without warmth or movement. Once again, the bishop applied holy water, and, this time, the cool water stirred up heat, and the man recovered his health. The poet's explanation that 'each thing rebounds at the sensation of its opposite' (*ad oppositi sensum res quaeque resultat*) could refer both to the expulsion of the unholy demon using holy water and to the reinvigoration of the man's body with the heat that was created through the application of cold. His interpretation of the madman's cure is indicative of the poet's interest in humoral medicine; sickness could be caused by imbalances in the bodily fluids – or humours – as a result of too much heat, too much cold, too much moisture or too much dryness. This chapter looks at records made in England between 1070 and 1220 of what were believed to be miracles performed by saints. Using representations of illnesses

1 *Importuna crisis febrem languentis acutam / Terminat in rabiem; geminat dementia vires: / Insanus sanis vix unus ab octo tenetur, / Quin velit et valeat pueris et conjuge vesci. / Praesulis ante pedes advolvitur, ut benedicta / Sanctus eum perfundat aqua; verbique rigore / Adjuratus abit daemon. Jacet ille soporem / Effigians mortis: color et calor ora relinquunt, / Lumen abit, sensusque vacant, pulsusque quiescit. / Exterius properat sensus revocare latentes / Praesul, et uberius benedicta proluit unda. / Spiritus in tepido discurrens sanguine frigus / Sentit; ad oppositi sensum res quaeque resultat, / Vimque caloris ibi contrarius excitat algor, / Sic pariter morbusque cadit patiensque resurgit: / Jam nec agit mentem rabies, nec corpus acuta: / Unde Deo grates, et sancto solvit Hugoni, / Compos homo nuper neutrius, nunc utriusque* (*Metrical Life* 1088–1105). Editions and translations used are listed at the end of the chapter. Where no translator is cited, the English translation is my own.

2 In this period, the term *rabies* was not always associated with a bite from a rabid dog, as it is today. In this record, *rabies* was used to denote frenzied madness.

in these records, it explores how ancient humoralism and classical ideas concerning holistic healing were incorporated into Medieval miracle narratives and what impact Christianity had on representations and understandings of physical, mental and spiritual suffering.

When we think of 'holistic medicine', we think of an approach to healthcare that treats the whole person as opposed to one specific part and that encompasses the complete bodily experience as well as non-corporeal aspects of the human condition (mental and spiritual health). Many elements of Medieval healthcare were holistic in this sense. Roman Catholicism taught that every human was made up of three parts (body, mind and soul), which were distinct yet indivisible, mirroring the Holy Trinity (Father, Son and Holy Spirit). At the end of the world, the mind (*spiritus*), soul (*anima*) and body (*corpus*) of each individual would be resurrected for the Final Judgement (1 Thessalonians 5:23). In the Bible, Christ acted as a physician (*medicus*) who came to Earth to heal sinners (Mark 2:17). The health of the soul was closely related to the health of the body and mind. Canon Twenty-Two of the Fourth Lateran Council (1215) decreed that

> physicians of the body, when they are called to the sick, [...] warn and persuade them first of all to call in physicians of the soul so that, after their spiritual health has been seen to, they may respond better to medicine for their bodies[3]
>
> *medicis corporum, ut cum eos ad infirmos vocari contigerit, ipsos ante omnia moneant et inducant, quod medicos advocent animarum, ut postquam infirmis fuerit de spirituali salute provisum, ad corporalis medicinae remedium salubrius procedatur.*

The canon acknowledged that bodily and spiritual illnesses were sometimes connected since 'sickness of the body may sometimes be the result of sin' (*infirmitas corporalis nonnumquam ex peccato proveniat*). After a soul was cleansed, 'when the cause ceases so does the effect' (*cum causa cessante cesset effectus*), meaning that spiritual impurity could be a contributing factor to physical suffering. Provision was also made for those patients who might have given up hope of recovery when a priest was summoned, believing themselves to be capable only of receiving the Last Rites before death. The soul was to be protected, first and foremost, in the hope that this protection could lead to a bodily cure but with the understanding that, were recovery not possible, the

3 Tanner (1990) I: 245.

soul should be prepared for the next life. The first model of holistic healing that I address in this chapter is this Christian model, in which physical, mental and spiritual health were intrinsically related and co-dependent.

The second model of holistic healing, which I refer to as the ancient model, is based on a Medieval interpretation of ancient texts and theories, which were discussed with renewed vigour in western Christendom in the twelfth century. Developing a concept first found in Hippocratic medicine, Medieval medical writers argued that health was achieved through the balancing of four bodily fluids, known as humours (*humores*): blood, red/yellow bile, phlegm and black bile. Excessive quantities of one or more humour could cause imbalance, which, in turn, could lead to sickness.[4] Medieval regimens – guides on how to live healthily – recommended maintaining humoral balance, which could be achieved in part through the regulation of the six 'non-naturals' (*res non naturales*): eating and drinking, sleeping and waking, evacuation and repletion, motion and rest, air, and emotions or passions.[5] The non-naturals were variants that affected the body and mind but were not part of their essential substance. To prevent illness, a person had to be careful not to over- or under-indulge in any of these six areas. Excess of any emotion – like anger, fear, pleasure and sorrow – was a risk-factor for ill-health. Sadness and anxiety, for example, made the body, and especially the heart, too cold and thus, upset a person's humoral balance.[6] According to the ancient model, then, health was holistic in the sense that humans were fundamentally influenced by their environment, that non-physical aspects of the human condition (like emotions) could have a corporeal effect and vice versa, and that health and sickness were experienced throughout the body as a whole because of its humoral make-up.[7]

1 The Classical Inheritance in Twelfth-Century England

Historians have, since the nineteenth century, been using the phrase 'twelfth-century Renaissance' to describe the period of cultural and intellectual change that took place in western Christendom from around 1070. Though he was not the first historian to use the term, Charles Homer Haskins's seminal

4 Johannicius, *Isagoge* 46.
5 For more on the 'non-naturals', see Siraisi (1990) 101 and 120–23 or Niebyl (1971).
6 Arnau de Vilanova, *Speculum medicinae* 83. For a summary of Medieval medical thought concerning the emotions and for more on Arnau de Vilanova, see Gil Sotres (1998) 113–14.
7 In P. N. Singer's chapter in this volume (chapter 6), holism is explored in relation to three aspects of ancient medicine: cosmic or environmental holism, mind-body holism, a holistic conception the human body itself.

book entitled '*The Renaissance of the Twelfth Century*', which was published in 1927, is credited with drawing serious historical attention to the concept in the English-speaking world. Haskins argued that, contrary to the popular belief that the Middle Ages marked a 'dark era' of intellectual ignorance and cultural stagnation, the twelfth century was an age of scientific and creative accomplishment.[8] Of course, knowledge of ancient medicine and science had not been completely lost in the period prior to 1100. Old English medical manuscripts circulated in significant numbers from at least the middle of the ninth century. Nonetheless, these manuscripts largely contained remedy collections with little or no attention to medical theory, though the unwritten theoretical basis behind such remedies indicates an understanding of ancient medical ideas.[9]

It was only from the middle of the eleventh century that Latin medical manuscripts began to circulate in England on a noteworthy scale. These Latin manuscripts contained a 'new medicine',[10] which dedicated considerable attention to humoral theory and drew on the established authority of ancient Hippocratic and Galenic medicine. One such 'new medical' manuscript (London, British Library MS Sloane 1621) has been associated with the eleventh-century Benedictine community at Bury in East Anglia.[11] Sloane 1621 was written entirely in Latin (including marginal additions), though the sophisticated medical vocabulary used was likely influenced by Greek.[12] The remedies in Sloane 1621 are also more complex than is typical of Old English medical texts and call on more exotic ingredients, like cinnamon.[13]

Moving into the twelfth century, many works of ancient origin, which had hitherto been unknown in the Middle Ages, were translated, reorganised and circulated, largely amongst monastic communities, like that in Bury. In the Benedictine monastery at Monte Cassino in modern-day Italy, the monks were engaged in the ambitious task of translating Greek and Arabic medical treatises into Latin so as to preserve and disseminate their contents. Perhaps the most famous Monte Cassino monk, Constantine the African, had spent the first part of his life in North Africa and used his knowledge of Arabic to translate

8 Haskins (1927) 4–7.

9 Banham (2014) 228.

10 Banham (2014) 228.

11 See Michael Gullick's analysis of the manuscript's physical and scribal features (190–225), and Debbie Banham's analysis of its contents (226–46) in Licence, ed. (2014) *Bury St Edmunds and the Norman Conquest*.

12 Banham (2014) 228. For example, use of the term *antidotum* for 'recipe' or 'remedy'. See Banham for full analysis of the terminology.

13 Banham (2014) 230–31.

into Latin the works of some of the great masters of Arabic medicine, including Abū Bakr Muhammad ibn Zakariyyā al-Rāzī (Latinised as Rhazes) and Abū Ja'far Aḥmad bin Abī Khālid Ibn al-Jazzār (Latinised as Algizar).[14] South-east of Monte Cassino in the city of Salerno was one of the most well-known medical schools of the Middle Ages, the *Schola Medica Salernitana*, where students could go to study medicine and where physicians and teachers produced a wealth of medical literature, which had its basis in Greek humoral medicine.[15]

The monasteries of Western Europe, especially those of the Benedictines, provided a network through which this new body of medical literature could be rapidly disseminated. Twenty-five percent of the surviving Latin medical manuscripts from this period were produced in England and Northern France, and English monasteries housed one of the largest collections of medical writings in Western Europe.[16] Nonetheless, the majority of England's monks were not physicians and had no or very little specialist medical learning. So great was the production of new texts in the twelfth century that it was almost impossible for one monk to master all fields of knowledge.[17] Although most Benedictine monks would have been familiar with 'new' medicine, they would have been 'by no means at its speculative cutting edge.'[18] Furthermore, medical and spiritual explanations for illness did not exclude each other. A case in point is the collection of the miracles of Saint Thomas Becket recorded by William of Canterbury, a monk of Christ Church Cathedral Priory in Canterbury who had a detailed understanding of contemporary humoral medicine, as evidenced by his use of sophisticated medical terminology to describe, for example, four types of leprosy (*tyria*, *leonine*, *elephantia* and *alopecia*) and three forms of epilepsy (*ephilensia*, *catalempsia* and *analempsia*).[19] Yet, William attributed over half the cases of madness he recorded to the activities of demons. In his records of madness, he made no reference to humoral imbalance and did not employ any of the specific terms used in contemporary medical texts (e.g. *frenesis*, *mania*, *melancholia*). Whilst he clearly appreciated 'new' medical ideas and was keen to impart them to the readers of his miracle collection (likely fellow monks), William did not consider ancient medical discourses and Christian theology to be incompatible. Therefore, in order to understand how ancient ideas concerning the interactions between body, mind and soul influenced Medieval Christian interpretations of sickness and healing, it is perhaps

14 Green (2018) 279.
15 Green (2018) 286–87.
16 Green (2009) 221.
17 Burnett (2013) 373.
18 Wilson (2014) 101.
19 Koopmans (2011) 186; William of Canterbury, *Miracula* IV.27 and II.6.

more useful to turn away from specialist medical manuscripts and to look instead at one of the most prolific forms of Christian writing of the Middle Ages, of which William's collection of the miracles of Saint Thomas Becket is just one example: miracle records.

The hundred and fifty years that followed the Norman Conquest of England (1066) saw a massive upsurge in the recording of miracles, which Rachel Koopmans has dubbed a 'miracle-collecting mania.'[20] Monks across England compiled written testaments to the miracles performed by their saints, which ranged from modest compendia of twenty to thirty miracles, to huge collections of almost five hundred miracles. These records provided enduring affirmations of God's favour, and they could also be put forward in support of a prospective saint's canonisation as evidence of his or her miracles. As papal canonisation processes were formalised during the twelfth century, culminating in 1234, when Pope Gregory IX made canonisation the exclusive prerogative of the pope, methods of verifying miracles became increasingly stringent. Of course, for an event to be considered miraculous, it had to be shown to have occurred in a way that was beyond the workings of nature. Nonetheless, to be perceived as credible, miracles had to stand up against contemporary theological, philosophical and medical standards.[21] Thus, when the poet who composed the *Metrical Life of Saint Hugh of Lincoln* (with which this chapter opened) explained that 'each thing rebounds at the sensation of its opposite' (*ad oppositi sensum res quaeque resultat*), he was not undermining the miraculous nature of the cure that Saint Hugh had provided. Indeed, the cure was recorded in Hugh's official canonisation report, from which the author of the *Metrical Life* drew his examples, as one of the miracles performed during the saint's lifetime. Instead, the poet aligned Hugh's miracle with contemporary understandings of human nature by demonstrating how the madman's physical, mental and spiritual suffering were interconnected.

2 Platonic Punishments

The works of many classical writers were reasonably well-known in Medieval monastic circles, and classical thought influenced almost all aspects of monastic writing from natural philosophy to dialectics. Whilst Medieval interest in the theories of Aristotle would not reach its peak until the thirteenth century, works of Platonic and Neo-Platonic origin began to take a more prominent

---

20 Koopmans (2011) 2.

21 Goodich (2007) 88.

place in Medieval theological debates from the late tenth century.[22] Plato's dialogue *Timaeus*, which had been translated into Latin in the fourth century by the philosopher Calcidius, played a central role.[23] Only the first part of the text, which described the formation and nature of the cosmos, was known in the twelfth century, and Calcidius's accompanying Latin commentary was highly influential.[24] Justin Stover has identified at least seventy individual twelfth-century writers who discussed the *Timaeus*, and he concludes that knowledge of Platonic ideas was becoming 'familiar, even commonplace' in the Latin West.[25] Particularly significant in Medieval philosophy was Plato's concept of a 'world-soul' (likened, by Christian writers, to the Holy Spirit), which encompassed all natural things and meant that human beings were holistically connected to the natural world around them.

In a collection of the miracles of Saint Edmund the Martyr, which was compiled in Bury in the 1070s and 1080s, a Platonic model of the cosmos was merged with a Christian interpretation of God's divine judgement. The miracle compiler, a Bury monk called Herman, took the Platonic concept of a 'world-soul' and aligned it with Christian understandings of God's presence throughout all of nature (Job 12:7–10). For example, one nobleman called Robert de Curcun had tried to seize a manor, which belonged to the monks of Bury, during the unrest that accompanied the 1088 rebellion against William Rufus. As de Curcun and his men rode towards the manor, a tremendous thunderstorm broke out.

> Struck with terror, they babbled among themselves, saying they were going astray and that God and the saint [Edmund], roused against them, had even planned this storm. They went off via the by-ways, hoping that the face of heaven would look upon them more kindly; and when after a while it did, they resumed their stupid journey. But at once a storm arose among the elements and followed them, restoring those fools to their previous mental confusion, until their master – namely the aforementioned Robert – fell into such a state of stupor that he retreated and dared not complete the journey he had begun. Afterwards his stupefaction was stamped on his face for everyone to see, for the state of his mind left a physical impression.

22 Gregory (1988) 54.
23 Dutton (2003) 184. For more on the post-Platonic debate regarding the parallel health of soul and body, see P. N. Singer's chapter in this volume (chapter 6).
24 Gregory (1988) 54.
25 Stover (2011) 13.

> *Perculsi terrore uerbositant inter se, dicentes ire se male, Deum et sanctum erga se commotos esse hanc tempestatem hoc etiam designare. Intrant ad diuerticula, si forte facies celi sit eis propitia; quod dum fit paululum, iterum iter intrant stolidum. Sequitur statim assurgens intemperies elementorum, eos hebetes reddens confusione mentium, donec retro cedens eorum dominus uidelicet predictus Rotbertus, stuporem mentis incidit iter inceptum perficere non ausus. Cuius signum stuporis in eius uisu denotare postea potuit omnis, cuius est mens aliquomodo physicalis.*[26]

Robert de Curcun's madness was evidently a divine punishment for his 'stupid' (*stolidum*) attempt to seize property from the monastery. Notably, his foolish plan was echoed in the chaos of the storm and reflected in the madness that was eventually his punishment. Additionally, de Curcun's madness was evident from his physical appearance, which meant that not only had madness prevented him from continuing his journey to the manor, it had also tarnished his reputation and made his divine punishment apparent to all. Thus, the natural world was intrinsically connected to the bodies, minds and souls of these sinners, which were themselves fundamentally united, and all were subject to the agency of God.

3 Physical, Mental and Spiritual Suffering

In Medieval Christian theology, divine punishment and God's wrath were understood to be just since they served to maintain a natural moral balance between right and wrong.[27] Furthermore, penal and penitential suffering on earth could pave the way for redemption at the Last Judgement, which would see the Second Coming of Christ and the resurrection of the dead to await their final judgement in the hope of eternal salvation in the Kingdom of Heaven (Matthew 7 and Luke 13). Historians have not found written references to purgatory as a distinct location in theological texts produced before the twelfth century.[28] As engagement between clergy and laity increased, thanks to the preaching movements of the twelfth and thirteenth centuries, purgatory emerged as a place where ordinary Christians (not just saints and monks) could attain salvation through suffering.[29] Therefore, when ancient ideas concerning

26 Herman, *Miracles of St Edmund* 36.
27 Freedman (1998) 176–77.
28 Le Goff (1981) 135.
29 Watkins (2002) 32–3.

pain as a diagnostic tool and as a symptom of illness were disseminated within a Christian framework, they had to ally with the concept that pain and suffering could sometimes be beneficial as instruments of redemption.[30]

Twelfth-century Salernitan medical texts placed a greater emphasis on theoretical understandings of pain than had previously been seen in western medicine.[31] Though experiences of pain appeared physical, for Medieval physicians, the ability to sense pain did not lie solely in one's physical faculties. Sensation was felt through the senses, which were experienced in the body and were interpreted in the ventricles of the brain.[32] Nonetheless, though pain was experienced via the body's corporeal senses, it was not caused by them. Ibn-Sīnā (Latinised as Avicenna), whose *Canon of Medicine* was translated into Latin by Gerard of Cremona in the mid-twelfth century and thence widely circulated, was the first known medical writer to classify pain as a *non-natura* (non-natural), which impacted upon the body and mind.[33] Since pain, in this sense, was contrary to nature, physicians were urged to assuage it as best they could.[34]

The classification of pain as a non-natural implied that, in its perfect state, humanity would not suffer pain.[35] This model was consistent with theological explorations of pain as an experience of the human soul brought about by mankind's Fall from innocence in the Garden of Eden (Genesis 3). In Medieval miracle records, pain, as a form of suffering, could be represented in various ways: as indicative of a problem in the body or as demonstrative of spiritual failings (these two causes of suffering were not necessarily incompatible). Accounts of how pilgrims suffered at the shrines of saints before being cured are, therefore, illustrative of the cohesion of physical and spiritual understandings of both illness and healing.

In the late twelfth century, a fisherman's daughter, called Ysembela, came to the shrine of the Apostle James in Reading, searching for a cure for the left-hand side of her body, which had become completely paralysed. She brought a candle with her, as an offering for the saint.

30 For a discussion of pain in Imperial Greek culture, see King (2018), particularly Part 2, which looks at representations of pain outside of the medical discourse.

31 Cohen (2010) 89.

32 Avicenna, *Liber canonis* 3.1.1.2. For more on the ventricles of the brain, see Siraisi (1990) 82–3.

33 Avicenna, *Liber canonis* 1.2.2.19, cited in Cohen (2010) 89.

34 For example, Constantine, *De morborum* VII.14. For a discussion of Medieval approaches to pain management, see Cohen (2010) chapter 3.

35 Cohen (2010) 89.

> Thus entering the church, when she had lit her candle, the hand of the Lord came upon her, and His spirit was troubled inside her. And so, stirred up for her cure, she collapsed on the pavement and, breaking forth in a sharp voice and the most high-pitched cries, she screamed in all directions. She shook her hair around, pounded her head and struck her body against the stone without consideration for herself so that one might have believed that she wished to pound herself to pieces and to extinguish what life remained.
>
> *Introiens igitur ecclesiam cum candelam suam accendisset, facta est super eam manus domini et anxiatus est in ea spiritus eius. Itaque in salutem suam conturbata super pauimentum corruit et in uocem clamoresque acutissimum prorumpens usquequaque ingemuit. Crines sparsit capud contudit corpusque suum ita absque sui respectu ad petram elisit putari posset se ipsam uelle conterere et que supererat spiritum extinguere.*[36]

The agony of the initial stage of her miraculous cure left Ysembela exhausted, and she was taken to the altar of Saint Mary Magdalene, where she fell asleep. The reason for moving Ysembela was not made clear in the account and may have been purely practical. However, the symbolic connections between Mary Magdalene and physical and spiritual contamination should be noted and give emphasis to the physical and spiritual nature of Ysembela's cure. Many leper hospitals across England were, because of these connections, founded in the name of Mary Magdalene, and one of them stood in Reading.

Upon awakening at the altar, Ysembela coughed up a 'bloody poison' (*virus sanguineum*), followed by more blood. This mixture of blood and poison was 'the humour that had harmed her' (*humor que nocuerat*) in the first place, and its removal completed her cure. The miracle compiler speculated that the girl's paralysis had started after she had slept overnight in the open air, and it is conceivable that poisons were believed to have entered her body at this time. Sleeping outside was associated with illness in other miracle narratives of this period, and it was commonly accepted that foreign substances could enter the body whilst a person slept. For example, in the *Life and Miracles of William of Norwich* (compiled in the 1150s), the miracle compiler recounted how a herdsman had become very ill after sleeping outdoors, which had resulted in a viper

36 *Miracles of the Hand of Saint James* 20. My transcription and translation from the manuscript. The miracles are not numbered in the manuscript, but each new miracle begins with a red or blue initial. I have followed Brian Kemp's numbering for ease of reference.

crawling into his mouth and taking up residence in his intestines.[37] Those who slept outside in remote locations also left themselves vulnerable to attacks from demons, just as Christ had been tempted by the devil in the wilderness (Matthew 4:1–11). One youth, who was travelling from Northampton to London sometime in the mid-1100s, decided to sleep in the woods and was driven mad by a demon in the form of a beautiful woman who placed a small bird in his mouth, probably as a representation of the demonic spirit entering the youth's body.[38]

Notably, Ysembela's paralysis occurred on the left side of her body. The fifth-century theologian John Cassian, whose writings were widely circulated in the Middle Ages, articulated a commonly-held belief when he explained that the left side was more open to temptations and attacks from demons.[39] That Ysembela's spiritually-weaker side had succumbed to harmful poisons perhaps explains the necessity for a spiritual element to her cure, through the Lord's possession of her. That it was necessary for the Lord to enter Ysembela could imply that His purity was used to counter the poisons inside her, which is in line with the Hippocratic principle that contraries cure.[40] Thus, spiritual and physical cleansing (the latter via the expulsion of harmful fluids) were combined in Ysembela's cure.

Ysembela's distress suggests that her cure affected her physically and mentally, though the cause of her illness was the physical presence of poisons in her body and its ultimate cure was brought about by miraculously purging the body through vomiting. The purging of harmful fluids or poisons from the body was a technique recommended by Medieval physicians and often required the use of emetics, diuretics or laxatives, which were, of course, not necessary for miraculous cures. For example, Gariopontus's *Passionarius* (an eleventh-century Salernitan medical treatise that was made up of interwoven section from three Galenic and pseudo-Galenic tracts, a copy of which was very likely held in Reading Abbey at the time that Ysembela's cure was recorded) recommended that manic patients be given a radish to induce vomiting, which would expel the excess phlegm and melancholy that were associated with mania.[41]

Experiences of purging comparable to Ysembela's can be seen in other miracles recorded in Reading and attributed to Saint James. The cure of a woman who was suffering from dropsy has striking similarities:

37 Thomas of Monmouth, *The Life and Miracles* V.3.
38 *Liber fundationis* II.9.
39 Cassian, *The Conferences* XI.10.
40 Demaitre (2013) 123.
41 Gariopontus, *Passionarius* I.9; Glaze (1999) 241.

> At about the first vigil of the night, as the monks were beginning matins, the aforesaid woman, falling on the pavement of the presbytery, became agitated and was disturbed to her marrow. Her bowels were indeed stirred up. Having passed some part of the night in this anxiety, behold, the pits of her stomach burst forth and the flood gates of her bowels were opened. She thus vomited and vomited again the venom, which had been built up for a long time, and removed all the putrefaction of the harmful fluid.
>
> *Circa primam uigiliam noctis monachis matutinos inchoantibus mulier prefata secus pauimentum presbiteri corruens cepit agitari, et in salutem suam medullitus conturbari. Commota sunt quippe uiscera eius. Decurso in hac anxietate aliquanto noctis spacio, ecce ventris eruperunt abissi et cataractae uiscerum aperte sunt. Vomuit itaque et reuomuit virus iamdiu conceptum, omnesque tabem noxii humoris exinaniuit.*[42]

Both Ysembela and the woman suffering from dropsy experienced extreme discomfort as part of their healing processes. Their suffering at the shrine contributed to the physical spectacle of their cures and visually represented their physical and spiritual healing. Notably, Ysembela had transgressed before she came to Reading to be cured. Despite receiving numerous visions of the Apostle James imploring her to come to Reading, she had first chosen to seek the assistance of other saints, including that of Saint Thomas Becket, whose cult in Canterbury was flourishing but who failed to provide Ysembela with a cure. It is therefore plausible that Ysembela needed to atone for negligently ignoring Saint James before her cure could be completed, though the written record of her cure did not specifically connect her healing experience with her moral misdemeanours.

For Ysembela and the dropsical woman, disturbed behaviour, pain and vomiting were not symptoms of the primary illness (the original state of ill-health) but nor were they considered indicative of a state of health. Once Ysembela had been miraculously cured, 'the things which are of the body were restored to the body and the things which are of the sense to sensibility' (*reddita sunt que sunt corporis corpori, que sensus sensibilitati*). The Lord saw fit not only to cure her illness but also 'to heal her distress' (*sanare contritiones*). A complete healing required not only recovery from corporeal suffering but also the restoration of emotional wellbeing. Alongside being made healthy, Ysembela was

42 *Miracles of the Hand of Saint James* 2.

made 'well and joyful' (*sana et hilaris*), which contrasts with the sickness and distress that she had previously suffered.

Physical and mental suffering were also interrelated in that either one could lead to the other. In a miracle record made sometime in the 1170s at the shrine of Saint Thomas Becket in Canterbury, we are told how the Dean of Lindsay's concubine, Alice, suffered such extreme agony in childbirth that she went mad.[43] Alice was given some of the holy water of Saint Thomas Becket (infused with the martyr's blood) to drink, and this remedy induced a deep sleep that allowed both her mind and her body to regain health (we do not know what happened to the baby). As well as having physical and moral elements, Alice's suffering had obvious spiritual connotations. Not only was childbirth the ultimate form of physical suffering to be endured by women because of their role in the Fall in the Garden of Eden, but Alice's own pregnancy had resulted from an illicit union with the Dean of Lindsay. Clerical marriage had been banned at the First Lateran Council of 1123, and this decree was reiterated at the Second Lateran Council in 1139.[44]

Another miracle record, from the same miracle collection as the account of Alice's cure, narrated the story of a sailor called Ralph who went mad after persuading his shipmates not to make a pilgrimage to Canterbury to visit the shrine of Saint Thomas Becket.[45] Ralph was told by a priest that he would remain mad until such time as he could be restored to God. He was then bound in chains and locked away. Ralph's mental incapacity led to his forced captivity and, in turn, had a physical effect on his body, since the squalor of his prison caused parts of his flesh to rot away down to the bone. Thus, Ralph's spiritual corruption and alienation from God were reflected in his physical and mental corruption. He was eventually restored to his senses (and to God's mercy) after making a vow of pilgrimage to Saint Thomas Becket, which he then fulfilled. Like the souls of the dead who awaited their salvation in purgatory, Ralph's prison, where he suffered physically and mentally, was a temporary place of torment, which cleansed him of his wrongdoing. We can compare Ralph's miraculous cure with the divine punishment of Robert de Curcun, which was recorded around one hundred years earlier in Bury. Whereas de Curcun's punishment restored natural balance in a Platonic fashion, with the suffering body and mind of the sinner echoing the chaos of the thunderstorm, Ralph's madness served to restore individual balance by enabling salvation through suffering. This shift in focus from macrocosm to microcosm can, in part, be attributed

43 William of Canterbury, *Miracula* VI.113.

44 Tanner (1990) I: 194–98.

45 William of Canterbury, *Miracula* III.47.

to increased theological interest in the morality of individuals. Nevertheless, it is also indicative of the declining influence of Plato in the second half of the twelfth century when the re-discovery and translation into Latin of Aristotle's works of natural philosophy, including his *Physics*, which was translated in the mid-twelfth century, sharpened conceptual distinctions between the natural and the supernatural worlds.[46]

Contention over these distinctions can be seen in a late-twelfth-century miracle text detailing the miracles of Saint Bartholomew, which were recorded in London. When a boy suffering from epilepsy was brought to Saint Bartholomew's church to be cured by the apostle, the miracle compiler elucidated that

> epilepsy is, the physicians say, a disease which compresses the ventricles of the brain and blocks the vital functions, takes away sight, hearing, and the other senses of the body, and wearies the body itself with terrible suffering.
>
> *Est autem epilepsia ut phisici tradunt morbus qui cerebri ventriculos compremens et animales actiones praecludit, visum, auditum, et ceteros corporis sensus tollit, ipsum que corpus dira passione fatigare consuevit.*[47]

Evidently, this miracle compiler was familiar with medical language and with contemporary medical theories that were derived from Galen via Avicenna. Avicenna argued that the brain was divided into ventricles, which were responsible for its various functions. The common sense or imagination in the front ventricle processed information obtained from the sense receptors of the face and body. This information was passed on to the central ventricle, which controlled the rational faculty and used sensory inputs to produce rational thoughts and judgements. The back ventricle stored memories as images, which were literally imprinted into the wet brain matter. If the ventricles of the brain became compressed, for example, by too much of the phlegmatic humour, information could not pass between them, and the pathways that sent messages between the brain and the body could become blocked, meaning that the 'vital spirit'[48] – produced in the heart and transported to the brain to be refined via the process of sensation and rationality – could not pass through.

46 Wilson (2014) 100.

47 *Liber fundationis* II.11.

48 For more on the bodily spirits (*pneumata*) in Galen, see Julius Rocca's chapter in this volume (chapter 11).

Hence, as the miracle compiler explained, the brain of someone suffering from epilepsy might not receive the correct sensory information and might not be able to send messages to the limbs, causing disordered movements.[49]

The boy's epilepsy was miraculously cured by Saint Bartholomew even though its aetiology was natural and was understood by contemporary physicians. Nonetheless, the same miracle compiler denied natural explanations for some of the other illnesses he recorded. For example, when a pestilence broke out among the oxen in Enfield, some people thought that the disease was caused by bad air, which was a theory in line with contemporary understandings of the non-naturals.[50] The miracle compiler, however, insisted that the pestilence had been 'inflicted from heaven for a reproof of men' (*ad correptionem hominum caelitus inflicta*). Of course, these causes were not incompatible; the bad air could have been brought about as a result of God's wrath. As Iona McCleery has noted, 'the relationship between Christ and Galen [in the Middle Ages] was really rather complex',[51] and descriptions of diseases in Medieval miracle texts present an amalgamation of ancient and contemporary aetiologies.

4 Holistic Healing

Miracles seem to have been perceived as a form of medicine in some respects, and it was not uncommon for hagiographers to refer to saints as 'doctors.'[52] Saint Thomas Becket, for example, was described as a 'good and faithful doctor' (*bonus et fidelis medicus*), who used 'celestial medicine' (*coelesti medicina*) to perform his miraculous healings.[53] There is evidence that miracles were understood to heal sufferers holistically, in body, mind and soul (in line with what I have termed the Christian model of healthcare). One pilgrim who came to Canterbury in the 1170s was a madwoman called Matilda, who was 'filled with a demon' and had travelled to the shrine of Saint Thomas Becket in the hope that she would be cured of her insanity. Matilda claimed that she was visited by the saint in a vision, in which she told him that she was suffering in body and in mind.[54] She later explained to the monks of Canterbury Cathedral that this physical and mental suffering had been brought about after her brother

49 Demaitre (2013) 129.
50 *Liber fundationis* II.5.
51 McCleery (2014) 128.
52 Bartlett (2013) 349.
53 William of Canterbury, *Miracula* II.6 and II.7.
54 Benedict of Peterborough, *Miracula* IV.37.

had killed her lover, which had led her to strike her newborn baby, killing it (the implication is that the baby was the product of an illicit union with the lover who, notably, was not described as Matilda's husband). Saint Thomas Becket, in Matilda's vision, promised to restore her to health and also assured her that she would receive absolution if she continued her pilgrimage either to the shrine of Saint James in Santiago de Compostela or to Rome itself, both prestigious Medieval pilgrimage destinations.

It was unusual, in a miracle record, for other shrines that were unconnected to the saint who was the subject of the text to be recommended as places of pilgrimage. After all, the miracle compiler's purpose in writing was to document the virtue of the subject saint and God's patronage of his or her shrine, not of another's. It seems that Matilda's extended pilgrimage was intended to be penitential since it would bring her absolution. The implication, then, was that, whilst Becket had restored health to her body, by expelling the demon, and to her mind, by restoring her sanity, Matilda's soul still in peril, and she thus required further healing. The sins for which Matilda required absolution were fornication (with her lover) and infanticide. Though the death of her baby had occurred when she was already insane, penance was still required, but to a lesser degree that it would have been had she committed this sin when in her right mind. Therefore, Matilda's condition was caused by a combination of physical possession by a demon, mental incapacity, possibly as a result of emotional trauma, and spiritual corruption brought about by sin. The physical, mental and spiritual elements of her suffering were intrinsically interrelated, and, therefore, she required holistic treatment to be restored to health.

Despite the striking suffering of sinners like Matilda, the majority of English miracle records from the twelfth century document the conditions and cures of innocent men, women and children, whose sickness was not explicitly related to sin. Earlier in the same miracle collection, the Canterbury monk who had recorded the case of Matilda's 'strange madness' (*mire insanientem*), made a comparison between physical and mental healing. As a preface to a miracle record in which he recounted the cure of a young man, called Henry, who was suffering from insanity (*insaniverat*), the compiler asked 'what is easier, to give health of the mind or of the body?' (*quid est facilius, dare salutem mentis an corporis?*).[55] His reason for asking was that this miracle record immediately followed, in his collection, a record of a man miraculously cured from blindness.[56] Of course, the question was rhetorical; Saint Thomas Becket was equally capable of healing both physical and mental afflictions. The compiler

55 Benedict of Peterborough, *Miracula* II.13.
56 Benedict of Peterborough, *Miracula* II.12.

explained that '[he] who brought light to these corporeal eyes [those of the blind man] also restored a youth of Fordwich, Henry, to his mind' (*Qui oculos hujus corporeos illuminavit, juvenem de Fordwico Henricum menti restituit*).[57] This very comparison reveals that, whilst the compiler understood physical and mental healing to be related, he also saw distinctions between them. Mental health had an impact on physical health, but the mind was not a part of the body, as the eyes were. Miracles then, as a form of Christian healing were holistic in the sense that saints were able to attend to the whole person, body, mind and soul. In this Christian model, there was some overlap with the ancient model of holism; all parts of an individual were connected, and factors external to the body could have repercussions for the body's internal balance. Medieval physicians were, of course, more limited than saints in the treatment they could provide. Although, for example, physical and spiritual wellbeing were believed to be connected, the council that gathered at Rome's Lateran Palace in 1215 felt that the physician's role was different from the priest's.[58] Whilst the Medieval physician was encouraged to acknowledge the co-dependence of body, mind and soul, most often, his own role in the healing process was to focus his attention on addressing a particular humoral imbalance through the application of its opposite or by purging the excess humour.

The interaction between earthly and celestial medicine is particularly notable in another miracle that was, like Matilda's and Henry's, recorded in the 1170s and attributed to Saint Thomas Becket.[59] A knight called Stephen of Hoyland had suffered from terrifying nocturnal visions for thirty years, and he believed that his condition was caused by demons. Stephen's physicians, however, were sure that his nightmares were *ephialtes*: a Greek medical term that referred to a condition in which a sufferer felt as though he were being crushed in his sleep. Though *ephialtes* (Latin: *incubus*) was frequently discussed as a condition influenced by demons in ancient and Medieval medical discourses,[60] the miracle compiler, here, seems to have been implying that, by diagnosing *ephialtes*, the physicians were rejecting Stephen's claim that his condition was demonic. It is likely that the miracle compiler shared the view held by fellow-clergyman William of Auvergne (Bishop of Paris, 1228–49), who admitted that physicians correctly diagnosed some cases of *incubus* as caused by compression of the heart, but who maintained that, more often, *incubus* was caused by demons,

57 Benedict of Peterborough, *Miracula* II.13.

58 Canon Twenty-Two of the Fourth Lateran Council is discussed above.

59 Benedict of Peterborough, *Miracula* I.13.

60 For more on ancient and Medieval medical and demonological discourses on *ephialtes/incubus*, see van der Lugt (2001), MacLehose (2013), Metzger (2018).

though he proposed no way of distinguishing between what he understood to be distinct causes.[61]

Of course, for the saint to emerge triumphant and for Stephen's condition to be shown to be healed miraculously, the healing techniques employed by the physicians had to fail, and they did. The very fact that Stephen had consulted with physicians, which was to be expected given his social status, enhanced the miraculous nature of his cure. The miracle compiler could prove that Stephen's cure was a miracle because the knight had already tried using physicians to no avail. Though the failure of incompetent physicians was a much-used trope in miracle stories,[62] here, the miracle compiler emphasised the miraculous nature of Stephen's cure by pointing out that even good physicians, who knew Greek medicine, had failed to correctly diagnose and treat his condition. The saint miraculously vanquished the demonic presence that Stephen had rightly identified was the cause of his suffering. This miracle is indicative of a multi-faceted approach to healing in Medieval England, which has been shown in all of the miracle records explored in this chapter. The close interaction between ancient medicine and Medieval Christianity meant that a holistic approach to healing reflected the connection between the divine and the material realms, and between the body, mind and soul. As the physician Avicenna explained when discussing the condition of *melancholia*, which was thought to be caused by excess black bile,

> we do not care if it happens by a demon or not because we teach medicine. Further, we say if it does happen by a demon, it is enough for us that it has changed the complexion to black bile, and the black bile is its immediate cause; then the cause of that black bile is a demon or not a demon.
>
> *nos non curamus cum physicam docemus, si illud contingat a demonio aut non contingat. Postquam dicimus quoniam si contingat a demonio sufficit nobis ut conuertat complexionem ad coleram nigram, et fit causa eius propinqua colera nigra. Deinde fit causa illius colere nigre demonium aut non demonium*[63]

61 William of Auvergne, *De universo* II.iii.24, cited in van der Lugt (2001) 192.

62 Bartlett (2013) 349–50.

63 Avicenna, *Liber canonis* 3.1.4.19, cited in Rider (2014) 55.

5 Conclusion

Though there has only been scope in this chapter to look at a handful of individual miracle records, these records are representative of wider developments in the twelfth century. As more and more ancient texts were translated into Latin, learned monastic men increasingly came into contact with the philosophies of their classical forefathers. Ancient ideas were not rejected because they were constructed outside of a Christian framework. Indeed, when a monk of Bury claimed that Saint Edmund's miraculous healings were more impressive than those of Hippocrates and Galen, he was not criticising these ancient medical writers; instead, he was using their prestige to enhance Saint Edmund's.[64]

Nonetheless, ancient ideas still needed to align with Medieval Christian theology. Christian understandings of a connection between the body, mind and soul were exemplified in records of physical and mental illnesses that were inflicted as divine punishments for spiritual failings. Similarly, physical and mental suffering could serve the purpose of spiritual atonement and bring absolution to the sufferer. In miracle collections, we can see how the materialistic fundamentals of ancient Graeco-Roman medicine were interpreted in relation to a Christian holistic understanding of suffering. Sickness, in the broadest sense, could have a delocalised spiritual cause, which required spiritual treatment regardless of the localised experience of suffering. Spiritual healing at the hands of celestial physicians (or saints) did not necessarily restore physical health but it could make earthly medicines more effective, since physical, mental and spiritual aetiologies were not incompatible. Medieval miracle compilers did not draw a sharp line between endogenous causes for ill-health such as humours and exogenous ones such as demons. Fundamentally, healing was about balance, whether it be the maintenance of physical balance by purging or avoiding harmful bodily excesses, the re-establishment of mental balance with happiness and joy, or the renewal of spiritual balance through penance.

Bibliography

Bartlett, R. *Why Can the Dead Do Such Great Things? Saint and Worshippers from the Martyrs to the Reformation*. Princeton and Oxford: Princeton University Press (2013).

Burnett, C. 'The Twelfth-Century Renaissance.' In *The Cambridge History of Science II: Medieval Science*, ed. D. C. Lindberg and M. H. Shank. Cambridge: Cambridge University Press (2013) 365–84.

64 Herman, *Miracles of St Edmund* 27.

Cohen, E. *The Modulated Scream: Pain in Late Medieval Culture*. Chicago: University of Chicago Press (2010).

Demaitre, L. *Medieval Medicine: The Art of Healing, from Head to Toe*. Santa Barbara: Praeger (2013).

Dutton, P. E. 'Medieval Approaches to Calcidius.' In *Plato's* Timaeus *as Cultural Icon*, ed. G. J. Reydams-Schils. Notre Dame: University of Notre Dame (2003) 183–205.

Freedman, P. 'Peasant Anger in the Late Middle Ages.' In *Anger's Past: The Social Uses of An Emotion in the Middle Ages*, ed. B. H. Rosenwein. Ithaca and London: Cornell University Press (1998) 171–88.

Gil Sotres, P. 'The Regimens of Health.' In *Western Medical Thought from Antiquity to the Middle Ages*, ed. M. D. Grmek, trans. A. Shugaar. London and Cambridge MA: Harvard University Press (1998) 291–318.

Glaze, F. E. 'The Perforated Wall: The Ownership and Circulation of Medical Books in Europe, ca. 800–1200.' Dissertation Duke University (1999).

Goodich, M. *Miracles and Wonders: The Development of the Concept of Miracle, 1150–1350*. Aldershot: Ashgate (2007).

Green, M. 'Salerno on the Thames: The Genesis of Anglo-Norman Medical Literature.' In *Language and Culture in Medieval Britain: The French of England, c.1100–c.1500*, ed. J. Wogan-Browne. Woodbridge: York Medieval Press (2009) 220–31.

Green, M. 'Medical Books.' In *The European Book in the Twelfth Century*, ed. E. Kwakkel and R. Thomson. Cambridge: Cambridge University Press (2018) 277–92.

Gregory, T. 'The Platonic Inheritance.' In *A History of Twelfth-Century Western Philosophy*, ed. P. Dronke. Cambridge: Cambridge University Press (1998) 54–80.

Haskins, C. H. *The Renaissance of the Twelfth Century*. London and Cambridge MA: Harvard University Press (1927).

Kemp, B. 'The Miracles of the Hand of St. James.' *Berkshire Archaeological Journal*, 65 (1972) 1–19.

King, D. *Experiencing Pain in Imperial Greek Culture*. Oxford: Oxford University Press (2018).

Koopmans, R. *Wonderful to Relate: Miracle Stories and Miracle Collecting in High Medieval England*. Philadelphia: University of Pennsylvania Press (2011).

Le Goff, J. *The Birth of Purgatory*. Trans. A. Goldhammer. Chicago: University of Chicago Press (1981).

Licence, T. (ed.) *Bury St Edmunds and the Norman Conquest*. Woodbridge: Boydell (2014).

Licence, T. (ed.) *Herman the Archdeacon and Goscelin of Saint-Bertin. Miracles of St Edmund*. Oxford: Oxford University Press (2014).

MacLehose, W. F. 'Fear, Fantasy and Sleep in Medieval Medicine.' In *Emotions and Health 1200–1700*, ed. E. Carrera. Leiden: Brill (2013) 67–94.

McCleery, I. "Christ More Powerful Than Galen'? The Relationship Between Miracles and Medicine.' In *Contextualizing Miracles in the Christian West, 1100–1500: New*

Historical Approaches, ed. M. M. Mesley and L. E. Wilson. Oxford: Society for the Study of Medieval Language and Literature (2014) 127–54.

Metzger, N. 'Not a *Daimōn*, but a Severe Illness: Oribasius, Posidonius and Later Ancient Perspectives on Superhuman Agents Causing Disease.' In *Mental Illness in Ancient Medicine: From Celsus to Paul of Aegina*, ed. C. Thumiger and P. N. Singer. Leiden: Brill (2018) 79–106.

Niebyl, F. H. 'The Non-naturals.' *Bulletin of the History of Medicine*, 45 (1971) 486–92.

Rider, C. 'Demons and Mental Disorder in Late Medieval Medicine.' In *Mental (Dis) Order in Later Medieval Europe*, ed. S. Katajala-Peltomaa and S. Nirranen. Leiden: Brill (2014) 47–69.

Siraisi, N. G. *Medieval & Early Renaissance Medicine: An Introduction to Knowledge and Practice*. Chicago: University of Chicago Press (1990).

Stover, J. A. *Reading Plato in the Twelfth Century: A Study On the Varieties of Plato's Reception in the Latin West Before 1215*. Dissertation Harvard University (2011).

Tanner, N. P. (ed.) *Decrees of the Ecumenical Councils*. Washington: Georgetown University Press (1990).

van der Lugt, M. 'The Incubus in Scholastic Debate: Medicine, Theology and Popular Belief.' In *Religion and Medicine in the Middle Ages*, ed. P. Biller and J. Ziegler. Woodbridge: York Medieval Press (2001) 175–200.

Watkins, C. S. 'Sin, Penance and Purgatory in the Anglo-Norman Realm: The Evidence of Visions and Ghost Stories.' *Past and Present*, 175 (2002) 3–33.

Wilson, L. E. 'Conceptions of the Miraculous: Natural Philosophy and Medical Knowledge in the Thirteenth-Century *Miracula* of St Edmund of Abingdon.' In *Contextualizing Miracles in the Christian West, 1100–1500: New Historical Approaches*, ed. M. M. Mesley and L. E. Wilson. Oxford: Society for the Study of Medieval Language and Literature (2014) 99–125.

Woolgar, C. M. *The Senses in Late Medieval England*. New Haven and London: Yale University Press (2006).

Primary Texts: Editions and Translations Used

Anon. 'The Canonization of St Hugh of Lincoln.' Ed. D. H. Farmer. *Lincolnshire Architectural and Archaeological Society Reports and Papers*, 6 (1956) 86–117.

Anon. *Liber Fundationis Ecclesie Sancti Bartholomei Londiniarum*. MS Cotton Vespasian B.IX, British Library, London. [The miracles are not numbered in the manuscript, but each new miracle begins with an initial written in blue and decorated in red. I have numbered them for ease of reference.]

Anon. *The Metrical Life of Saint Hugh of Lincoln*. Ed. C. Garton. Lincoln: Honywood Press (1986). [I have amended the translation in places so as to be more faithful to the original Latin terminology.]

Anon. *The Miracles of the Hand of Saint James*. MS 1, Gloucester Cathedral Library.

Arnau de Vilanova. *Speculum Medicinae*. In *Opera Omnia Medica*. Barcelona: University of Barcelona (1985).

Avicenna. *Liber Canonis Avicenne Revisus et ab Errore Mendaque Purgatus Summaque cum Diligentia Impressus*. Hildesheim: Georg Olms (1507, repr. 1964).

Benedict of Peterborough. *Miracula Sancti Thomae Cantuariensis*. In *Materials for the History of Thomas Becket, Archbishop of Canterbury*. Ed. J. C. Robertson. London: Longman (1876) II: 21–281.

Cassian, J. *The Conferences*. Trans. E. C. S. Gibson. In *A Select Library of Nicene and Post-Nicene Fathers of the Christian Church: Second Series*. Ed. P. Scaff and H. Wace. Grand Rapids: W. B. Eerdmans (1894) XI: 356–57.

Constantine the African. *De Morborum Cognitione et Curatione*. In *Opera Omnia*. Ed. H. Petrus. Basel: Henricus Petrus (1539) II: 1–167.

Gariopontus. *Passionarius Galeni*. Lyon: Bartholomeus Trot (1526).

Goscelin of Saint-Bertin[?]. *Miracles of St Edmund*. In *Herman the Archdeacon and Goscelin of Saint-Bertin. Miracles of St Edmund*. Ed. T. Licence. Oxford: Oxford University Press (2014) 127–303.

Herman the Archdeacon. *Miracles of St Edmund*. In *Herman the Archdeacon and Goscelin of Saint-Bertin. Miracles of St Edmund*. Ed. T. Licence. Oxford: Oxford University Press (2014) 1–125.

Johannicius. *Isagoge ad Techne Galieni*. Ed. G. Maurach. *Sudhoffs Archiv*, 62 (1978) 148–74.

Thomas of Monmouth. *The Life and Miracles of St William of Norwich*. Ed. and trans. A. Jessop and M. R. James. Cambridge: Cambridge University Press (1896).

William of Auvergne. *De Universo*. In *Opera omnia*. Ed. A. Praland. Frankfurt am Main: Minerva (1674, repr. 1963) 593–1074.

William of Canterbury. *Miracula Sancti Thomae Cantuariensis*. In *Materials for the History of Thomas Becket, Archbishop of Canterbury*. Ed. J. C. Robertson. London: Longman (1875) I: 137–546.

CHAPTER 16

'Treating the Patient, Not Just the Disease': Reading Ancient Medicine in Modern Holistic Medicine

Helen King

Abstract

This chapter explores the uses made by modern holistic medicine of Hippocratic texts and of a broader idea of what they contain. Both orthodox and alternative medicines use Hippocrates either to project an ideal of what medicine should be, or to create a story of medical progress. The term 'holistic' is used in a wide range of ways, often seen as a quality of the past which has been lost as modern medicine has become more specialised; related to this are both the holistic healer's combination of a variety of different forms of healing, and the claim that ancient Greek medicine is valid for all times and regions. Those claiming Hippocratic origins for their method of healing demonstrate how authority is constructed both in print and online; online, the Wikipedia Hippocrates page continues to have enormous impact for orthodox medicine as well. Plato's representation of Hippocrates giving priority to 'the whole' has surprisingly little overt influence, while wording often attributed to Osler, about treating the patient rather than the disease, has shifted to being something said by Hippocrates. While in previous generations the focus has been on finding the Hippocratic treatise that best fits one's own views, and presenting this as the work of Hippocrates himself, today there is less interest in the texts and more in the supposed personality of Hippocrates and his attention to the powers of 'Nature.'

In this chapter I want to extend our reflection on a central theme of this book: namely, models of disease which go beyond localising it in an organ, or a set of organs. In what forms part of a larger project on how Hippocrates is used in contemporary medicine and beyond, I shall consider various approaches which operate under the umbrella of 'holistic medicine' today and outline their reception of Hippocratic medicine.[1] I shall then locate some of the claims made, in relation to the texts of the ancient Mediterranean world and to the earlier history of holism. This means addressing the value and the shortcomings of

1 King (2019).

 | DOI:10.1163/9789004443143_018

some of the basic models we apply to the history of medicine, and particularly the models used by those who claim to be practising 'holistic' medicine today. What do they mean by 'the whole', and how do they enlist ancient sources in support of their arguments?

I find useful here the model of 'projection.' Thomas Rütten has pointed out that any biography of Hippocrates, including those created or repeated today, is a way to 'give concrete form to the concerns of professional politics and religion, to theoretical concepts, and to ethical-moral claims', so that Hippocrates becomes 'the projection screen for all the medicinal utopias that since the Roman Republic have taken him and his writings in tow.'[2] This recalls James Davidson's comments on ancient Greek sexuality, when he challenged the modern view that it was all about who was penetrated and who did the penetration: 'The Greeks did not award points for penetration ... they certainly did not structure the whole of society let alone the entire world according to a coital schema. The whole theory is simply a projection of our own gender nightmares on to the screen of a very different culture.'[3] How does the holistic Hippocrates fit into this practice of projecting utopias or nightmares? Whose Hippocrates is he: does he belong to orthodox medicine or to alternatives to this? What versions of holism are currently being projected back on to the classical past, what does this tell us about current views of what medicine should be, and how are the classical texts used to reinforce what their users mean by holism? In this chapter I shall be examining these questions mostly through that key figure of Hippocrates, the screen upon whom western medical systems have long projected their various visions.

In this volume, P.N. Singer has identified three possible meanings of holism in Galen and his near-contemporaries: one focused on the relationship between mind (or soul) and body, another considering the body as a whole, and the third concerned with the body's unity with the cosmos; this last meaning was the one chosen by Paul Carton, one of the French naturopaths who promoted what he considered Hippocratic holism in the 1920s as part of a return to simplicity as an 'antique virtue.'[4] Singer has demonstrated how Galen emphasises the importance of correctly identifying the 'affected part' (Lat. *locus affectus*), but also provides evidence that the Methodist approach to medicine rejected any interest in parts on the basis that,[5] even if one part of the body suffered more badly than others, this would have no effect on the mode of

2 Rütten (2010) 439.
3 Davidson (1997) 176.
4 Weisz (2002) 264.
5 See Leith in this volume.

treatment, since this was aimed at the body as a whole.[6] Hynek Bartoš has offered a different three meanings in the context of the Hippocratic treatise *On Regimen*: one involving treating all parts together with the whole; another concentrating on the influence of the environment on the body; and a third considering the body as mimicking the tripartite structure of the cosmos.[7]

Modern holistic medical approaches, rarely constrained by any of these meanings, tend towards the larger, 'cosmic' interpretations. Often combined with using the name of Hippocrates, they promote better ways not only to treat illness, but also to live. For example, when we read on a website advertising the Apivita cosmetics range that its founders were inspired by 'the holistic approach of Hippocrates to health, beauty and well-being' and that this approach influences their 'make-up, fragrances, soaps, hair products and sunscreen, all of their unique products are designed to act beneficial [sic] to the body, spirit and soul',[8] the word 'holistic' is being used in a deliberately imprecise way; what is most important is, firstly, that whatever it means it is supposed to be a Good Thing and, secondly, that its credibility is somehow enhanced here by its attribution to Hippocrates.[9]

Why Hippocrates? In her chapter, Brooke Holmes has raised the question of what is at stake in going back to the ancients, asking whether 'ancient' is seen as a marker of value, or of irrelevance.[10] In the case of the invocation of the holy name of Hippocrates, the message is almost always one of value: tracing the lineage of a treatment or approach back to Hippocrates is usually a winning move in a power game. Writing about medicine in the United States in the period before the Civil War, John Harley Warner described a key benefit of invoking Hippocrates as being that 'At a time when a multitude of irregular healers were competing successfully for recognition and clients, recounting an historical story that displayed two millennia of enduring tradition was a tool that orthodox physicians could use to set themselves apart.'[11] New is bad: traditional, having a history, is good. As that example from contemporary cosmetics advertising shows, however, Hippocrates, 'Father of Medicine' – although that

6 *De sectis* 7, 1.86–87 K.; Singer in this volume.

7 Bartoš in this volume, 113–15.

8 https://greekcitytimes.com/2018/07/22/greeces-leading-natural-cosmetics-brand-taking-the-world-by-storm/; unless otherwise stated, all websites accessed 24 August 2020.

9 Sellars and Yeatman (1930) used the capitalized phrase 'A Good Thing' to describe historical events which are universally accepted in schoolbook history as having had a net positive effect. So, for example, the signing of the Magna Carta was A Good Thing.

10 Holmes in this volume, 48–54.

11 Warner (2002) 201–2.

was not one of his earliest titles – is not the sole preserve of either mainstream or orthodox medicine.[12]

1 Hippocrates in Contemporary Holistic Medicine

In looking at how ancient Greek medicine features in holism today, the website 'Greek Medicine' is a good place to start, not least because it is so widely used by other online materials, whether or not they credit it as their source.[13] It is run by David K. Osborn, who describes himself as 'Master Herbalist – Astrologer – Holistic Health Consultant and Educator' and who explained its genesis as 'a website about traditional, holistic, Greek Medicine'; note the capitals here, and those two very powerful adjectives.[14] He is also a trained acupuncture practitioner and certified yoga instructor. Holism, in terms of its current practitioners, often involves one person using a range of methods, making the contrast to specialism, where one person is an expert on a very narrow field. Healers project their range of healing methods back in time so that the sanctuary of Asklepios in Cos becomes 'a holistic healing centre' which 'contained infirmaries, temples, hot springs, hostels, a school for physicians and much more';[15] taken from a Greek tourism website, this wording picks up and gives a 'holistic' spin to an older scholarly view that healing sanctuaries were much like modern health spas frequented by 'health tourists.'[16]

Osborn's online bio describes how his life changed when he found a book which

> correlated the astrological signs and planets with the four temperaments and humors of Greek Medicine. This gave David the Golden Key to medical astrology; he was then able to relate everything he had learned and studied in holistic healing to astrology. This key to medical astrology also started David's study of Greek Medicine.[17]

12 King (2002).
13 http://www.greekmedicine.net/whos_who/Hippocrates.html.
14 http://www.greekmedicine.net/blog/events/celebrating-ten-great-years.html.
15 http://www.discovergreece.com/en/greek-islands/dodecanese/kos/hippocrates-asclepeion-a-holistic-healing-centre accessed 10 September 2018; with a fine disregard for chronology the current version of the site, https://www.discovergreece.com/experiences/feel-healing-energy-asclepion-kos, presents the temple as built to 'further the teachings of the father of medicine, Hippocrates' and as promoting 'a holistic approach to wellbeing.'
16 Graf (1992) 199; Israelowich (2015) 111.
17 http://www.greekmedicine.net/whos_who/Hippocrates.html.

His basic approach is that 'Truth is one, but the sages of these different traditional medical systems call it by different names.' Holism, then, is broader than anything we have so far encountered: for him, it concerns a single medical truth which connects all forms of medicine. Greek medicine is 'truly a natural healing system for the whole world' and is 'the traditional healing system from which modern medicine grew and evolved.'[18] One truth: whole world. Here, holism is about more than treating the body as a whole: it's about treating medicine as a whole, with different local models expressing the same truth, and being the ancestors of 'modern medicine.' In his history of naturopathy, Whorton called this trend 'world medicine.'[19]

While there is no reason why users of the site would necessarily read Osborn's bio, he also writes a blog, on which in March 2017 he celebrated ten years of the greekmedicine.net site.[20] In the same blog post, he explained that the book which gave him that Golden Key was *L'Astrologie Médicale* by Sylvie Chermet-Carroy, an astrologer and graphologist.[21] This is an example of how the greekmedicine.net site adds to its image of authority by Osborn's practice of giving 'acknowledgements' of some of the books he has used, a common internet strategy which plays into a model in which books must surely be (even) better than online materials. Robson and Baek's *Engines of Hippocrates* similarly notes how many 'Hippocratic' quotes there are online but alludes to 'following the scholarly tradition of reporting back to published, print-on-paper sources', which means we need to find these quotes in a *book* before using them.[22] This strategy often backfires, however, as books and articles in print may take seriously something thoroughly untrustworthy which originated on the internet.[23]

On the greekmedicine.net site, Osborn does not use the standard printed works we would perhaps expect; those deriving from scholarship on ancient medicine. What is his position on Hippocrates and his works? He considers that we can be 'fairly certain' that some of the works of the corpus can be attributed to him; specifically, *Airs, Waters, Places*, *Aphorisms* and *Ancient Medicine*. He

18 http://www.greekmedicine.net/blog/events/celebrating-ten-great-years.html.

19 This 'strives to embody the healing wisdom and techniques of all civilizations from antiquity onward and to overcome the spiritual poverty of the biomedical model of disease'; Whorton (2002) 305.

20 http://www.greekmedicine.net/blog/events/celebrating-ten-great-years.html.

21 Chermet-Carroy (1998).

22 Robson and Baek (2009) 57. Note that this is not the most reliable of sources; for example, it has 'Celus' for Celsus.

23 See King (2020) for the internet origin, and print afterlife, of the story of Hippocrates' jail sentence.

writes that Hippocrates led a 'band of renegade physicians' who moved with him from Cnidos to Cos. His source here is acknowledged as another printed work, Ghulam Chishti, *The Traditional Healer's Handbook: A Classic Guide to the Medicine of Avicenna*.[24]

That 'band of renegade physicians' phrase is repeated widely; greekmedicine.net was cited in 2009 by a chiropractic blog using it.[25] Not just the 'band of renegade physicians' sentence, but the entire section of greekmedicine.net in which it appears, was copied with attribution by Jim Putnam in his blog *The Colton Points Times*, 31 January 2017, as part of a piece on the Hippocratic Oath.[26] The phrase also features extensively without attribution; for example, on a site selling nutritionals, *Tested Nutrients*, which proudly proclaims 'We are people in search of science.'[27] It features in supposedly academic publications, including those 'published, print-on-paper sources.'[28] A 'band of renegade physicians' sounds almost like Robin Hood ('riding through the glen/ … with his band of men'), and immediately identifies Hippocratic medicine with the forces of the Resistance; Hippocrates himself can become 'The medical renegade who came to be called the Father of Medicine.'[29] The resistance story has other internet variations, most notably the myth that he was imprisoned for 'opposing the infrastructure' of ancient Greece, on which I have published elsewhere.[30]

In Chishti's and Osborn's narrative, holism is used to account for the alleged move from Cnidos to Cos. Both say that Cnidian medicine 'considered the body to be merely a collection of isolated parts, and saw diseases manifesting in a particular organ or body part as affecting that part only, which alone was treated.' So, a focus on an organ or part is seen as wrong.

This part of the Osborn/Chishti model is repeated on the website of Red House Australia, an independent centre for the treatment of eating disorders majoring on superfoods eaten in a community environment, where it appears on a page on 'Hippocrates' Influence on Red House Philosophies, Principles,

24 Chisthti (1988) 11.

25 http://doctorscrubs.blogspot.co.uk/2009/04/hatred-of-tmb-and-tma-against.html accessed 25 March 2020.

26 https://coltonspointtimes.blogspot.co.uk/2017/01/.

27 https://www.testednutrients.com/en/story/; also in the author's response to a comment on http://jamesmalloy.blogspot.co.uk/2013/07/nietzscheaphorism-120-gay-science.html.

28 Much of the page of greekmedicine.net is copied without attribution in Cacciafoco (2012) 20–2 where, bizarrely, the words 'band' and 'renegade physicians' are marked by quotation marks when the rest of the plagiarised text is not.

29 http://www.unani.com/hipporcates.htm.

30 King (2020).

and Practices.'[31] The Osborn/Chishti idea that 'The Cnidian school considered the body to be merely a collection of isolated parts' is quoted, alongside what was then the opening of the Biography section of the Hippocrates page on Wikipedia:

> Historians agree that Hippocrates was born around the year 460 BCE on the Greek island of Kos. He is renowned as the 'Father of Modern Medicine' – in recognition of his lasting contributions to the field as the founder of the Hippocratic School of Medicine. It was Hippocrates who finally freed medicine from the shackles of magic, superstition, and the supernatural.[32]

Use of the Wikipedia line 'Hippocratic medicine was humble and passive' (still showing on the page in August 2020) also betrays the origins of this Red House page. While I have not yet been able to work out the origin of this widely-repeated line – it could simply be the creation of a Wikipedia editor – it proves a particularly useful marker for reliance on what holistic practitioners often wrongly call the 'wonderful Hippocrates wikipedia page', which was created in May 2001 and currently running at a daily average of over 1300 hits.[33] One indication of just how widely used the Wikipedia Hippocrates page is comes in Ian Learmonth's ('MBChB(Stell), FRCS, FRCS(Ed), FCS(SA)Orth, Professor Emeritus') opening address to the European Hip Society Meeting in 2010 which began with 'Hippocratic medicine was humble and passive. Treatment was gentle, kind to the patient, and emphasised the importance of keeping the patient clean and sterile.'[34] Every word there is taken straight from the Wikipedia Hippocrates page.

For Chishti and Osborn, holism thus characterises Cos and marks its superiority over Cnidos. As it is from Cos, it must also be the approach of Hippocrates. The logical next move would be to cite the Hippocratic whole/parts claim from Plato's *Phaedrus*, where priority is given to 'the whole.'[35] In modern discussions

31 http://www.redhouseaustralia.org/hippocrates, which also claims that the philosophy owes something to 'Louis Pasture.'

32 https://en.wikipedia.org/wiki/Hippocrates.

33 Acknowledged as the source for the 'humble and passive' on http://www.isabellehutton.com/Hippocrates.FatherOfMedicine.html (domain now expired). For the statistics on the page, see https://xtools.wmflabs.org/articleinfo/en.wikipedia.org/Hippocrates and https://tools.wmflabs.org/pageviews/?project=en.wikipedia.org&platform=all-access&agent=user&range=latest-20&pages=Hippocrates.

34 http://www.scielo.org.za/pdf/saoj/v10n4/v10n4a03.pdf.

35 270c1-4, suggesting that both for the soul and for the body one cannot know their nature unless one learns 'the nature of the whole.' Tsekourakis (1991–1993) 164 suggests that any

of holistic medicine, however, this is rarely cited explicitly: it tends to linger in the background. For example, consider Robson and Baek's 'Hippocrates held the belief that *the body must be treated as a whole and not just a series of parts*, which is the underlying concept of the recently emerging *systems biology*';[36] by omitting any mention of Plato, this gives the impression that the whole/parts point can indeed be traced to a specific Hippocratic text.

As other contributors to this volume have shown, what is meant by 'the whole' in Plato is in any case far from clear. Is it, as Galen and subsequently Littré thought, the universe, or is it the whole body?[37] Is it 'all external factors that influence health'?[38] And does the passage tell us more about Plato than about what the Hippocratic writers, let alone Hippocrates himself, originally meant? For Wesley Smith, what was meant was 'the nature of the whole man', 'the nature of the cosmos' and perhaps also 'the nature of all body.' Smith argued, 'As always, Plato uses his language precisely and self-consciously, and if he is purposely ambiguous he will take account of all the meanings he has suggested.'[39] So, rather than either/or, perhaps we should see this as both/and: the 'whole' is all of these things.

Chishti himself clearly had Plato's *Phaedrus* in mind, although not naming this as the source: 'He [Hippocrates] viewed the human body as a complete, integrated whole (as opposed to a collection of parts) and his system of treatments was of a general nature, rather than a specific treatment against one set of symptoms.'[40] So, we also learn here that, in addition to being opposed to specialisms, holism supports treating the whole person rather than 'specific' treatments. And here is Osborn's development of this: 'As a holistic healing system, Hippocratic medicine treated the patient, and not just the disease.'

This is interesting wording. In 2013, in one of his assaults on alternative medicine, Edzard Ernst – formerly Chair in Complementary Medicine at the University of Exeter – noted that when he asks alternative practitioners 'What do you treat effectively?' he was given answers like 'Alternative practitioners, unlike conventional clinicians, do not treat diseases' or 'I treat the whole person, not just the disease.' In response to these answers, Ernst argued that 'any good medicine always has been and always will be holistic. High-jacking [sic]

---

attempt to tie this passage to a single Hippocratic treatise is doomed, as Plato was referring instead to Hippocratic medicine in general.

36 Robson and Baek (2009) 57.

37 Tsekourakis (1991–1993).

38 Wellmann (1929) 16–21, cited in W. D. Smith (2002) 38 n. 40.

39 W. D. Smith (2002) 46. See also Smith (2002) 48: 'Plato left 'the whole' ambiguous because both 'man as a whole' and 'cosmos' are comprehended in the Hippocratic science.'

40 Chishti (1988) 12.

holism as a specific characteristic for alternative medicine is misleading and an insult to all conventional clinicians who do their best to practice good medicine.' Ernst's concern is that, by claiming a monopoly on holism and saying that they treat the whole person, alternative practitioners are given what Ernst calls 'a 'carte blanche' for treating any disease or any condition or any symptom.'[41]

The answers Ernst received and Osborn's statement about Hippocratic medicine are, whether consciously or unconsciously, echoing the quotation I have used in the title of this chapter. Found on many holistic medicine internet sites, often simplified into 'treat the (whole) person, not the disease', it is a saying associated with one of the greatest physicians of the modern era, Sir William Osler (1849–1919): 'The good physician treats the disease; the great physician treats the patient who has the disease.'[42] It has however so far proved impossible to source it in Osler's writings; the nearest quotation may be 'Care more particularly for the individual patient than for the special features of the disease.'[43] Hippocrates does not have a monopoly on 'fake quotes.'

Unlike many other modern users of Hippocrates, practitioners of holistic medicine tend not to give 'quotes' but instead simply invoke the name of Hippocrates in support of their beliefs. For example, Sandra Sigur, a practitioner from Florida of reflexology, yoga, reiki and aromatherapy, and a former doula, author of *Healing Groovy* (2015),[44] was interviewed for the blog *Windermere Sun* in 2016:

---

41 http://edzardernst.com/2013/10/alternative-practitioners-treat-the-whole-person-not-the-disease/. See also the earlier post, 'Integrated medicine makes no sense', http://edzardernst.com/2012/12/integrated-medicine-makes-no-sense/ and the later post, http://edzardernst.com/2014/10/the-disgraceful-abduction-of-holism/ which dates 'clinical holistic medicine' 'as far back as Hippocrates.'

42 See http://www.osler.org.uk/osleriana-2/oslers-aphorisms/; claimed as the key principle of Chinese medicine on https://www.chinesemedicineliving.com/acupuncture/cancer-chinese-medicine-part-3 or used on the website of a natural healer in several traditions on https://www.drlaurenpolm.com/.

43 I owe this reference to Dr Mary Hague-Yearl, Head Librarian of the Osler Library at McGill University, pers. comm. 24 September 2018; the source is Osler (1899). Dr Hague-Yearl checked with one of the compilers of *The Quotable Osler* (Silverman et al. 2003), Charley Bryan, who 'wrote that he was 99% sure that it was merely attributed to Osler, and agreed that an investigation of these attributions would be very interesting indeed.' Those who attribute the words to Osler sometimes date them to 1895, but the best I have been able to find here is Shorter (1996) 144, with 381 n. 45 citing the aphorism as being quoted by Clarence B. Farrar in a 1959 article. Shorter later repeated this footnote, in Shorter (2005) 9–10.

44 On how 'dis-ease can become disease if left unresolved': https://www.amazon.com/Healing-Groovy-Realistic-Holistic-Self-Care/dp/1505613256.

> Natural or holistic medicine has been around for over 5,000 years. Hippocrates, who is considered the Father of Modern Medicine, emphasized a holistic approach to medicine, warning doctors not to interfere with the body's ability to heal itself, as well as to treat the body as a whole – mind, body and spirit. The early Hippocratic Oath was revised to exclude the word 'spirit' because it was thought to mean religion, when in actuality our spirit is what defines us as unique individuals (i.e., how we respond differently to life's circumstances).[45]

Holistic here becomes another word for natural. That exclusion of 'spirit' is, I think, a reference to those versions such as the Revised Hippocratic Oath proposed by the British Medical Association in 1997, which have dropped the opening invocation of the Greek gods.[46]

A now-deleted page on the site *Natural Wellbeing* went into more detail. It used to feature a page on 'The History of Holistic Medicine: The Ancient Greeks and Holistic Medicine', by Paulina Nelega.[47] Written in 2009, this was part of a short series on the allegedly-long history of holistic medicine, all written by Nelega, in which the ancient Greeks provide 'another forebearer [sic].' Nelega is a clinical herbalist based in Vancouver who describes how her passion for 'exploring our relationship with nature and the healing properties of plants' developed from growing up surrounded by 'majestic cedars [which] shared their timeless wisdom as I sat beneath them.' She went on to explain on the *Natural Wellbeing* site that she then took a 'conventional path', becoming a medical laboratory technologist, which taught her 'the benefits – and shortcomings – of allopathic medicine' and encouraged her to understand 'our body's innate wisdom and profound intelligence to heal – *vis medicatrix naturae*.'

This phrase features heavily in alternative medicine, sometimes in the mistaken variant *vis mediatrix naturae*; Latin looks good, even if it is not

45 http://windermeresun.com/2016/03/08/natural-healing-with-sandra-sigur/ Sigur supports other myths about Hippocrates, such as 'Hippocrates said 'let food be thy medicine and medicine be thy food.' So, since food is your medicine, I would say there are many deficiencies leading to illness in America.' I discuss this further in King (2019).

46 This and other modern versions are discussed by Hurwitz and Richardson (1997).

47 http://www.naturalwellbeing.com/blog/the-history-of-holistic-medicine-the-ancient-greeks-and-holistic-medicine/ accessed 3 September 2018. Nelega can now be found on https://blog.naturalwellbeing.com/author/paulina-nelega-rh-agh-clinical-herbalist. According to the Wayback Machine the now-defunct site was updated until 2018, https://web.archive.org/web/20180101000000*/http://www.naturalwellbeing.com/blog/the-history-of-holistic-medicine-the-ancient-greeks-and-holistic-medicine/.

correct.[48] The Wikipedia page on 'Vis medicatrix naturae' presents this as the Latin form of a Greek phrase, 'Νόσων φύσεις ἰητροί ('Nature is the physician(s) of diseases').'[49] The origin of the phrase in its Latin form may lie with the eighteenth-century William Cullen.[50] While it has been seen as something entirely un-Hippocratic,[51] it does in fact translate the three opening words of the fifth section of the Hippocratic *Epidemics* 6 although, as Wesley Smith pointed out, 'the text of the manuscripts shows signs of commentators' interference' and *physis* here seems to mean both the nature of the body, and *physis* as opposed to *logos*.[52] The Latin phrase was reclaimed by some orthodox practitioners in the nineteenth century, perhaps in reaction against the excessive interventions of 'heroic medicine', but from the 1830s to the 1860s at least, 'art' was still believed to trump 'nature.'[53]

In holistic circles, the phrase may be taken to mean that there is a natural healing force in everybody, that nature tends towards health and should either be left alone or should be given encouragement to get on with it: or it may be used to suggest that healing depends on actual contact with 'nature', whether that is growing a plant in a pot or being in a forest. Nelega not only learned from the cedars, but also trained at Coastal Mountain College of Healing Arts in Vancouver.[54] This does not appear to be operating any more, but at one point it was merged with Wild Rose College, a school which offers individual online courses at around $200–300, and is currently running a 'Wholistic [sic] Therapist Diploma' one-year extension course in which for a mere $100, acting as far as I can tell as a top-up after taking the Practical Herbalist Diploma which

48 See Neuburger (1944) for an overview; see also Warner (1986) 21 on the reluctance of some physicians to give Nature a 'personality', and Warner (1977–1978). Naturopathic sites often just repeat the phrase as if we all knew what it meant; http://www.foundationsproject.com/documents/NDNR-reprint%20oct2010%20Turner-Snider.pdf and 'Hippocrates, 460 BC–370 BC, who is considered to be the father of medicine, introduced Vis Medicatrix Naturae – the concept of the healing power of nature', https://eatbreathegarden.com/horticulture-and-health-according-to-three-wise-men/.

49 https://en.wikipedia.org/wiki/Vis_medicatrix_naturae.

50 G. Munro Smith (1909) 321 attributes ('as far as I can discover') the Latin phrase to William Cullen.

51 Hiroshi (1998) is often cited as evidence that 'The power, called vis medicatrix naturae, has been traditionally asociated [sic] with Hippocrates in spite of the fact that he did never mention it anywhere clearly in his writings', https://web.archive.org/web/20080610160955/http://sciencelinks.jp/j-east/article/199907/000019990799A0162403.php.

52 W. D. Smith, *Hippocrates Vol. VII* (Cambridge MA: Loeb edition) 255 n. a.

53 Whorton (2002) 6–7.

54 https://ca.linkedin.com/in/paulinanelega.

costs from $149.70 a month for ten months.[55] For a mere $97, you can submit a 'Wholistic Therapist Thesis' and 'you have one year from date of approval to complete your thesis.'[56] 'Our emphasis is on the wholism of the individual – the integration of the body, mind, and spirit. We believe wholistic healing is an art to be cultivated through a sound investigation.'[57]

Wild Rose College's 'wholistic' medicine with a 'W' deserves some attention, as other holistic sites too prefer this spelling. One institution which used to favour this version of holism is Loma Linda University, a Seventh-Day Adventist school in California, its motto being 'To make man whole.'[58] This concerns the body's natural tendency to heal 'when given the right resources from the outside … to look beyond the one part of the body that is diseased and to see a person as a whole.'[59] Adventists 'believe the key to wellness lies in a life of balance and temperance' and recommend – although do not insist on – a vegetarian diet.[60] Ellen G. White, revered by Adventists as a prophet whose writings are second only to the Bible in their relevance, wrote *The Desire of Ages* (1898), where she retold stories from the gospels: about Jesus as the Great Physician who taught that 'health is the reward of obedience to the laws of God.'[61] 'For the sick we should use the remedies which God has provided in nature, and we should point them to Him who alone can restore.'[62]

Loma Linda University's children's clinic, opened in 2010, was originally labelled 'Wholistic'; at the opening, the director of the clinic 'differentiated 'wholistic' from the more commonly used 'holistic', to emphasize the whole-person care the clinic strives to provide.'[63] In 2008, Loma Linda had stated that the adoption of this spelling was 'to distinguish it from some of the things that have happened in the field of holistic health … There are many quacks and false promises, and some are simply interested in making money.'[64] This spelling, now no longer used at Loma Linda, has become widespread. There are Wholistic Medical Centres in Sydney, Melbourne, Atlanta, Marylebone; at the last of these 'the Wholistic Journey, led by Dr Shamim Daya and her team

55 https://wildrosecollege.com/; https://wildrosecollege.com/product/wholistic-therapist-diploma-extension/ accessed 25 March 2020. These prices are those valid until August 2020.
56 https://wildrosecollege.com/product/thesis-wholistic-therapist/.
57 https://wildrosecollege.com/home/wild-rose-college-about-page/.
58 https://lluh.org/about-us/mission-vision-and-values.
59 https://www.pearlywhitesdds.com/holistic-providers.html.
60 https://www.adventist.org/en/vitality/health/.
61 White (1898) 824; http://www.thedesireofages.com/The_Desire_of_Ages_text/DA.pdf.
62 White (1898) 824.
63 https://myllu.llu.edu/oncampus/story/?id=3290.
64 https://www.redlandsdailyfacts.com/2008/01/09/wholistic-for-kids/.

of highly skilled practitioners, incorporates other important modalities' including 'bio-meridian testing' (£695 for an initial appointment which checks your 'toxic load'), 'functional biochemistry' and thermal imaging.[65] Not all of these invoke the name of Hippocrates to support wholism, but a holistic healer who does – and whose approach has been challenged – is Rebecca Carley, who developed what she calls 'the Hippocratic protocol' which she says can cure autoimmune diseases, autism and cancer.[66] Suspended as an MD in 2003, Carley – who believes she can reverse what she identifies as vaccine-induced diseases – repackaged herself as a 'holistic' healer. As her archived website for 'the Hippocrates Academy Protocol' puts it, 'Note that Dr. Carley does NOT practice medicine, and does NOT give medical advice. Rather, she teaches her students what she would do if she were you after reviewing your individual history of assaults to your immune system.'[67]

Picking up this imagery of 'assaults', it is clear that today holism also involves the belief that other forms of medicine cause harm, and that it does not, because it waits on 'Nature' rather than 'interfering.' As we saw above, Sandra Sigur's comments on 'natural medicine' included the statement that Hippocrates 'emphasized a holistic approach to medicine, warning doctors not to interfere with the body's ability to heal itself.'[68] This language of interference recalls that other Latin tag of Hippocrates, *primum non nocere*. Many websites stating that Hippocrates wrote 'First, do no harm' will elaborate that originally this was *primum non nocere*, without noticing that this is Latin while Hippocrates was Greek. A two-part episode of the hospital drama *Holby City* broadcast in June 2018 used the Latin phrase as its title.[69]

This is one of the popular sayings which the medical profession has now realised cannot be found in its supposed Hippocratic source, the *Oath*; it does not

65 https://www.wholisticmedical.co.uk/ accessed 25 March 2020; fees for these services on https://0be15daa-e522-484c-a268-6f028995b8a7.filesusr.com/ugd/01457c_207dfa3b6f6b4787894029a40eb8d270.pdf.

66 http://www.agreenroadjournal.com/2012/05/dr-rebecca-carley-md-now-holistic.html; on her suspension and the revoking of her licence, https://www.quackwatch.com/11Ind/carley1.html.

67 https://web.archive.org/web/20130925081055/http://www.reversingvaccineinduceddiseases.com/services; also quoted on https://quackwatch.org/cases/board/med/carley/order_2004/.

68 http://www.windermeresun.com/2016/03/08/natural-healing-with-sandra-sigur/.

69 https://www.imdb.com/title/tt8490842/: the 'trivia' for the episode on IMdb read 'The episode title, "Primum Non Nocere", is Latin for "First, do no harm", an important ethical rule in the medical profession, meaning "even if you can't make the patient any better, at least make sure you don't make him any worse".'

say this, 'just as nobody says "Play it again, Sam" in "Casablanca".'[70] In 2005 the *Journal of Clinical Pharmacology* published a piece by Cedric Smith in which he tried to trace its origins.[71] Smith, as a pharmacologist, was keen to consider potential adverse drug interactions. One of his key findings was 'Who was the author? Not Hippocrates.'[72] He wrote that 'like a proverb ... it is a crystallized bit of wisdom ... this maxim has several levels of meaning and can be applied to a wide range of situations ... It also *sounds* true, especially with its combination with the Latin.'[73] In 2013 Daniel Sokol found 393 articles in PubMed with 'do no harm' in their title; his conclusion was that it is an unhelpful axiom for today, when 'Clinicians inflict harm all the time, whether it is by inserting a cannula, administering chemotherapy, performing a tracheotomy ...'[74] Wider discussions of what Hippocratic medicine involves, and wider criticisms of mainstream medicine, thus lie behind holistic medicine's current versions of Hippocrates.

2 Invoking Hippocrates through History

These examples show how references to Hippocrates support a range of alternative healing practices which operate under the 'holistic' – or 'wholistic' – umbrella. Historically, the relationship between western biomedicine ('allopathy') and alternative and complementary medicine has involved many groups engaging with Hippocrates and claiming him as their ancestor, meaning that holistic medicine's current use of his name is far from being an isolated example. In the repeated reclaiming of the true Hippocrates from the hands of a mistaken or deliberately-distorting orthodoxy, while the imagined moral core of the man remains intact, many different versions of 'his' views have been constructed. Those who have called on Hippocrates show enormous confidence that he was, or would have been, one of their number. In the late nineteenth century, when dosimetry was invented by Adolphe Burggraeve at Ghent, it was placed 'under the protection of a great name' by being associated with him; 'had he had the benefits of modern medical knowledge, Hippocrates

70 Fabre (1997).

71 An online account of the non-Hippocratic nature of the phrase is available in an October 2019 piece by N. S. Gill at https://www.thoughtco.com/first-do-no-harm-hippocratic-oath-118780.

72 C. M. Smith (2005) 371.

73 C. M. Smith (2005) 375–76.

74 Sokol (2013); Smith is not listed in the references, but they are the ones used by him.

would have been favourable' to it.[75] More recently, if Hippocrates 'were living today, no doubt he would be labelled a Naturopath.'[76]

One of the patterns of engagement with the image of Hippocrates, found throughout the history of medicine and still strong today, is to contrast him with whatever the speaker or writer perceives as most negative in mainstream medicine: 'appeals to Hippocrates were explicitly and most fundamentally appeals to the past which expressed considerable discomfort with contemporary science and, more generally, with the world that science had created.'[77] This clearly happens with contemporary holistic medicine websites. The various binaries implied by appeals to Hippocrates today have been summarised by David Newman:

> Hippocrates was a holistic practitioner intent on treating the complete person, whereas today we tend to specialize in exquisitely narrow fields of anatomic and physiologic knowledge, leaving the balance of the human body to our colleagues. Hippocrates was a devoted and objective empiricist, while most modern doctors spend so little time with each patient that it's absurd to claim serious observational skills. Hippocrates was a consummate communicator, while today's doctors (ask our patients) are walking communication nightmares. Hippocrates felt and demonstrated sympathy, while we've chosen a colder, more 'scientific' model for doctor-patient interaction ...[78]

Patients today, apparently, even 'wonder aloud at how nice it might be to have Hippocrates as their doctor.'[79]

What, then, is really new in the current image of the holistic Hippocrates? Perhaps not as much as we may think. In the second century CE, Galen set himself up as the prophet pointing to the god Hippocrates,[80] who 'was selected to personify medical authority.'[81] Since then, Hippocrates has consistently stood for a balance of reason, detailed observation, caring bedside medicine, experience, honesty, patriotism and what William Osler referred to in a lecture delivered in 1913 as 'the note of humanity.'[82] Galen's creation of this Hippocrates

75 Haller (1981) 272; Weisz (2002) 261, author's italics.
76 http://www.rethinkingcancer.org/resources/articles/who-was-hippocrates.php.
77 Weisz (2002) 272.
78 Newman (2008).
79 Newman (2008).
80 Harris (1973) 267.
81 Rocca (2014) 285.
82 Osler (1921) 62–63.

'seduced' succeeding generations into seeing the Father of Medicine as 'the source of true science perversely misunderstood by those after him.'[83] In the second century as much as in the mid-twentieth century, we see that pattern of 'discomfort with contemporary science' versus the true science of Hippocrates.

In the history of medicine – in contrast to contemporary claims about Hippocrates and holism – claims for the true Hippocrates have traditionally been combined with a quest to identify his 'genuine works': the treatises the man himself wrote.[84] Various forms of medicine promoted across the early modern and modern periods show how important it used to be to find a Hippocratic treatise that fitted your view of medicine, one which revealed the true Hippocrates: a few examples must suffice here. In the second half of the sixteenth century, the 'Paris Hippocratics' favoured the treatises *Coan Prognoses* and *Epidemics*; the case history format of much of the *Epidemics* sits particularly easily with a Hippocrates who is all about observation and a good bedside manner.[85] At the same time, Petrus Severinus argued that occult philosophy and the chemical ideas of Paracelsus were closer to true Hippocratic medicine, which meant that *Ancient Medicine* and *Regimen 1* had better claims to Hippocratic authorship.[86] In the seventeenth century, Thomas Sydenham, who studied epidemic disease, presented an empirical, theory-averse Hippocrates and favoured not only *Epidemics* but also *Prognostics* and *Aphorisms* as genuine works, so that 'the Hippocrates that Sydenham perceived in those works was the Hippocrates most like himself.'[87]

What is different in the present uses of Hippocrates is that none of this concern for a 'genuine work' seems to interest those promoting holistic medicine today, who construct their own claims about Hippocrates with very little reference to any texts. This partly stems from the period between the World Wars, when the neo-Hippocratic movement developed as 'a revolt against the system, formalism, academics, professionalism, materialism, and analysis of the nineteenth century', favouring instead 'vitalism, humanism, individualism, and synthesis, a return to Hippocratic doctrine.'[88] There were regional vari-

83 W. D. Smith (2002) 106.

84 Difficult, or perhaps impossible, because of the lack of good external evidence, this quest may be on the resurgence among those studying ancient medicine in the academy; for example, considering *Fractures* and *Joints* and noting their 'remarkable' prose style, Craik (2010) 233 wonders 'perhaps indeed we have the words of Hippocrates' here. See also Craik (2015) 289.

85 Lonie (1985) 162.

86 Shackelford (2002) 63 and 69.

87 Cunningham (2002) 103.

88 Crookshank (1932) 123, cited in Cantor (2002) 280.

ations: in Britain, the neo-Hippocratic movement was about Hippocrates as generalist rather than specialist,[89] while in France it provided support for both homeopathy and naturopathy.[90] Homeopathy has had a particularly strong relationship with Hippocrates as 'an ancestral figure worth of veneration' but also as a practitioner of direct observation of the patient,[91] which is not always a feature of current holism, as the practitioners discussed in the previous section of this chapter demonstrate. Through 'selective reading', the different treatises of the Hippocratic corpus could be called upon to support homeopathy's practice of curing like with like as well as allopathy's cure by opposites.[92]

Analysing why the name of Hippocrates was so important for the emerging holistic movement in 1920s and 1930s France, George Weisz argued that 'The notion that was most identified historically with Hippocrates was that of 'nature' or 'natural' healing'; Emile Littré, the great editor and translator of the Hippocratic Corpus, defined 'hippocratisme' as 'the doctrine which attempts to imitate Hippocrates, giving to this imitation the particular sense of following nature, that is to say of studying the spontaneous effort that it makes and the crises that it produces.'[93]

Ideas of the healing power of nature, used not only in past forms of holism but also today, could find plenty of support in the Hippocratic Corpus; for example, 'The body's nature is the physician in disease. Nature finds the way for herself, not from thought … without instruction, Nature does what is needed' (*Epidemics* 6.5.1). Such ideas had also been widely discussed in American medicine of the 1860s. John Harley Warner has argued that the mid-nineteenth-century interest in Nature was a reaction to changing therapeutic interventions, as doctors moved from trying to reduce fever and inflammation by attacking with bleeding and purging, to seeing their role as being more about building up the strength of the patient.[94] The conclusion reached was that while 'bloodletting had indeed been carried to absurd excesses greatly impeding nature's work … this did not mean that bloodletting was necessarily bad in principle.'[95] Nor did believing that diseases were self-limiting mean that the answer was to do nothing, as the role of the doctor could be to support the body in healing itself. By warning against violent interventions, Hippocrates has long been elided not only with nature but also with safety, providing an

89 Cantor (2002) 284.
90 Weisz (2002) 268.
91 Warner (2002) 222–23.
92 Weisz (2002) 260.
93 Weisz (2002) 270, 278 n. 82.
94 Warner (1977–8) 301–6.
95 Warner (1977–1978) 307.

antique seal of approval for methods concerned with maintaining a balance with a 'nature' seen either as an external factor or as something deep within us.

In response to western biomedicine's increased focus on pharmacological solutions from the nineteenth century onwards, various alternative 'drugless systems' of healing arose.[96] As James Whorton has charted for the United States (and to a lesser extent for Britain), in the mid-1990s 'alternative' medicine (used as an alternative to orthodox medicine) became 'complementary' (used alongside orthodox medicine) and then moved towards 'integrative' as a range of methods were employed together.[97] The warmth of that word 'integrative' is unusual in the history of the relationship between allopathy and other medical approaches because, formerly, 'alternatives' oscillated between trying to graft themselves on to the Hippocratic family tree and wanting to annihilate the established system. At the 1911 party for Andrew Taylor Still, the founder of osteopathy, the toast included: 'The name that shall be blazoned out of the Skies of Science will not be Hippocrates, the Father of Medicine, but Andrew Taylor Still, the Father of the Healing Art.'[98]

James Whorton has noted that alternative practitioners often consider Hippocrates to be 'their doctrinal father.' The Hippocrates of orthodox medicine, Whorton argues, was designated the Father of Medicine because he had rejected supernatural phenomena as the causes of illness. The 'alternative' Hippocrates, however, is valued for his 'natural' methods of healing, and belief in an 'inborn ability of the human body to respond to the insult of illness or injury and restore itself to health.'[99]

Today, alleged Hippocratic holism does not even have to be an 'alternative': mainstream medicine wants to claim it too. For example, in 2000, the Royal Society of Medicine held a conference on the topic 'Healthcare for the Whole Person: Is Holistic Medicine More Healthy?'[100] An article by a medical student in the 2008 edition of the American Medical Association's *Journal of Ethics*' online section, *Virtual Mentor*, argued for the humanistic integration of Hippocratic holism with modern knowledge. The author gave a view of the history of medicine which suggested that medicine has moved 'from prescientific holistic approaches to modern, scientifically supported explanations of pathology', and contrasted 'the integrative Hippocratic view ... [with] the specialization view.'[101] This, apparently unconsciously, echoes the concerns of

96 Gevitz (1988) 125.
97 Whorton (2002) 299; Barrett et al. (2003) 938.
98 Quoted in Whorton (2002) 300.
99 Whorton (2002) 3, 6.
100 Robson and Baek (2009) 267.
101 Mantri (2008).

inter-war British neo-Hippocratics, who emphasised Hippocrates as generalist rather than specialist and, looking back at the First World War, criticised what they saw as the specialisation of German education and the centralisation of its institutions, as opposed to the greater focus on the individual and on personal initiative in British society.[102] They saw the unity of the organism as a key principle, and – according to the leading neo-Hippocratic Alexander Cawadias – a focus on the 'whole individual patient' was essential.[103] Mantri ended with a call for fuller integration to take into account 'both the individuality of illness and the universality of disease etiology.'

What we often find in constructions of the medical past is something like the pattern hinted at here: a shift from integration, or holism, or Hippocrates, towards fragmentation and then back again to a new holism; or, perhaps, from holism, to fragmentation, and then to a merger giving the best of both worlds. In this model, which is usually only implicit in the material, medicine in the past is inevitably presented as holistic, until 'the turn away from holism in medicine allowed diseases to be located in specific organs, tissues or cells.'[104] Holism today, whether as a goal of orthodox medicine or a claim for an unorthodox system, thus presents itself as a return to a superior past. This is of course a tried and tested strategy for convincing an audience of the value of a 'new' thing: claiming that it is 'old', or ancient, or just traditional.

Mantri's contrast between 'the integrative Hippocratic view' and 'the specialization view' is worth exploring further. The history of medicine has long been interested in the history of specialisms. Vanessa Heggie's 2010 article in *Medical History*, 'Specialization without the Hospital: The Case of British Sports Medicine', summarized the main approach as follows: 'Specialization in medicine acts to normalize categories of health and sickness that, once constructed, can appear to be obvious and rational divisions of the body, of disease, or of populations.'[105] This underlines the point that, while decisions on how we divide the body into organs or systems or other sorts of 'part' are arbitrary, once these categories exist they can then take on a life of their own.

102 Cantor (2002) 284, 286.
103 Cantor (2002) 289.
104 Heggie (2010) 458.
105 Heggie (2010) 457. Sports medicine, Heggie showed, was a particularly unpromising area to become a specialism due to the breadth of what it covered: it is 'a holistic practice, covering everything from gross musculo-skeletal injuries to dietary advice to genetic testing. It has virtually no unique diseases or injuries (one can get tennis elbow cleaning floors) nor any unique treatment modalities or technologies.' On medical specialisation more broadly, see Weisz (2003) and (2006).

As Roger Cooter argued for the emergence of fracture treatment under the control of orthopaedics, a specialism also needs 'professional interests and aspirations' to propel it into existence; its emergence was partly due to World War I leading to a greater interest in accidents and trauma, and partly to orthopaedists 'enlarg[ing] their professional space.'[106] Cooter argued that 'accidents and trauma cut across the 'organ geography' of medical and surgical specialties' and, in an interesting parallel to what I am doing here with holism, argues against the claim that orthopaedics can trace its lineage to 'traditional bone-setting [which] appears to legitimate orthopaedic surgeons as the rightful menders of broken bones';[107] nevertheless, that claim of antiquity was important. Cooter subsequently argued not only that orthopaedics emerged 'as a specialized branch of general surgery ... in the early twentieth century in terms of a holistic physiological vision of the structures and functions of the musculoskeletal system – a naturalized division of labor' but also that it later became fragmented into separate smaller branches: 'the surgery of the hand, the foot, the ankle, the spine, and so on.'[108] This increasing fragmentation was at least partly due to the various technical developments in the field, in which 'knowledge appeared to increase year after year';[109] 'There is no mind so comprehensive that it can keep pace with all the requirements of modern surgery', as Robert Jones had said in a lecture delivered in May 1925.[110] So, here we have spurious claims of historical continuity (those traditional bone-setters), then the emergence of specialisms due to social and economic factors and also to new techniques, further division into sub-specialties, and then – perhaps – a return to holism?

While mainstream medicine can now claim to be holistic, hits on search engines suggest that there is still more *popular* interest in holism than *mainstream* medical interest.[111] I have already alluded to the veiled criticisms of allopathy: holism is seen as a 'whole life approach' rather than being about 'fragmented (i.e. nonholistic), episodic (i.e. lack of continuum of services), and external symptom-based (as opposed to dealing with the root cause of illness)

106 Cooter (1987) 306.
107 Cooter (1987) 307.
108 Cooter (2003) 467–68.
109 Heggie (2010) 458.
110 Quoted in Cooter (1987) 314.
111 Robson and Baek (2009) 267. In 2009 they reported nearly 3 million hits for 'holistic + medicine', half a million for 'holistic medicine.' In March 2020 I had over 4 million for the first search, and only a few less for the second. They had 154,000 hits for holistic + 'managed care' (a key term in US medicine): I had over 2 million. Even taking into account the vagaries of search engines, I suspect that this means the word is moving further into the mainstream.

diagnostics and treatment, mostly depending on the one-fits-all approach and yet on the trial-and-error for treatments.'[112] Here holism comes a little closer to 'personal medicine' – individualised and empowering to the patient[113] – but, as ever, holism is defined by what it is *not*: it is not about fragmentation, or about specialists clinging to their little empire of one organ or system.

3 Conclusion

Everyone – in biomedicine and in various branches of alternative medicine – wants Hippocrates on their team. The term 'holism' is always used in a positive way, but in its alternative medicine uses it often contains a barely-veiled criticism of western biomedicine. Considering the whole, whether that is the whole body rather than an organ or system, or the body in relation to its wider setting, clearly has a long history. But contemporary holistic medicine goes well beyond arguing that a knowledge of the whole body is essential to understanding what is wrong with a part of it. Holistic medicine presents Hippocrates as its ancestor, using the strategy of the claim to be returning to the 'original', the 'ancient.' The past is a time of integration, holism and Hippocrates, and the answer to our present problems is to reject fragmentation and return to this holistic Hippocrates. Comparing this with other current uses of Hippocrates as a projection screen on to which we place our ideals of medicine, they usually start from a 'quote' – for example, 'Let food be thy medicine' – which may or may not have its origins in any text of the Hippocratic corpus. Yet, despite having a rather promising potential source text in Plato's *Phaedrus*, very few holistic medicine sites referencing Hippocrates make any use of this. I wonder if the problem is that it is in Plato, not the Hippocratic corpus, that the key sentence about the whole and the part is found?

Several medicinal utopias are currently held under the umbrella of 'holism.' The holistic Hippocrates conjures up nightmares of excessive specialism with a vision both of the individual as being heard and understood and of participating in a worldwide natural healing system. While not the sole preserve of either mainstream or orthodox medicine, here as elsewhere Hippocrates remains a trump card to be played in any medical competition.

---

112 Robson and Baek (2009) 20.

113 Barrett et al. (2003) 940–41.

Bibliography

Barrett, B. et al. 'Themes of Holism, Empowerment, Access, and Legitimacy Define Complementary, Alternative, and Integrative Medicine in Relation to Conventional Biomedicine.' *Journal of Alternative and Complementary Medicine*, 9.6 (2003) 937–47.

Cacciafoco, F. P. *Food as Therapy: Elements of the History of Nutrition in Ancient Greece and Rome*. Pollenzo: Università degli Studi di Scienze Gastronomiche, Teatro Vocali Edizioni (2012).

Cantor, D. 'The Name and the Word: Neo-Hippocratism and Language in Interwar Britain.' In *Reinventing Hippocrates*, ed. D. Cantor. Aldershot: Ashgate (2002) 280–301.

Chermet-Carroy, S. *L'Astrologie médicale*. Paris: Editions Guy Trédaniel (1998).

Chishti, G. M. *The Traditional Healer's Handbook: A Classic Guide to the Medicine of Avicenna*. Rochester, VT: Healing Arts Press (1988).

Cooter, R. 'The Meaning of Fractures: Orthopaedics and the Reform of British Hospitals in the Inter-war Period.' *Medical History*, 31.3 (1987) 306–32.

Cooter, R. 'The Evolution of Orthopaedic Surgery (Review).' *Bulletin of the History of Medicine*, 77.2 (2003) 467–68.

Craik, E. M. 'The Teaching of Surgery.' In *Hippocrates and Medical Education: Selected Papers Presented at the XIIth International Hippocrates Colloquium, Universiteit Leiden, 24–26 August 2005*, ed. M. Horstmanshoff. Leiden: Brill (2010) 221–34.

Craik, E. M. *The 'Hippocratic' Corpus: Content and Context*. London: Routledge (2015).

Crookshank, F. G. 'The New Psychology and the Health of the People.' *Purpose*, July-September (1932) 122–7.

Cunningham, A. 'The Transformation of Hippocrates in Seventeenth-century Britain.' In *Reinventing Hippocrates*, ed. D. Cantor. Aldershot: Ashgate (2002) 91–115.

Davidson, J. N. *Courtesans and Fishcakes: The Consuming Passions of Classical Athens*. London: HarperCollins (1997).

Fabre, J. 'Medicine as a Profession: Hip, Hip, Hippocrates: Extracts from The Hippocratic Doctor.' *British Medical Journal*, 315 (1997) 1669–70.

Gevitz, N. 'Osteopathic Medicine: From Deviance to Difference.' In *Other Healers: Unorthodox Medicine in America*, ed. N. Gevitz. Baltimore: Johns Hopkins University Press (1988) 124–56.

Graf, F. 'Heiligtum und Ritual: Das Beispiel der griechisch-römischen Asklepieia.' In *Le sanctuaire grec*, ed. A. Schachter. Vandoevres: Fondation Hardt (1992) 159–99.

Haller, J. S. *American Medicine in Transition 1840–1910*. Urbana, Chicago and London: University of Illinois Press (1981).

Harris, C. R. S. *The Heart and the Vascular System in Ancient Greek Medicine from Alcmaeon to Galen*. Oxford: Clarendon Press (1973).

Heggie, V. 'Specialization without the Hospital: The Case of British Sports Medicine.' *Medical History*, 54.4 (2010) 457–74.

Hiroshi, H. 'On *Vis Medicatrix Naturae* and Hippocratic Idea of *Physis*.' *Memoirs of School of Health Sciences, Faculty of Medicine, Kanazawa University*, 22 (1998) 45–54.

Hurwitz, B., and R. Richardson. 'Swearing to Care: The Resurgence in Medical Oaths.' *British Medical Journal*, 315 (1997) 1671.

Israelowich, I. *Patients and Healers in the High Roman Empire*. Baltimore: Johns Hopkins University Press (2015).

Jones, R. 'Lady Jones' Lecture on Crippling Due to Fractures: Its Prevention and Remedy.' *British Medical Journal*, 1 (1925) 909–13.

King, H. 'The Power of Paternity: The Father of Medicine meets the Prince of Physicians.' In *Reinventing Hippocrates*, ed. D. Cantor. Aldershot: Ashgate (2002) 21–36.

King, H. *Hippocrates Now*. London: Bloomsbury Academic (2019).

King, H. 'Hippocratic Whispers: Telling the Story of the Life of Hippocrates on the Internet.' In *Medicine and Markets in the Graeco-Roman World and Beyond. Essays in Ancient Medicine in Honour of Vivian Nutton*, ed. R. Flemming and L. M. V. Totelin. Cardiff: University of Cardiff Press (2020) 143–60.

Lonie, I. M. 'The 'Paris Hippocratics': Teaching and Research in Paris in the Second Half of the Sixteenth Century.' In *The Medical Renaissance of the Sixteenth Century*, ed. A. Wear, R. K. French and I. M. Lonie. Cambridge and New York: Cambridge University Press (1985) 155–74.

Mantri, S. 'Holistic Medicine and the Western Medical Tradition.' *Virtual Mentor*, 10.3 (2008) 177–80, http://journalofethics.ama-assn.org/2008/03/mhst1-0803.html.

Neuburger, M. 'An Historical Survey of the Concept of Nature from a Medical Viewpoint.' *Isis*, 35.1 (1944) 16–28.

Newman, D. H. 'What Would Hippocrates Do?' In *Hippocrates' Shadow: Secrets from the House of Medicine*. New York: Simon & Schuster (2008).

Numbers, R. L. *Prophetess of Health: A Study of Ellen G. White*. 3rd edition. Grand Rapids: Wm. B. Eerdmans (2008).

Osler, W. 'Address to the Students of the Albany Medical College.' *Albany Med Ann.*, 20 (1899) 307–9.

Osler, W. 1921. *The Evolution of Modern Medicine: A Series of Lectures Delivered at Yale University on the Silliman Foundation in April, 1913*. New Haven: Yale University Press. Online, https://biotech.law.lsu.edu/books/osler/modern_medicine.htm.

Robson, B., and O. K. Baek. *The Engines of Hippocrates: From the Dawn of Medicine to Medical and Pharmaceutical Informatics*. Hoboken: Wiley (2009).

Rocca, J. 'Present at the Creation: Plato's 'Hippocrates' and the Making of a Medical Ideal.' In *Attitudes towards the Past in Antiquity. Creating Identities. Proceedings of an International Conference Held at Stockholm University, 15–17 May 2009*. Acta

Universitatis Stockholmiensis, Stockholm Studies in Classical Archaeology 14, ed. B. Alroth and C. Scheffer. Stockholm: Stockholm University (2014) 285–99.

Rütten, T. 'Hippocrates.' In *The Classical Tradition*, eds. A. Grafton, G. W. Most and S. Settis. Cambridge MA and London: Harvard University Press (2010) 438–9.

Sellars, W. C., and R. J. Yeatman. *1066 and All That: A Memorable History of England, Comprising All the Parts You Can Remember, Including 103 Good Things, 5 Bad Kings and 2 Genuine Dates*. London: Methuen (1930).

Shackelford, J. 'The Chemical Hippocrates: Paracelsian and Hippocratic Theory in Petrus Severinus' Medical Philosophy.' In *Reinventing Hippocrates*, ed. D. Cantor. Aldershot: Ashgate (2002) 59–88.

Shorter, E. 'Primary Care.' In *Cambridge Illustrated History of Medicine*, ed. R. Porter. Cambridge: Cambridge University Press (1996) 118–53.

Shorter, E. 'The History of the Biopsychosocial Approach in Medicine: Before and After Engel.' In *Biopsychosocial Medicine: An Integrated Approach to Understanding Illness*, ed. P. White. Oxford: Oxford University Press (2005) 1–11.

Silverman, M. E., T. J. Murray and C. S. Bryan. *The Quotable Osler*. Philadelphia: American College of Physicians (2003).

Smith, C. M. 'Origin and Uses of *Primum Non Nocere* – Above All, Do No Harm!.' *Journal of Clinical Pharmacology*, 45.4 (2005) 371–77.

Smith, G. M. '*Vis Medicatrix Naturae*: Inaugural Address at the Annual Meeting of the Bath and Bristol Branch of the British Medical Association.' *Bristol Medico-Chirurgical Journal*, 27.106 (1909) 321–36.

Smith, W. D. *The Hippocratic Tradition*; revised electronic edition, http://www.biusante.parisdescartes.fr/ressources/pdf/medicina-hippo2.pdf (2002).

Sokol, D. K. "First Do No Harm' Revisited.' *British Medical Journal*, 347 (2013) 23.

Tsekourakis, D. 'Plato's *Phaedrus* and the Holistic Viewpoint in Hippocrates' Therapeutics.' *Bulletin of the Institute of Classical Studies of the University of London*, 38 (1991–1993) 162–73.

Warner, J. H. "The Nature-Trusting Heresy': American Physicians and the Concept of the Healing Power of Nature in the 1850s and 1860s.' *Perspectives in American History*, 11 (1977–1978) 291–324.

Warner, J. H. *The Therapeutic Perspective: Medical Practice, Knowledge, and Identity in America, 1820–1885*. Cambridge MA: Harvard University Press (1986).

Warner, J. H. 'Making History in American Medical Culture: The Antebellum Competition for Hippocrates.' In *Reinventing Hippocrates*, ed. D. Cantor. Aldershot: Ashgate (2002) 200–36.

Weisz, G. 'The Emergence of Medical Specialization in the Nineteenth Century.' *Bulletin of the History of Medicine*, 77 (2003) 536–75.

Weisz, G. *Divide and Conquer: A Comparative History of Medical Specialization*. Oxford: Oxford University Press (2006).

Weisz, G. 'Hippocrates, Holism and Humanism in Interwar France.' In *Reinventing Hippocrates*, ed. D. Cantor. Aldershot: Ashgate (2002) 257–79.
Wellmann, M. 'Hippokrates des Herakleides Sohn.' *Hermes*, 64 (1929) 16–21.
White, E. *The Desire of Ages*. Mountain View CA: Pacific Press Publishing Association (1940; original 1898).
White, E. *The Ministry of Healing*. Mountain View CA: Pacific Press Publishing Association (1942; original 1905).
Whorton, J. C. *Nature Cures. The History of Alternative Medicine in America*. New York: Oxford University Press (2002).

Primary Texts: Editions and Translations Used

Galen, *De Sectis ad eos qui Introducuntur*, Kühn I.
Hippocrates, *Epidemics* 6, *Hippocrates Vol. VII*. Trans. W. D. Smith. Cambridge MA: Harvard University Press (1994).
Hippocrates, *Oath*. Hippocrates Vol. I. Trans. W. H. S. Jones. Cambridge MA: Harvard University Press (1923).
Plato, *Phaedrus*. Trans. A. Nehamas and P. Woodruff. Indianapolis: Hackett (1995).

Index Rerum

Index Locorum

Corpora and adespota

Index Verborum (selected)

www.ingramcontent.com/pod-product-compliance
Ingram Content Group UK Ltd.
Pitfield, Milton Keynes, MK11 3LW, UK
UKHW022225051026
15624UKWH00002B/354

9 789004 443082